THE CONVERSATION, TALKS, LIFE & TIMES OF
HERING

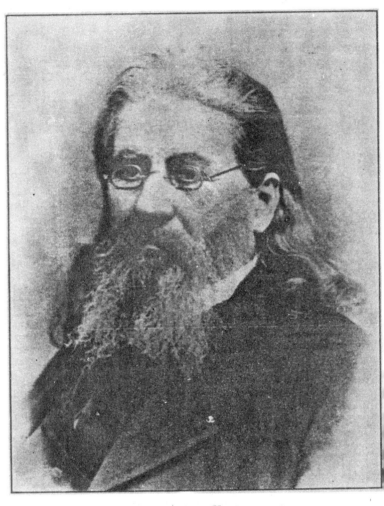

CONSTANTINE HERING.
REPRODUCED FROM A PHOTOGRAPH IN THE
POSSESSION OF HERMANN S. HERING, HIS SON.

THE CONVERSATION, TALKS, LIFE & TIMES OF
HERING

by

CALVIN B. KNERR, M.D.

B. Jain Publishers (P) Ltd.
New Delhi

First Edition : 1992
Reprint Edition : 2000

Price : Rs. 100/-

© Copyright with the Publisher

Published by :
Kuldeep Jain
For

B. Jain Publishers (P.) Ltd.

1921, Street No.10, Chuna Mandi
Paharganj, New Delhi-110 055 (INDIA)
Phones: 3670430; 3670572; 7536418
FAX : 011-3610471 & 7536420
Email : bjain@vsnl.com
Website : www.bjainindia.com

Printed in India by:
Unisons Techno Financial Consultants (P) Ltd.
522, FIE, Patpar Ganj, Delhi- 110 092.

BOOK CODE : B-3662

To the Memory Of

My Wife, Melitta Pauline Hering,

Her Mother, Therese Buchheim Hering,

Hermann Siegfried Hering,

and to the Rising Generation of

Physicians In All Parts of the World

This Book Is Dedicated

INTRODUCTORY REMARKS

In the Fall of 1867 I came from my home, near Allentown, Pennsylvania, to Philadelphia to attend Hahnemann College, which was then entering upon its first year under reorganization and amalgamation with the older Homoeopathic College of Pennsylvania, with a new faculty, of which Dr. Hering was dean.

On visiting Dr. Hering, whose name had become a household word in my father's home, owing to his affiliation, at the Allentown Academy, with my great uncle, the Rev. John Helfrich, I was warmly received with a handshake and the greeting: "Welcome, descendent of my old friend." I was invited to call at the house where occasionally I spent an evening, or made a visit on a Sunday afternoon, during my winter's course at the College.

Shortly after my graduation, in 1869, I made my home with the family to fill the position of assistant to the venerable doctor, who had, for a time, been without such help.

Realizing that the years, in which I was to sit at the feet of the Master, were to be years of golden opportunity from which to gather precious knowledge, such as nowhere else could be obtained, I thought this might afford an opportunity, to share at some future time, with others of my profession among coming generations, the advantages so enjoyed. I resolved, from the beginning, to record in a diary the conversations of the great teacher, his tabletalk, the daily incidents that occurred in the home life, and his interviews with other physicians who came to consult, or to be instructed and entertained, by the sage so widely known and respected.

I believe that now, at an advanced age, near the dawn of another life is the time to share with the profession these notes, held in sacred keeping so many years—more than fifty; I have in mind, particularly the younger generation of homoeopaths who have come too late to enjoy personally the intimacy and inspiration of the great teacher.

I feel it, not only to be a privilege, but a great and pleasant duty to share with the profession, and also the laity, including the few remaining ones who, at one time or another, have benefitted by his personal treatment, as well as the many with whom Hering's *Domestic Physician* is still a household word, a friend and a help at home to those who needing first aid live remote from a homoeopathic physician.

From the day of my return from Europe in 1873 the notes in my diary were resumed, at intervals, not always dated, and were continued to the time of Dr. Hering's death, in July of 1880. Soon after, almost before the ink had dried on the page of Vol. 4 of the Master's lifework, his *Guiding Symptoms of Our Materia Medica*, a ten volume book, it fell to my lot assisted in part by Doctors Raue and Mohr, to prepare for the press this monumental work, from the mass of material accumulated through years of labor by Constantine Hering.

If, by publishing these notes, I have, in a small way, contributed to the edification and instruction of my colleagues, and especially to the many who will come after me, my pleasant duty will have been accomplished.

These records, religiously kept for a number of years, eleven in all, were made openly, by permission and approval of the Master, on tablets in longhand, and regularly copied into a book which grew to a fair sized volume, from which these pages are transcribed.

After graduation from Hahnemann Medical College in the spring of 1869, there followed two years of uninterupted application to an extensive practice under Dr. Hering, together with arduous labor at literary work, which helped to break down my health, none too robust. I was called the pale student. Realizing that I began to suffer under the strain of trying to keep up with the man of iron constitution, who never seemed to tire, or to need time for rest and recreation, a vacation was planned for the duration of a year, in which to go abroad, a part of which time was to be spent in travel and sightseeing and later, with health restored, to attend lectures and to take some special courses in medicine in the hospitals abroad.

I left in my place Dr. Claude R. Norton, a recent graduate from the New York Homoeopathic College, a bright and able young man.

After several months in Germany, spent in visiting friends and relatives of the Hering family, there followed some special courses of study at the University in Berlin, under Helmholtz, who taught physics, and Dubois Reymond, noted physiologist. There was also a short course in Archaeology describing the ruins of Herculaneum and Pompeii, places to be visited later on a tour through Italy.

During a winter course at the hospitals in Vienna I attended the clinics of Schroeder and Stoerck, throat and lung specialists, and some lectures on anatomy by the venerable Hyrtl, also some on skin diseases by Hebra and Skoda.

The rest of my stay on the continent was devoted to sightseeing with occasional visits to some of the eminent early homoeopaths, prominent among whom were Rueckert in Herrnhut, Aegidi near Berlin, Hartlaub in Thuringia, and Heermann in Paris. To all of these intimate friends of Dr. Hering I had letters of introduction.

When in Leipzig, for a short stay, I called upon the widow Moosdorff, eldest daughter of Hahnemann, practising in her father's house in Coethen, near Leipzig. From this gracious lady I received some interesting relics which included pellets of *Aconite* from a vial used by her father. She had nothing kindly to say of Melanie, the second wife who lured her father to Paris and separated him from his family and home ties to be exploited in a lucrative practice in the great metropolis.

I spent a week or two in Salzburg, ancient city in Bavaria, which had been the home of Theophrastus von Hohenheim, better known by the name of Paracelsus, in whose life and labors Dr. Hering was deeply interested, to the extent of accumulating what is probably the largest collection of books, by and on Hohenheim, in the country;

which library, after Hering's demise, was placed in a fire-proof vault in the Hahnemann College of Philadelphia together with souvenirs carefully catalogued and kept under glass.

My efforts to obtain admittance to the museum in Salzburg were made successful through the courtesy of the curater of that institution and I was allowed the privilege of making photographic copies of portraits of Hohenheim, including a picture of the fractured skull exhumed from St. Peter's graveyard, in Salzburg, by the German anatomist, Soemmering, confirming the legend that Hohenheim was killed by enemies by being thrown from a cliff at the foot of the castle, on a hill, late one night when returning home from a banquet.

After Salzburg came Vienna, the hospitals, and later a trip to Italy, in company with two young American doctors, one of them my friend, Dr. Charles M. Thomas from Philadelphia, skilful surgeon and oculist who later became dean of Hahnemann College. After a visit to Paris and Dr. Charles Heermann, by whom my friend and I were hospitably received and entertained, and seeing some of the sights, and making a fruitless search for the burial place of Hahnemann, in Montmartre cemetery, we sailed for England. We spent a few days in London and went on to Edinburgh, Scotland, where three more months were profitably spent in reading the medical books we had accumulated, and in visiting historic places of interest in the vicinity of Edinburgh, and in the Highlands.

In the summer of 1873, with renewed health and vigor and a deeper rooted belief in the principles of homoeopathy, I returned to my place by the side of Dr. Hering, where, soon after, I became united in marriage to his daughter Melitta, to whom I had become engaged before leaving for Europe the previous year. This happy union lasted for fifty-three years, blessed by three sons and a daughter.

It is my fervent wish that the seeds of wisdom gathered and thus disseminated may fall upon fertile ground and bear a rich harvest in the years to come; in the time, when we hope, that homoeopathy will have become the dominating School of Medicine.

I wish to thank the members of the Hering family for their kind offices in helping to make the publication of this book possible; and all others who have assisted in any way.

— CALVIN B. KNERR, M. D.

Philadelphia, Pa.

October, 1939.

TABLE OF CONTENTS

PAGE

THE HOUSE OF HERING.

The house in which Dr. Hering lived at the time of my association with him in 1869 and to the end of his life, in 1880, was located centrally between Arch and Cherry Streets, on the west side of North Twelfth Street. It was a double house of three stories built of brick; the numbers were 112 and 114, and there were white marble steps leading to the front door, which was heavy and had a silver-plated knob and bell-pull. There came a roomy vestibule, then another door which led into a long hallway which separated the rooms on the first floor. The door at the far end of this hallway led into a large garden with an elm tree, shrubbery, flowers and grapevines on a trellis. At the rear of the garden was a stable of brick, large enough to house a carriage and pair of horses. The entrance to the stable gave on Budden's Alley, so named after a sea-captain by the name of Budden. Over the stable lodged George, the German coachman.

On the first floor of this double house were located, to the North, two large rooms separated by heavy mahogany doors, the one in front serving as reception room for patients, and the rear room for private consultation in office hours, which were from 10 to 12 in the morning, and from 4 to 6 in the afternoon. It was here that the doctor's friends foregathered about the round table on Sunday afternoons and on those especial evenings so well-remembered by the many who were guests and visitors at the house, when hours sped by and were never long enough for host or company. This large room held some of the doctor's books and papers, particularly his clinical notes which filled shelf upon shelf behind a red curtain, running along the wall and reaching to the top of the ceiling on the South side of the room. At the rear end were two large windows which gave into the garden. Before one of these stood an aquarium, oblong in shape, in which were kept goldfish and the usual aquatic plants,

pebbles and objects shaped from stone. There, too, in
the corner, was a large cabinet which contained the Zent-
mayer microscope, with slides and appurtenances used in
mounting specimens; also books explaining the wonders
of the microscope. Before one of the windows stood the
doctor's easy chair, with gothic back and arm-rests, in
which he spent an occasional half hour reading or medi-
tating when patients had been dismissed or while waiting
for the supper hour.

In this room Dr. Hering's intimate friends gathered on
Sunday afternoons, for long talks over coffee and cigars,
discussing homoeopathy, science, art, and the affairs of
the nation; conversations in which Dr. Hering led and
which called to mind the classic Addison and the Round
Table. In this familiar room Dr. Hering received visiting
colleagues and talked to a class of students on Saturday
nights.

On the South side of the hallway, nearest the street, was
located a smaller room, the doctor's office in which he
received male patients and which held his medicines, books
of reference, and his account books. There were two
desks, in this room, at one of which sat Dr. Hering, at
the other his assistant who put up the prescriptions, and a
table, by one of the windows, at which, after consulting
hours, sat the doctor's whitehaired German secretary, Dr.
Knabe, whose duty it was to copy Dr. Hering's manu-
_cripts in handwriting so neatly done as to resemble steel-
engraving. Next to this room to the West, was a passageway leading to the stairs and to the dining-room.

The doctor's family was large, requiring a long table,
running the length of the room, generally seating eight
or ten, and on extra occasions as many as eighteen or
more people. On the walls of this room were hung wood-
engravings representing scenes from the hunt, made by
an artist friend named Traubel. Back of the dining-room,
was a small room into which was built a large refrigera-
tor, containing a coil of lead-pipe on which rested a block
of ice which served the double purpose of cooling the
drinking water, and keeping fresh the contents of this

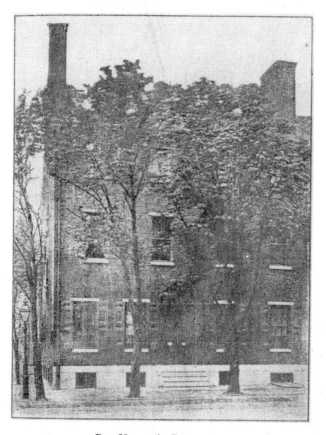

DR. HERING'S RESIDENCE
112-114 NORTH TWELFTH STREET
PHILADELPHIA

receptacle built of wood and lined with metal. Back of this pantry was a short passageway which led past the back stairs to a roomy kitchen, with a large old-fashioned coal-range, the one which figured in giving such prompt relief to the doctor's left hand and arm when poisoned by the fangs of a dead rattlesnake, a circumstance to be mentioned later. Both the cook and waitress were German girls who had been in the family for a long time. There was a third servant, the door-girl, who spoke both languages and sat in one of the offices making powders in spare moments. This raised the number of help in Dr. Hering's family to four; three women and George, the coachman, all of them German, excepting the office girl, who was American born.

———————

NOTES FROM MY DIARY.

April 21, 1869.

Dr. Hering speaks of an extraordinary man, a Professor Roehrig, who has a great talent for acquiring foreign languages. When a boy Roehrig found an Arabic grammer, in Dr. Hering's library. He seized upon it and took it away with him to study the language along with his other work. In a short time he had mastered Arabic. Later, in Europe, he encountered some Arabs and Turks at a Fair, whom he addressed, to their great astonishment, in their native tongue, which brought him into notice. He had already mastered a number of other languages, including German, French, Italian, etc., which knowledge secured him a position on a Prussian expedition to Russia. He was then only fourteen years old. While visiting Constantinople he learned the Persian and Chaldean languages. Wherever he saw an outlandish person he made his acquaintance and very soon was able to speak the language. While in Russia he committed the innocent blunder of writing sonnets to the sultan, in the Russian language, for which offence his Prussian embassy sent him home. Although said to speak twenty languages fluently, he is unable to speak the Pennsylvania German dialect.

Roehrig placed documents in Dr. Hering's hands from which a history of his life might be written. He has a wife, at present engaged as a seamstress in the Hering family, while her husband is in New York trying to earn some money. The wife speaks in the highest terms of her husband, who seems to neglect her.

Jahr's Therapeutic Guide.

In the evening I am occupied with scissors cutting symptoms copied by the secretary from Jahr's *Therapeutic Guide*. These are intended to go into the work on *Materia Medica*. These symptoms, written on slips of paper, Dr. Hering pastes on sheets of brown manila paper, in an order

which, he says: "Enables him to look behind the scenes."
He says he has done this with Guernsey and Raue's books;
claims "that Raue did not like this so well."

MacFarlan.

Dr. Malcolm MacFarlan is elected to give a course of
lectures at the College on operative surgery in the coming
fall. Both Koch and Raue were opposed to MacFarlan's
election. Doctors Gause, Thomas, Martin and Hering,
likewise Morgan, who specialized in surgery, were in his
favor. MacFarlan was married yesterday to a rich florist's
daughter.

Flowering Plants. Has their color any relation to the
spectroscope? Acids.

Hering is trying to find out if the way in which the
flowers of medicinal plants are coloured has any relation
to the spectroscope. He presumes that red-flowering
plants act upon one side of the body, while blue-flowering
ones affect the other side.

In certain combinations the mineral acids have a predominating number of symptoms, leaving those from
organic acids in the background.

Primary colours, red, blue and yellow, are represented
in a diagram as occupying the three corners of a triangle,
red standing for *Lithium,* blue for *Kali,* and yellow for
Natrum.

John Hering.

While at table Dr. Hering received a letter from his
oldest son, John, who lives in Surinam, South America.
He said jocosely: "Oh! this is from my oldest, good-for-
nothing son, John! Take it to my wife and let her read it!"

Houatt's Provings.

"Houatt, a Frenchman, has made provings of *Kali hydri-*
odicum, Sarracenia, etc. It is questionable if his provings
are reliable."

This Houatt made an experiment which Hering had
proposed to Hahnemann twenty-five years ago, viz: to
select for proving twelve medicines, in the 200th potency,

the names of which were to be carefully sealed to the observer, only to be revealed by symptoms obtained from the provings. Houatt proved *Belladonna* in the manner prescribed, obtained about three hundred symptoms, two-thirds of which showed the character of the remedy.

April 22, 1869.

Hegel.

"Hegel, who wrote books on philosophy, did not know the difference between the two electricities."

Kill or Cure.

"A young man who had suffered a long time from inter-mittent fever came to me with a doleful tale. He wished to marry the daughter of a rich manufacturer. He could only get her on condition that he would be able to fill the position of fireman in her father's establishment. This, he said, was impossible on account of his being harassed by chills and fever. The young fellow was desperate; said he would either drown or shoot himself if he could not be relieved of the malady. He demanded of me a prescription which would either 'kill or cure!'

"I hesitated a moment, then gave him the following advice: Go to the Schuylkill River when again you feel the attack coming on. Undress. Get some of your friends to tie a rope under your shoulders so that they can suspend you in the water up to your mouth. Jump into the river and force yourself to stay there during the chill. When the fever, which follows the chill, comes on remain there until the sweat appears, then leave the water.

"My directions were followed to the letter. The patient soon became blue in the face; his friends thought he would die, but he motioned to them that he wished to stay in the water. Soon the fever took hold of him and the poor fellow became so weak that he could scarcely utter a word. His friends again motioned to pull him out, but he decided to stand the ordeal. He had been in the water two hours when the sweat came on. He now consented to be taken from the river and his friends pulled him to the shore, wrapped him into warm blankets and took him home. From that day he had no return of chills or fever, was married to the girl of his choice, and supposedly lived happily ever after.

"If again I should be moved to advise such heroic treatment I would urge the patient to get out of the bath as soon as the fever came on.

"The remedy, in good faith, is one of kill or cure!"

Case of the Cuban.

"A young Cuban was brought to Philadelphia for treatment. I was called in consultation with an allopathic physician who had the case in hand. I found a young man, with black eyes, a mere skeleton filled with air, unable to swallow a morsel of food without vomiting it up directly after. He cursed at doctors in general and swore that he would take neither homoeopathic nor any other kind of medicine.

"I sent to the nearest shop for some plain cream, of which I ordered a teaspoonful to be taken, with a little sugar every half hour. The patient took it. Next day he said he had not vomited once. I then increased the quantity of cream to dessert spoonful doses, every hour. On the following day he complained of severe pain in the stomach. I felt a large lump there the size of a fist. This his physician had pronounced to be a cancer. It was none.

"I gave him two globules of *Hyoscyamus* on the tongue. He had no more pain after this. I now ordered a tablespoonful of beef-tea to be taken on the one-half hour, and the same quantity of arrowroot on the next half-hour, turn about. The young man kept on gaining weight steadily and in a short time he returned to his island a well man.

"When he received my bill, in the amount of one hundred dollars, he paid it promptly, telling me that I was the most sensible doctor he had ever met, and at the same time the most stupid, because he had expected to pay me no less than a thousand.

"This patient recommended a great many others to me, from Cuba. Homoeopathy flourished there until it was spoiled by another physician, a colleague."

Unpaid Advice.

"Later, while still living on Walnut Street, there came to my office, a father and son. The son was in almost the same condition as the case just described. The father asked me what he should do. I told him to give his son small quantities of food, and often. When I had turned my back the two slipped out from my office without paying a fee. I subsequently learned that the father said: 'Anybody could have given him the same advice!' And yet it cured his boy! There is much truth in small suggestions like these, often overlooked, or disregarded by reason of their apparent insignificance."

Imagination.

"This plays a strong part in the getting well, or being made worse, with many sick people. Well people who yet imagine themselves to be ill should be punished."

Ungrateful Patients.

"I was asked the other day whether it was not very provoking, as well as discouraging, to meet with ungrateful patients. Ingratitude we meet with every day, said I. Our Lord and Master was covered with it. Surely God has more cause to complain of ingratitude than have I!"

More of the same Medicine.

A patient, one morning, sent his man to "get some more of the same medicine," but to get it from the young doctor; who had probably prescribed it on the advice of the older one.

Charity.

One morning a man was waiting in the reception room. When I came in he asked that both doors be closed. He then told me that his name was B..............., a young doctor from Boston, on his way to West Chester, where he had an uncle. He said he was without a penny in his pockets, so asked me to lend him sixty cents, to go by the noon train. I gave him seventy-five cents, which he promised to return on the following day. I never saw him again. He had

said that he had expected his uncle to meet him at the
American House. He smelled of rum and wore shabby
clothes. Dr. Hering is frequently approached by mendi-
cants; by some honestly, mostly otherwise. I am supposed
to stand between him and these to shield him from unworthy applicants, but he is often imposed upon in one
way or another, in spite of my efforts.

Natural History. The Ichneumon Fly.

The Icheumon Fly lays its eggs into the body of a live
caterpillar. After the caterpillar is converted into a
chrysalis there emerges from it, not a butterfly but the
Ichneumon Fly.

April 23, 1869.

Aloes.

"I went to a druggist in Philadelphia by the name of
Morris to buy some *Aloes.* He showed me two kinds. I
told him that both of them were adulterations. He sent
his boy out to all the drug stores in town for more samples.
An immense heap of *Aloes* was collected, all of them
bogus. The druggist was chagrined. He sent to New
York for more samples. I came to examine this large
assortment bu did not find a single genuine specimen
among them. At last I noticed that the druggist held back
a small package, carefully wrapped in paper, which he
did not seem willing to show me. I asked to see it. He
handed it over, smiled as I said: 'This is genuine aloes.
Where did you get it'' He confessed that he had stolen
it from a collection in the Academy of Pharmacy, of which
he was a trustee. The sample had been brought into the
country by an expedition that had sailed around the world
and had received the specimen from the Sultan of Muscat,
who grew the plant from which the substance is derived.
When you break a piece of *Aloes* the fracture must show
a purplish golden tint, almost transparent. The adulterated specimens were boiled in certain oils to such a degree that they made the paper, in which they came,
greasy.

"*Aloes* has its sphere of action in the pelvis. There is great congestion there, with a feeling of fulness as if everything was tending there; *hemorrhoidal tenesmus.*"

Inflammation.

"Inflammation is the result of overaction of the serous membranes. If these become overactive the natural vacuum which exists in the serous sacs is increased and a congestion of blood to the part results. Vertigo is due to diminished action of the serous membranes of the brain, causing diminution of blood there. Overaction of the serous membranes of the heart produces violent palpitation and other heart symptoms. When the pendulum swings back we have the opposite symptoms; depressed heart-action, etc. They wish to prove this theory by experiments. This cannot be done."

Anecdote. Disobliging Help.

"Whenever others do not wish to do a thing for me I always go and do it myself. At one time a heavy snow fell. It snowed as if there were huge bags of feathers in the clouds which were ripped open and emptied of their contents upon the earth beneath. The family wash hung on the line, on the stable roof. The coachman had been asked to take it down. He refused. I pulled on a pair of heavy boots said: "Hahnemann geh du voran, du hast die grossen Stiefel an." (Hahnemann, you take the lead, the biggest boots are on your feet) and plunged to the shoulders into the snow. After me rushed the whole pack of servants; with them one of the young ladies who had some valuable clothes among the lot, and who was most eager to press forward, following close at my heels. At last, after great exertion, we reached the stable. Having first lifted the heavy trap-door, laden with snow, I made my way to the roof where I cut down the line upon which the clothes were suspended, brought it down to the ground where those below took them off. When we got back to the house everybody exclaimed: "Oh, but this is outrageous! Just think of the doctor!" The coachman had hidden angrily in some corner.

"A man who wished to have some letters taken to the Post Office, on finding that his errand boy was busy, asked his coachman to carry the letters. The coachman replied: "It is not my business!" "Ah, yes!" said the man, "I forgot. Excuse me. You may hitch the horses and bring the carriage around to the door." The coachman opened his eyes wide in surprise when the boy-of-all-work stepped into the carriage, letters in hand and asked to be driven to the Post Office in style, there to deposit the letters."

Often in life the doctor had to take the burden upon his shoulders, without thinking it too hard to bear if thereby he could serve the cause.

Martin. Co-Editor of Journal.

Today Dr. Martin came to ask for copy. He asked for more characteristics, such as were being printed in the College Journal. Dr. Hering said that he had thousands of them up-stairs; that he had only waited for Martin to ask for them. It seems that at one time the co-editor had shown reluctance to printing more of the keynotes which had become so popular with the students and subscribers to the Journal.

Work on the Repertory.

Dr. Hering asked me today, to make a further classification of the symptoms from Jahr's *Leitfaden* (Therapeutic Guide). He said that Jahr gave some remedies, like *Aconite* and *Su.,.hur* almost universally; *Kali bich.* only once or twice; *Gelsem.* not at all, and some of the other remedies very rarely. It is a great piece of work to dissect a book of this kind, but it "gives one a look behind the curtain," as Hering expresses it.

April 25, 1869.

Ferrum. Digitalis.

"*Ferrum* has great similarity to *Rhus tox.* It would be interesting to know if there is much iron in the soil where the *Rhus* grows. I could hardly tell the difference in the cough peculiar to the two remedies. There is also great similarity in the asthmas and neuralgias.

"Does *Digitalis* grow on calcareous soil? The plant grows in large patches as though sown, in the Schwarzwald near Wildbad. I do not know if it is found growing near the *Belladonna*, but think it is; at least so says Dr. Koch, Sen."

The Man who hired a Mule. Anecdote.

"A man from ancient Greece hired a mule to ride. It became very warm, the mule sweated, became tired and stood still in the sun. The man got off the mule to rest in the animal's shadow. The driver, who followed at the mule's heels, claimed that the shadow belonged to him and not to the man who hired the animal. A quarrel was the result and the case went to court. Query. If a man hires a mule, does he also hire his shadow?"

Odd Fellows.

Today there was a parade by Odd Fellows. Hering says that the Odd Fellows do a great deal of good.

Morgan. Theories.

Professor Morgan preaches his pet theory on spinal centrics and excentrics to Dr. Hering, who does not seem to favor it much. Morgan was the son of a school teacher.

Euphrasia and Cepa.

Hering calls attention to a comparison between them.

April 27, 1869.

Sugar Cane.

"Sugar Cane is planted in beds intersected by canals. The water which is let in at high tide drives the mills. Negroes float the cane to the mills where it is pressed. The men get drowsy over the work at the machines and sometimes are drawn in. An axe is kept ready to hand with which to sever their limbs, when caught."

"The liquid pressed from the cane is boiled and the crystallized mass is put into barrels. The leakage is termed Plantation molasses. The sugar cane is soaked and pressed a second time, when it yields a good deal more of sugar. The dry cane should be burned and the ashes put back into the soil. An old farmer once told me, 'Everything that my acre gives, it must have again.' "

College. Jealousy.

Professors Martin and Koch, of the College, conspire against Professor Gause. The green-eyed monster, jealousy.

Palpitation.

Palpitation, worse from motion, is hard to find in the *Materia Medica.*

April 28, 1869.

A Curse upon Secretmongers.

Hering says he has written down a terrible curse against all persons who keep secret things that would be of benefit to the world.

The curse is to be printed. He says: "It was written before my acquaintance with Fincke, who kept secret his process of potentization."

The terrible curse condemns offenders to everlasting perdition, in the lowermost depths of hell, to the second and third generations. Hering calls it the most terrible curse ever pronounced.

A Fair.

A Fair is to be organized for the benefit of a Homoeopathic Hospital in Philadelphia. The first meeting is to be held at the College. The attendance of two hundred and fifty ladies is expected at the initial meeting.

Museum.

"I suggest that a museum be established in which, for adornment, there will be columns decorated with designs taken from natural trees, in leafwork, branches and flowers; from the coca tree, the camphor tree, etc. Designs for Grecian columns were taken from nature."

Nitrum.

"A keynote of *Nitrum* is: drinking often but little at a time. The patient drinks little at a time because the act of swallowing interferes with respiration. This is Grauvogl's observation."

Pictures.

Hering is opposed to the hanging of certain pictures of skin diseases on the College walls. It makes the place look like what he quaintly calls a show-shanty.

April 29, 1869.

Newspapers.

"*The New York Herald* was begun in Philadelphia and went to New York. It was a sensational paper which published scandals under the management of Bennett. *The Tribune*, under Horace Greeley, became an opposition paper. Whatever in the way of editorials appeared in Bennett's paper, was contradicted in the *Tribune*, on the following day. This rivalry continued for many years. If the *Herald* condemned homoeopathy, the *Tribune* was in favor of it. If the *Herald* disapproved of spiritualism, the *Tribune* defended it. The *Tribune* gained ascendancy over the *Herald* when that paper got into bad repute.

"A certain geologist predicted that the waters going over the Falls of Niagara would in time wear away, or undermine. the rocks over which they flow and there would no longer be a Niagara. The story was a hoax, which the *Herald* printed as news. The *Tribune* had the laugh on its rival.

"Yesterday the Philadelphia *Press* printed an article which said that Greeley had been swindled for the 86th time, by a story that a young man, who had an accomplice in Philadelphia, had induced a certain candidate for office to pay him money for advertising him in the *Tribune*."

Ancestors. Moravians.

Hering's ancestors were Moravians who spelled their name Hring. They had come from their home in the mountains to settle on the banks of the river Elbe where they became sailmakers and fishermen.

Hering likes the custom of the Moravians which, at sunrise, on Easter morning, brings them to the churchyard where they hold religious services. They keep holy All Saint's Day, which comes on the second of November. He believes that the Moravians honour men as Saints who have been of great use to the world.

Schiller.

The doctor asks me to remind him to tell the story of Schiller in the role of a Saint. The story is about a farmer who prayed to the statue of Schiller. He was put up to it by a student.

Plays for the benefit of the Hospital. Gaertner. Septette of Beethoven. Formes. A Fire.

A project for raising funds to build a homoeopathic hospital is under way. Tonight there is to be given a theatrical entertainment for this purpose in Dr. Hering's house, in which members of his family will participate. The sum of twenty-four dollars was raised by this performance, which is to be devoted to the buying of material to be used at the Fair. Two plays were given, one of them *Der Geburtstag der Geister* (Birthday of Ghosts) by the children; one of whom, Walter was to play the part of the boy who boasts before the other children that he is not afraid of ghosts. For this he is ridiculed by his playmates. To take revenge upon his tormentors he disguises himself as a ghost, and as such makes his appearance. When the real ghost comes upon the scene the bogus one becomes so frightened that he tears off his mask and sheet, and has to face the ridicule from the other children who call him "Hasenfuss" (coward).

In a second play, *Die Hochzeitsreise by Bendix*, Rudolph, the oldest son, took the principal part, that of the Professor; Bertha, a niece, the part of the wife Antonia; Melitta played the part of the Famulus; in men's clothes. The Professor's assistant, or student, was played by William Boericke, who later became prominent among homoeopathic physicians. He took the comedy part of Hahnesporn, a man-servant. Miss Raue, niece of Professor Raue of the Hahnemann College, took the part of the chambermaid across the way from the Professor's house.

The Professor, in white vest, black coat and pants and a high hat was excellently portrayed by Rudolph. The Professor has peculiar notions of a wife's duties in the home, and after the wedding, is seemingly more in love with his books than with his wife who finds herself in a cheerless house, without servants; no cook, not a decent bedroom, no household comforts, while the Professor, interested to know how the ancient Greeks and Romans treated their wives, forgets that he is a husband. His pretty and determined wife does not relish this and sets about converting her indifferent spouse. She at first succeeds in arousing his jealousy, after which she proposes a wedding-trip. He agrees to this and just before the curtain falls he is seen awkwardly trying to take her into his arms.

The large communicating rooms, with wide folding-doors of mahogany, separating the doctor's private office from his reception room, afforded an excellent opportunity for a stage setting in the back room, and for places for about forty or fifty friends of the family, who, after enjoying the German play, adjourned to the dining-room across the hall, where ale, tapped from the wood, and pretzels were served by the German maids. All became merriment and German *gemuethlichkeit*.

Private theatricals were of frequent occurrence in the home, in which the writer took part. There were musical events, programs of strictly classical music, rendered by prominent musicians, who thought it a pleasure to play for Dr. Hering, whenever invited. His friend Carl Gaertner, a Swede, a fine violinist, who was among the first to introduce classical chamber music to Philadelphians, was always ready to oblige. On several occasions the Septette of Beethoven was performed, which required seven instruments for its rendition. A musician by the name of Schneider played the horn.

This particular composition, arranged for four hands

on the piano, was played nightly, after the dinner hour, by myself and one of the daughters, Melitta, who became my future wife. This was done to entertain the doctor who sat at his work in the adjoining study humming his favorite melodies.

The celebrated opera basso, Carl Formes, was a frequent guest at the house, where he was entertained whenever his performances in grand opera brought him to Philadelphia. He was then the world's finest basso, who, in his roles of Sarastro, Leperello, Rocco and Marcel had no equal. To the famous aria, sung by Leperello from Mozart's *Don Giovanni*, Dr. Hering had made words in accordance with the rapid increase in members of homoeopathic physicians throughout the world. This aria Formes rendered with great *eclat* and gusto on occasions when friends were assembled in the house.

After some of the guests had departed, a small party of the gayest who remained, adjourned to the stage back of the curtain to play the game of *Heraus wers hat* (Button, button, who has the button) with great hilarity. Mrs. Hering, as gay as her daughters, and Hering's niece Bertha, joined in the fun and Carl Gaertner, violinist and wife, Mr. and Mrs. McGeorge, Mr. Faber, artist and wife, Mr. Midnight, Rudolph Hering, Miss Tafel, William Boericke and myself, enjoyed the party, which lasted into the small hours. Dr. Hering had retired to his study.

Before the party ended there was an alarm of fire in the neighborhood. We looked out of the windows. The sky to the North was lurid. We all rushed to the top of the house, better to see. Some crying, some laughing, "Is it our Church?" (The Swedenborgian Church at Broad and Brandywine Streets.) Others said, "It is the great velocipede-ring close to the Church." Who will run to the fire? "I and I"—even the ladies are ready to go. We rushed madly down stairs to the second floor. There stood the gray-haired doctor. "No! Ladies, you shall not run to a fire. Gentlemen," he said, "when I was as young as you, I was first at a fire." We made a dash for it, Professor Koch and myself in the lead. We encountered a stream of

water from a hose that had sprung a leak; Koch was completely drenched, I almost as badly. We were in our best
clothes. We arrived in time to see a large and beautiful
building almost a heap of ashes. We stood against a
brick-wall, almost red-hot, whence we had a good view
of the fire, there to dry our wet clothes. No ill effects
followed.

April 30, 1869.

A Concert.

I went with Mrs. Hering and some of the younger folks,
to attend Carl Gaertner's Fifth Classical Concert. Miss
Bertha Hering sang in a duet from *Der Freischuetz;* also
in a trio. Gaertner played a solo on the violin, *The
Soldier's Farewell,* his own composition, with great effect.
These concerts are truly appreciated by the music lovers
of Philadelphia. There is to be a grand introductory
concert, to be given by Gaertner, for the benefit of the
Fair fund.

Wedding Trips.

Dr. Hering is opposed to wedding trips, which he condemns in the strongest terms, as "Eine, verruchte Sitte," an
outrageous custom. He believes it to be deterimental to
health to be travelling at such a time. Thinks it is the
time, of all times, when young married couples should
stay at home instead of philandering about the country.
He says the mode was introduced by the German nobility,
and claims that the custom had a questionable origin
morally, like the coming into fashion of the crinoline
among the French.

May 1, 1869.

Gambling. Gaertner.

Carl Gaertner dined with us. He spoke of the vice of
gambling; how it obsesses its victims, even more powerfully than the abuse of narcotics; how men in Europe have
staked their honour, that of their wives, and the liberty of

their children for the sake of material gain.

Fairs.

Dr. Hering wishes Fairs to become general. People must work for an end *(zweck)*. Money is an equivalent for work. Work therefore is money, and money work. Each and every worker for the Fair must set an estimate upon his labor, whose equivolent it must bring. No more, no less. Homoeopathic Fairs should be an annual occurrence, like the *Jahrmarkt* in Germany.

Character Building.

Hering's teachers were mild, genial, loving men. His father, a teacher, was of the same disposition. He had great respect for etiquette, and a yielding disposition, Hering's grandfather not quite so much. Hering is different, straight forward and unyielding when on the side of truth. Children should not be obliged to imitate their parents, at least not their faults. He says he would not advise his sons to go through with all he had experienced. Yet, he says, he has had great luck in his life.

A man from the Pfalz. De Nusky.

I conversed with one of the doctor's patients this afternoon whose name is Koch, formerly from Allentown. He is a German, originally from the Palatinate. He has great admiration for the Pennsylvania German people. He thinks them hospitable and kind, and admires their honesty. He remembers my great uncle, the Rev. John Helfrich, who was associated with Dr. Hering at the Allentown Academy. He saw him at a convention of ministers at Norristown. Also the Reverends Bibige and Miller. He knew De Nusky, a resident of Kutztown, who had also been a minister, and originally came from Hamburg, in Germany; left his country on account of religious persecution. Everything he did was for money. He married a rich but very ignorant woman. He had suffered shipwreck on his way to this country, arriving at New York, poor, almost naked. He became very rich, in later life, while living in Allentown.

Bethlehem. Moravians.

"Bethlehem in Pennsylvania was founded more than 200 years ago by Moravians under a certain Count Zinsendorf, who left Saxony on account of persecution. The Indians around Bethlehem stood in great awe of this man who they thought was sent to them by the Great Spirit, and they prostrated themselves before his shadow. They could not have been moved to do him harm. The Count lies buried in the graveyard by the Moravian Church in Bethlehem."

Pennsylvania German Dialect.

"A good part of the dialect was brought from the Palatinate in Germany. Many immigrants came from Switzerland. Those who came from Holland had been greatly persecuted by the Spaniards. A stipend was given to young men who wished to study for the ministry, afterwards sent as missionaries to America. Michael Schlatter was one who was sent to Pennsylvania. It was the Prince of Orange, whose forces won a victory over the Spaniards, who saved Protestantism in Holland. The dreadful Spanish Inquisition spread over Europe. In Paris thousands of Protestants were put to death; King Charles himself fired upon them from the windows of his palace, the Luxembourg. The Huguenots secreted themselves in the catacombs, under the city. The Spanish put to death many of the Protestant Moors, in their country, who were a modified race of Caucasians, very skilful in the art of architecture."

May 2, 1869.

Keeping the Sabbath.

Rainy and cold in the morning. I helped Rudolph make forms of crystals from pasteboard. He has no special regard for the Sabbath, which he estimates like any other day in the week. This at first affected me strangely.

In Europe, where Rudolph received his education, some of the people go to church in the morning, and others,

young and old, take their pleasure in the afternoon which
is devoted to enjoyment of every kind. He does not go to
church, says he does not derive any benefit from it. He
visited Oschatz, in Saxony, the birthplace of his father:
also Dresden, which has 150,000 inhabitants. Philadelphia at the present time, 1869, has but 100,000.

Oschatz.

Oschatz, a small town in Germany, was destroyed by fire
and rebuilt, so it no longer bears much resemblance to the
birthplace of Dr. Hering. His father moved his family to
Zittau, a picturesquely situated small town in Saxony.
None of the relations are living in the former place at the
present time.

Different stories are told of the way in which the town
received its romantic name. Hering's secretary, Dr.
Knabe, also a Saxon, told the tale in the following way:
The count who governed the domain, was on a hunting
party with his lady-love, on horseback, when they halted
and overlooked the few houses that were built. "What
shall we name the place, my dear?" said the count. "*O
Schatz*," modestly said the lady, "how should I tell?"
"*Oschatz* it shall be then," said the count. *Schatz* being
German for sweetheart.

Travelling in Europe.

Rudolph Hering thinks it would cost two thousand
dollars to make the tour of Europe at the present time.
Three years later, when visiting abroad and giving some
time to the hospitals, besides touring, I found that this was
about the sum required for an eighteen month's stay, devoted to study and to travel.

A Sunday afternoon. Round Table. Allopathic Doctors.

I read to the ladies a delightful article, from the Gartenlaube, entitled *Ohne Dornen, keine Rosen* (Without
Thorns, no roses). In it four characteristics, peculiar to
women, are described:

1. Roses with but few thorns.
2. Roses with many thorns.

3. *Klatschrosen* (red ones) for the gossipy kind.
4. *Eva-Roeschen*, roses named after mother Eve.

Then came some of the Sunday visitors to gather about the round table, in the back room, with Hering in the center of the circle, and Mrs. Hering pouring delicious coffee. The younger women sat with their *Handarbeit*, knitting, embroidery, or some light occupation, listening to the wisdom of the men as German women are wont to do.

Dr. Hering on the subject of allopaths says: their ways are mean, cunning and underhand; they deceive, they cheat, they steal, they kill. He relates the case of a lady, who hid in the closet of a room while allopathic doctors were holding a consultation over the case of one of her women friends, who was employing Dr. Lingen, a homoeopath. In a revengeful mood the doctors declared that this patient should not, dare not be permitted to get well and live under homoeopathic treatment. The lady in the closet overheard the conspiracy. Under some pretext the patient was removed, taken to England, away from her homoeopathic physician, where after five or six weeks, she died.

Macfarlan. Surgery.

Dr. Malcolm Macfarlan accepted the position of Professor of Operative Surgery in our College, which Hering thinks will ultimately make it a successful institution, since surgery is the point of the augur *(Chirurgie ist die Spitze des Bohrers)*.

Dr. Macfarlan had become popular as surgeon in the army during our Civil War. He was particularly successful with operations for hernia.

Fairs.

Dr. Hering aims to raise American Fairs to the standard of the European *Volksfest*. He thinks Fairs will have a good moral influence upon people. Children will work with an end in view. He contemplates writing articles for the papers on the subject of "Fairs and their Philosophy."

Some years ago, Miss Hering says, her father was desperately opposed to Fairs. He is now prepared to de-

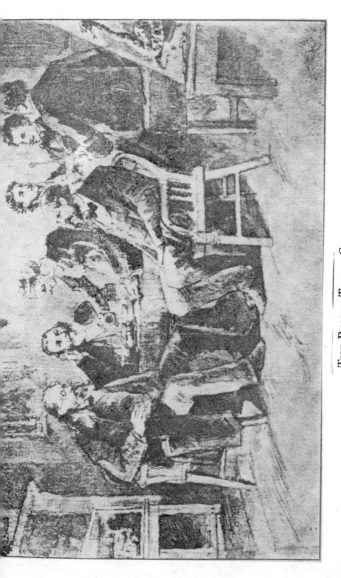

THE ROUND TABLE GROUP.

COPY OF A DRAWING BY HERMANN FABER OF A FAMILY GROUP IN DR. HERING'S HOME IN PHILA-
DELPHIA. THE PERSONS REPRESENTED ARE, FROM LEFT TO RIGHT: CONSTANTINE HERING; DR.
AUGUST KOCH, PHYSICIAN; MRS. HERING; DR. OSWALD SEIDENSTICKER, PROFESSOR; MELITTA
HERING (DR. KNERR'S WIFE); DR. C. B. KNERR; HERMANN FABER, ARTIST.

fend them. Also Dr. Guernsey, who is said to be opposed to Fairs, *in toto*, has had his name placed on a circular letter to be sent to the doctors.

The Sabbath.

Hering observes that Dr. Gause never stays a minute over 12 o'clock, midnight, at any of the faculty meetings, on a Saturday night. He says: "Now my Sunday begins!" To which Hering replies: "That's right, Dr. Gause, keep your Sunday. I like you for that. You are honest." Dr. Morgan, too, keeps his Sunday strictly. Dr. W., who is opposed to keeping the dispensary open on Sunday, says it will bring us into bad repute. He is the one who told Hering, "Every man ought to go to church for appearances sake!"

Hering says it is an old story that when Christ was asked: "Is a man justifiable to break the Sabbath?" he answered: "If he knows what he is doing." *(Wenn er weiss was er thut)*. The saying is Godlike enough to have come from Jesus' lips. Hering seems to think that Christ instituted the Sabbath for the Jews, who needed some such formal arrangement.

May 3, 1869.

Fair.

In the evening a preliminary meeting was held by the Professors of the College, seconded by Dr. Williamson, to discuss Fair matters; the principal meeting is to be held tomorrow.

Temperance.

Hering talked on the subject of temperance. Said he had treated two prominent lecturers on the subject, for *mania potu.* They gave as a reason for drinking; that "they could lecture better under the influence of liquor!" Wine is sacred, he thinks, and whosoever says anything against its proper use, commits a sin against the Holy Ghost. Alcohol is injurious, therefore a bad thing to be addicted to. Wine is an antidote to drunkenness.

He thinks that beer, in moderation, serves a good purpose, but that in those parts of Germany where beer is
taken to excess the people become fat, gross and slothful
and lack ambition. Horace Greeley remarked that he had
seen about as much drunkenness in those parts of Europe
where wine is used as in other places. Henry Ward
Beecher denied this, saying that he found very little, or no
drunkenness, in places where the use of wine is customary.
Hering says: "One ass comes out and says, 'I saw drunkenness,' and the other one says: 'I saw none!' "

The Tribune.

A man by the name of Young, who wrote contributions
in the form of letters, for Greeley's paper, sued Dana, the
proprietor of another paper, in the sum of .one hundred
thousand dollars, for publishing his letters which revealed
a certain swindling plot.

_____

May 4, 1869.

The Fair. Richard Koch's opposition.

Dr. Hering received a letter from Dr. Pulte, in Cincinnati, where they also are getting up a Fair for the benefit of a homoeopathic hospital. Pulte is to conduct pioneer
tables and is asking Hering to contribute a dozen of his
pictures. Hering says he must do something to help them,
then maybe they will do something for us. Pulte was
associated with the Allentown Academy. While there he
wrote a biography of himself in which he quoted a memorial poem, written after the death of Schoenlein, the
German pathologist. Although Pulte has done much for
homoeopathy he is of such an overbearing disposition
that he is hard to get along with. He wrote of a certain
man, whom Hering respected, "he is unscientific, ignorant
and unworthy of confidence!" The elder Miss Hering,
Odelia, was quite indignant over Pulte's behavior.

Richard Koch predicts that the Fair will be a failure, by
reason of a certain member being on the committee,
(meaning Morgan) who "from selfish motives will hinder
its success." He thinks that Morgan will arrogate to him-

self directorship of the hospital. Koch says "he will eat
his shirt" if the Fair realizes more than five thousand
dollars, and offers to bet five hundred to back his opinion.
It netted seventeen thousand. The bet was not paid.

Somehow everything Hering proposes, Koch opposes.
If Hering asks to have the plates representing diseases of
the skin removed from the walls of the College building
on visiting days, Koch insists on having them remain. This
morning the Janitor at the College, and myself, removed
these pictures to a floor above, on account of a Ladies'
meeting to be held in the lower room. When Koch found
this out he made complaint because they were not put in
the chemical room, down stairs. Hering threatens to play
the madman. Should Koch hang the pictures again in the
objectionable spot, he says he will "break them up!"

A Caller.

A certain doctor, living not far from Hering's house, a
man not of very good repute in the neighborhood, called
at a late hour to see Dr. Hering, who had retired to his
room on the second floor. The visitor gave the bell a violent pull. When the servant had admitted the gentleman
I stepped into the vestibule and there met a man of middle
age, who grasped my hand, squeezed it, almost lifting it
to his face. His eyes were blue and twinkling, holding
one firmly while he bowed low. Dr. Hering has retired,
I told him, but he will send you a note in the morning.
"Oh no! I will call again. I am not going to Europe before the first of J .e." Another bow, as I opened the
front door; two more bows and he was gone.

The Fair. Dr. Martin.

A ring at the door. In came Dr. Martin. "Professor,
what makes you come so late, the doctor has retired." He
sits down. "I had business," he said. "It is getting so that
I can't see the doctor any more."

"Do you wish to leave a note, Dr. Martin?" "No; it is
nothing in particular."

I explained that Dr. Hering had been up until half after
twelve the evening before and was tired. Prof. Martin

asked, "Who was here?" "Doctors Morgan, Williamson and Gause were here, talking about the Fair."

"Oh, that's the way things are done! Well the whole thing will go to ruin. The dragon's teeth were sown today. There were things done today that will ruin the whole undertaking, perhaps break up the College, too. Many ladies who were present thought so, too."

"Why, Professor, don't be downhearted; I thought a good deal was accomplished today at the meeting."

The Professor gets up and walks to the table. "Ah yes, you have no experience in such matters."

Dr. Martin said: "Well, good night," and walked off in a hasty manner, as if out of humor.

The object of the Ladies' meeting, called for today, was to organize for work to be done for the Fair. The meeting opened at four o'clock. Professor Gause made a short address. The constitution and by-laws were read and discussed; some of the ladies requested that several articles should be changed, or omitted therefrom, after which the constitution and by-laws were adopted. The ladies had brought some men-friends with them who acted as spokesmen and all were enthusiastic over the prospects. About seventy ladies signed their names for membership in the Association.

Student Days.

In the evening, Dr. Farrington present, Hering related the history of his early student days in Leipzig, when he was poor, and struggling to maintain a living.

"On account of leaving the ranks of the allopaths, in which school I had graduated at the University of Wuerzburg, and joining the homoeopaths, I was in sore straits. I occupied a room but poorly furnished, for which I paid twenty-five cents per week; a cold place, where, without fuel, I almost froze on bitter cold days. I was invited to meals at a students' free eating-house (a kind of soup house), but only at such times when other boarders had skipped their meals because they did not think them good enough. Here the bread was good, whatever might be

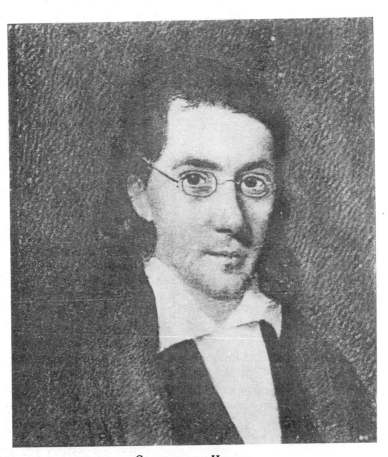

CONSTANTINE HERING.
REPRODUCTION OF A MINIATURE OIL PAINTING ON IVORY,
MADE ABOUT THE TIME OF HIS ENTERING THE
UNIVERSITY OF LEIPZIG.

said of the rest of the food. Often I took home with me scraps of rye bread, which, stale and dry, I soaked in weak broth, or ate them, hard as they were, which made my gums bleed, but in this way I thought I obtained some organic matter for my system! One day a student friend told me of a woman who kept a boarding house, a believer in homoeopathy and in need of treatment.

"My friend coaxed me to go with him to see the woman, who needed *Ignatia;* she invited me to stay to supper. The kind woman soon learned of my condition. She provided me with some spare pieces of wood for a fire and some milk. One day, when she came to my room, she noticed some of the dry bread heaped up on my desk, and wished to know what I intended to do with it. I told her I was saving it for sustenance. She asked me if I had a mind to exchange some of it for milk; that she had some cows and pigs for whom stale bread was very good food. She took some of the hardest pieces. Later, in exchange for treatment, she boarded me until better times came. Shall not one, in remembrance of all this, be enthusiastic for homoeopathy?

"All this is nothing compared to the sufferings Hahnemann experienced when living in Leipzig, persecuted by the old school doctors and apothecaries. His wife upbraided him daily for not doing like other doctors, whose equal he was in learning, and who made money with which to keep their families from starving.

"Hahnemann's son Frederick had become a hunchback in consequence of a wagon overturning with him when a child, on one of the many movings, from place to place, the father was forced to make.

"Also my hand, my *right* hand, I owe to Hahnemann. Why should not I be grateful and enthusiastic for homoeopathy?"

"Should we not be kicked," I (Dr. Knerr) said to Farrington, "if we open our mouths to complain?"

At Raue's House.

In the evening I called for Mrs. Hering, who was visiting at the house of Dr. and Mrs. Raue, on Tenth Street. I there met Dr. Starkey and Mrs. Peltzer, the wife of a student at Hahnemann. Mrs. Raue entertained us by playing exquisitely on the piano. How well these dear German people know how to enjoy themselves! We had wine and cake, laughed and sang, and there were "good nights" and good-night kisses, at parting, with invitations soon to come again.

Berridge.

Hering wrote a letter to McClatchey, editor of the Hahnemann Monthly magazine, calling attention to Dr. Berridge's repertory, which he thinks is the clearest and best, so far. "As many of us," he says, "as do not wish to eat what others have chewed, ought to get the book!"

Motion.

There are four kinds of motion: (1) Up and down; (2) From side to side; (3) Forward and backward—the motion of the rocking chair, and (4) the swing.

The first is the motion of health, enjoyed by babies. The baby-jumper is an excellent invention for the nursery.

The second is not health, but not quite as bad as the third, which is most detrimental to women and children, causing all manner of diseases with them. No person can stand a rocking chair in the long run.

A fourth motion, that of swinging around in a circle, is the worst of all motions.

The Fair.

An old lady suggested that Dr. Hering get some oak wood from the old Lutheran Church at Fourth and Cherry Streets, where reconstruction is going on, and make relics out of it to be sold at the Fair. I went to a Mr. W. and bespoke a load of the wood to be used for this purpose, from which were fashioned brackets, paper knives, etc., which brought a good price at the Fair.

In the evening Dr. Gause brought printed copies of an *Appeal to Homoeopathic Physicians for Aid for the*

Fair. The word *Similia* was misspelled, and one thousand copies had to be corrected!

Raue.

We went again to Dr. Raue's house to celebrate his wife's birthday. It happened to be a rather dry affair and Dr. Hering slept through the better part of the evening. We could not get warmed up, on this occasion.

May 6, 1869.

Hempel. Arsenic. Aconite. Lippe.

"Hempel posed as a scholar in *Materia medica.* He was extremely ignorant in general practice and scarcely knew the difference between two medicines. He did a lot of translating and brought out a huge volume on *Materia medica.* At a meeting of the Institute, held in St. Louis, he boasted that he had studied the subject *considerably!*

"When he was Professor of *Materia medica,* in Philadelphia, he wrote a *New Organon,* in which he defended free love. There were but a limited number of copies printed, some twenty or forty, which later went for waste-paper.

"In Canada there was a certain married man by the name of King, who fell in love with another woman and gave his wife powders for the ostensible purpose of making a proving. The woman died from arsenical poisoning. The man was arrested and put on trial. Hempel was subpoenad to give testimony in the case. He went to Canada for this purpose, and appeared in court where he was to give his opinion. He was asked: 'What constitutes an allopathic dose of arsenic?' He mentioned some mistaken quantity and an authority, quoted at random, and obscure names, which disgusted the jury. He was asked whether large doses of the poison were permitted under homoeopathic treatment, and whether patients ever died from them. Hempel answered: 'Oh, we *try* not to kill them!' The witness was removed from the trial in disgust and the jury unanimously found King guilty of murdering his wife, whose body had been exhumed and found full of arsenic. The murderer was hung. Hempel's testimony was not mentioned in the Judge's summary. His own lawyers were disappointed in their witness.

"In the Michigan University there was to be instituted a chair for homoeopathic *Materia medica*. A lady living in the town, who had been a patient of Dr. Lippe, in Philadelphia, was appointed to look for a genuine homoeopath to fill the vacancy. She was taken ill and sent for a young physician in the town, a homoeopath, who came to see her. The patient asked for tumblers in which to prepare the medicine. The young doctor said: 'I will have no use for the tumblers!' 'Why not?' 'Because I wish to treat my patients, as Hahnemann did, with powders.' 'You are the right one,' said the lady.

"She then wrote an account of this to Dr. Lippe, who on learning that Hempel was trying for the professorship at Michigan, promptly consulted Dr. Hering in the matter, who then showed to Lippe the papers from Canada, containing an account of the trial of King, revealing the ignorance and disgrace of Hempel. Lippe sent the papers to the lady, whose husband was influential in politics. Hempel's standing was investigated by the physicians who attended the wife, also through correspondence with Lippe, which brought down the wrath of Hempel upon his head."

Some years later, when the Institute was to meet in New York, a man from the West came to Hering to enlist his influence in making Hempel president of that association. The man mentioned the opposition from Dr. Lippe. Hering said: "It was I who gave Lippe the papers and told him to send them."

It was reported, later, when Hempel was in the West, that he had an affair with a divorced woman, which resulted in the birth of twins, that these soon died after being taken to Hempel's home, with symptoms of *Aconite* poisoning. Not long after, the mother also died of similar symptoms.

At one time Hempel tried to introduce this woman to Mrs. Hering, which was "No go," the doctor says. For which reason, and the sending of the papers, Hempel opposed everything that came from Dr. Hering; even the

Lachesis was condemned as being "no remedy," an assertion made by Hempel in his *Materia medica*.

History.

"The first inhabitants of Europe were a barbarous race
of people which came from Asia. They were followed by
the Gauls, also from Asia. These destroyed the barbarians
which gave rise to the Epistle to the Galatians. The French
are descendents from these. After the Gauls came the
Aryans, who came from the Caucasus and from these were
the Teutons and other Germanic races. After them came
the Slavs. The Anglo Saxons were a modification of
Aryans as also are the Normans. After the Slavs came
the Moors, who were opposed by the Catholics, which
opposition caused a religious war. Later came the Huns,
who settled in Hungary, and many centuries later the
Turks, who were scattered by King Charles".

College. The Fair.

There is now a great disturbance going on among the
members of the Faculty over a disposition to be made of
the money realized from the Fair. Professor Morgan
came to say that the money must not go into an endowment
fund for the college, but must be put out at interest, at six
per cent, which is contrary to Hering's idea, also opposed
to the wishes of Professors Koch, Gause and Martin, all of
whom are dissatisfied with Morgan's attitude, such contention being likely to ruin the Fair. All that the Ladies,
who work for the Fair, are interested in is raising as large
a sum of money as possible for the purpose of building a
hospital, caring little about the form of investment of the
capital. In order to bring the quarrel to an end and save
the enterprise, Hering, with great determination, says: "I
will see that my plans are carried out and put through!"

One is here reminded of the attitude of Marcus Pontius
Cato, the Roman Senator, of whom Hering says: "When
his mind was made up, he allowed nothing to stand in the
way of accomplishment." When Cato had decided that
Carthage must be destroyed he never missed an opportunity to make known his will. When he voted "Yea" in

the forum, he always finished with: "And Carthage must be destroyed." If he voted "Nay" he added: "But Carthage must be destroyed." And Carthage was destroyed! Cato was a negative man. Our Benjamin Franklin, also a man with a determined will, was a positive man, also thrifty, who, when he saw a piece of rag lying on the street, picked it up and said: "It cost a deal of work to make it!"

Hering often says concerning the last drop of wine in the bottle: "We must count the drops. There is an ancient saying among people in Germany that every drop of wine costs seven drops of sweat, to grow it. Wine cannot be manufactured. It must grow." So Hering, too, is a positive man who has to fight a great deal with the rest of the faculty.

The Fair.

Gause made a misstatement, in a circular concerning the Fair, in which he asks for a hundred thousand dollars to be raised; an amount out of reason and not to be expected.

College. Macfarlan.

Dr. Hering is bound to have Macfarlan in the Faculty. In this he succeeded against great opposition from some of the members.

Satire.

Hering, when an allopath, before coming over to homoeopathy, wrote a skit against Hahnemann, a burlesque. The theatrical manager of the town could not get his company to play it. They were all staunch homoeopaths! Hering says he never told Hahnemann about this.

Theatre. Beauty.

Hering once saw the famous play, *Kaetchen von Heilbronn*, played by a very homely girl who won her laurels by her meekness and modesty.

May 9, 1869.
Herbariums. Botany.

Hering helped his friend Weigel in Suriname to press three thousand plants. The plants were sent to South

America from the Academy of Natural Sciences, in Philadelphia, to be assorted and pressed.

Instructions, "The plants are first laid carefully upon
some sheets of blotting paper. Newspapers will do. Parts
of the plant must not touch. A leaf must not touch a
stem; slips of paper must be put between, also between
the petals of flowers. Lay the sheet of paper containing
the plant between two pads of brown, or any common
paper, and these upon a board, or a table, with a weight
on top. Proceed in this manner until you have a pile of
them. Pass a string around the parcel and draw it mod-
erately tight. The important thing is to press the plants
gradually. At intervals of a few days the string will bear
tightening, while the plants shrink and begin to dry.
Should moist plants get mouldy take them out of the paper
to dry, and also dry the paper before putting back the
plants."

Gradual Force. The Story of the Tick. Prolapsus Uteri.
Hering's principle in all mechanical operations is to
go to work gradually: which is illustrated by the following story told by Hering:

"While still a boy, going into the woods berrying with
my sister, she got a tick fastened upon her back. Later
she came to me crying, saying: 'She had a tumor on her
back, which hurt, and she did not wish to tell father because he would send for a doctor to whom she would have
to expose her body, and she would rather die than consent
to this.' I went to work on the offending insect to pry it
loose, but sister said: 'If you pull off its body, its head
will remain in the flesh and I will die!' I took hold of
the insect, pressed its body gently, but very gradually, as
you might when holding a pen. At first the tick pinched
harder, as all living things will do when attacked, but the
pressure, applied slowly, unflinchingly, as moves the
minute hand on a clock, compelled the insect to let go
and my sister was relieved. I had performed my first
surgical operation!"

"Mrs. L. . . . . , a patient with *prolapsus uteri* sent for me to give her medical treatment but objected to an examination, thinking that her obstetrician was the one to perform this. When finally persuaded to allow me to make an examination I found the womb low down. I touched the *os uteri* very gently, but firmly, and exerted very gradual pressure, diverting her attention the while from the operation by conversation, when, all at once, the womb went back into its place and the patient experienced great relief. Eminent medical talent is sometimes unable to succeed in similar cases of wedged-in *uteri*, which may be quite painful. I prescribed *Belladonna*, and there was no further trouble. This remedy overcomes spasm of the shpincter muscles in all orifices of the body."

Fish. Taxidermy.

"The bodies of fishes may be beautifully prepared for preservation in the following manner. Take a perfect specimen, lay the fish upon a board on its side, the best side uppermost; the one you wish to preserve. Cut the under side of the fish, from tail to head, with a sharp knife, remove the body and scrape the skin carefully and rub it with lime, or common wood-ashes, stuff the skin with cotton and sew it into shape. When the fish is dried you can mount it upon a board. If the colours have faded they can be revived by suitable pigments applied with a brush."

St. Peters Cathedral in Rome. Prophecies.

"The cupola of the world-famous cathedral will fall, and the Cathedral at Cologne one of whose spires has remained unfinished for a couple of centuries, will soon be completed and at the same time Germany will become united, two problems which in the minds of the people have long been considered improbable, if not impossible of solution. The cupola of St. Peters, as is known, has had a crack, ingeniously mended by heavy bands of iron placed around it. These were heated then allowed to cool, which caused them to shrink and hold tight the damaged structure."

When the writer made a tour of Italy in 1872-3, he visited the Dome of St. Peters in Rome, was given permission to mount to the roof of the immense structure, and found there the iron-band described by Hering, while on the inside of the cupola were seen men at work, on a scaffold, repairing cracks in the ceiling.

At the same time, when visiting Cologne on the Rhine, he beheld the completed spire pointing aloft, while Germany had become united under Bismarck, as predicted by Hering.

Hering thinks he has inherited a gift for foretelling events, from an ancestor in Saxony, who was known as the Prophet on the Elbe, about whom a book was written under the title of the *Man from Prossen*, in which is foretold the fortification of the Lilienstein against the invasion of Napoleon's army, a feat then believed impossible of accomplishment by strategists.

Obelisk.

"A fallen obelisk in Egypt had to be raised and no one knew how to go about it. A young man who thought he had a plan which would do the job, went to the king and offered to raise the obelisk, or lose his head if failing in the attempt. He made the trial with new ropes made wet, which, by causing a shrinking, gradually lifted the obelisk to its place."

Parentage. Birth. Inherited Characteristics.

"From my father I learned uprightness and truth. From my grandfather Schroeder I learned humour and drollery He was wont to say, 'Here, boy, is threepence; run and buy me some snuff! Run; tuck your feet under your arms, and don't let the grass grow under you!' "

"My father was an organist, second to none in all Germany. He was headmaster at the school in Oschatz and played the organ in the church there. He often played in Leipzig, on which occasions the church was crowded. They ca.ed him Magister, a title signifying Master of Arts, or in later times Doctor of Philosophy.

"On the first of January, 1800, about midnight, when my father was playing-in the New Year at the church organ, in Oschatz, it happened that my mother was in childbirth and I was being born. Our neighbor, Zoellner by name, was walking up and down before the house, which adjoined the church, waiting for the maid to bring word as soon as the child had arrived, so that he could carry the news to father, who was seated at the organ. He had not long to wait when godfather Zoellner hurried to father's side and whispered in his ear, 'Herr Magister, it is a boy!' Thereupon pealed forth a burst of praise in the good old Chorale of Martin Luther: *Nun danket alle Gott,* (Let all give thanks to God) so dear to every German heart. The trumpet-angels, attached to the organ, sent forth their hallelujahs, heralding the advent of a new century and with it the birth of a son.

"On the following day, when there was snow on the ground, the parents believing in the hardening process, the child was carried out of doors. My grandmother told me that the child was blue when he was brought into the house. My father, who had lost his first-born son, said: 'This one must live! The other one was weakened by too much coddling!' "

May 11, 1869.

Biography.

I received from Mrs. Hering a biographic sketch of Hering in pamphlet form.

Norton. A Patient.

I called this morning on a wealthy patient of Dr. Hering, who lives in a brown-stone mansion on Arch Street; a banker. This man has been a patient for a number of years, suffering from a chronic neuralgic affection of the head. Of late it was reported that this patient had, contrary to Hering's advice, been taking sulphur baths. The object of my visit was to invite him to the Fair. Mrs. Hering had tried to induce the doctor to make this visit himself, hoping thereby to keep the man for a patient, but Hering proudly said: "On no account will I make a visit

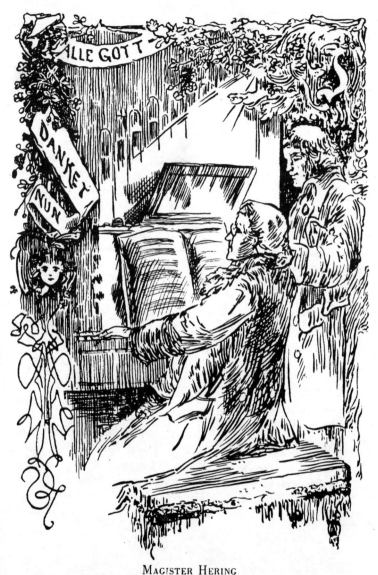

MAGISTER HERING
SEATED AT THE ORGAN PLAYING-IN THE CENTURY ON THE
OCCASION OF THE BIRTH OF HIS SON, CONSTANTINE,
JANUARY 1, 1800, AT OSCHATZ, SAXONY. THIS
DRAWING WAS COPIED FROM AN ORIGINAL
SKETCH BY HERMANN FABER, ARTIST,
OF PHILADELPHIA.

to a patient unasked. Never! Even if I had no practice at all!"

College Journal.

Hering has trouble with Martin, co-editor on the College Journal, who arrogantly writes things which Hering neither hears of, nor sees, until they get into print.

Mortgage.

Dr. Hering speaks of placing a mortgage upon his property for the benefit of the College and Hospital. He fears he might die and his family get the money. He says: "My family shall not have it. I do not wish it so. It is for the cause." For the cause he would sacrifice all.

Laws in History.

"In history there are laws. The laws bring about events. These laws are just as harmonious as those governing astronomy. Their workings are as certain as the motion of the planets. To what end, otherwise, are the countless multitudes of insects, called men, placed upon the earth!"

Martha Washington. Hahnemann.

"One time, in a debate, I maintained that America would never have been freed if it had not been for Martha Washington.

"Mrs. Washington was a rich young widow belonging to one of the noblest families in the Colonies when she married the young lieutenant whose fine traits she admired. At Valley Forge, when almost dead from hardship, and loss of spirits, Washington declared that he would not give up, but if necessary would retire with his army beyond the Rocky mountains, and keep fighting while retreating. It was Martha Washington who had the courage to make a long and dangerous journey from Virginia, through winter snows, to the camp at Valley Forge. She said to her husband: 'You must keep on. You dare not lose courage!'

"We must always take into account the hardships people endure while working in the interest of a great cause. We think of Hahnemann flying from his persecutors in Leipzig with his family, in a wagon, which upset, killing one of his boys outright and making a cripple of another (Frederick) for life."

Revolutionary War. The Ginger Bread Baker.

"Before the revolution a German baker came to this country to make his gingerbread. He had a ready sale for his ware and made quite a sum of money. He used to peddle his stock on the streets. He was an amiable man who talked a mixture of languages. At the time Mrs. Washington came to Valley Forge the impossibility to succeed stared everyone in the face, for there was no money. A meeting was held in the State House, in Philadelphia, where the Gingerbread Man came and sat on a barrel listening to a report that General Washington could not carry on the war because there was no money in the treasury. The Gingerbread Man jumped on top of his barrel and made a speech in which he said: 'Here is a hundred pounds, all the money I have; it is for General Washington to do with as he pleases.' When he had finished his speech he dismounted from the barrel, swore like a trooper, and asked the men who were present to follow his example. All present followed his example, not the swearing, but the contributing of money for the cause. When Washington found out about the gingerbread baker's act, he looked him up and thanked him in the Pennsylvania German dialect, which he had learned to speak, and offered the baker a position to bake for the army.

"The story is told that in contracting for bread to be delivered for the army, Washington asked that an equivalent in weight of a pound of bread for as much flour, should be given. Again the Gingerbread Man began to swear, now, more than before, at the dishonesty of such a contract. He said to the General: 'You have been tricked by a lot of scoundrels in accepting such a dishonest bargain.' He explained the matter to Washington; how the weight of the water and other ingredients that go into the baking would have to be estimated as additional weight. which would demand a larger supply of bread. Washington patted him on the back, called him an honest man and admitted that he had been cheated."

Hering thinks it likely that Martha Washington herself may have gone to Philadelphia to talk with the Gingerbread Man. "It would have been like her," he says.

Married Life.

"I have often observed that if a man loses his wife by death, who has given him a great deal of trouble during their married life, he will mourn her loss more than if their union had been a happier one. *Vice versa* also obtains."

Thomas.

Dr. Thomas, who has been seriously ill, with typhlitis, is recovering, but looks haggard and is weak. Hering has a very high opinion of Thomas and would have been at a loss to replace him, in the chair of anatomy, if he had passed on. Dr. Martin had suggested McClatchey as a substitute.

College. Carpenter.

I never saw Hering so pleasantly excited as he is this evening while telling the following story: "Dr. Koch hired an old carpenter to fix up the College museum. The old carpenter hired two more men to help him. They took it easy. The writer can testify that he never came to the museum but he found one, or all of these men resting or lounging about, and Dr. Hering says he sometimes found them asleep when he went there. In short they had worked six long weeks on a job that three carpenters could have easily done in half the time. Their contract called for the sum of one hundred and twenty-five, to thirty dollars. An order for some additional cases was given, which annulled the contract, so the carpenter now demands three hundred and fifty dollars for the entire job and threatens the college with a lawsuit if his demands are not complied with."

This afternoon the landlord of the carpenter came to Dr. Hering to ask if any money had been paid. "One

hundred and fifty dollars," was the answer. The man became furious. "So he has lied to me," he said. "I will turn
him into the street tomorrow morning!" "Wait," said the
doctor, "I will tell you how we can prevent two lawsuits!
In the first place you will not sue the carpenter for his
rent, and in the second the carpenter will not have to sue
the college; for if he does, the college will have to pay
him the balance on the three hundred and fifty, since
Judge and Jury, in America, generally decide in favor of
the workingman. So do not turn the man out, for in that
case you will receive nothing. Send him to me and I will
pay him seventy-five dollars, the amount of rent he owes
you, and he must give us a receipt in full for the amount
received." The landlord gave Dr. Hering a look as if to
say, "After all you are a business man!" He went home,
said he would talk to the man.

After supper I heard a medley of voices in the front
office. First Dr. Koch's, then Dr. Hering's, also the carpenter's and that of his landlord.

The carpenter: "You promised so and so. I'll go to
court."

The landlord: "You may! I'll throw you out."

Dr. Hering: "Go to court and be dammed!"

The carpenter was obstinate, would not give a receipt
in full for his excessive bill, and still threatened to go to
court. After the combatents had gone, there was a tableau
in the hall, of which Dr. Hering formed the centre; about
him his wife, sons and daughters, all displaying the greatest anxiety. The old man fairly shook with laughter,
mainly at Dr. Koch, who had bungled the matter, saying:
"This perhaps will teach him a lesson, and take him down
a peg!"

"Our reverses," he said, "are as valuable to us as our
gains!"

An Aspirant for a Diploma.

A strange thing happened to Dr. Hering this morning
in his office hours. A young woman, recommended by
Dr. Farrington, came and wished to know if she might

attend the summer course of lectures at the College. Dr.
A. from New York State had sent her to F., who sent her
to Hering. She was in poor health, had suffered all
through the winter with cough and spitting of blood, for
which she had taken *Phosphorus;* she also had a continuous coryza, still she desired a diploma. Dr. Hering was
surprised, because at that time women were not co-eds,
as now, but he referred her to the Registrar.

In spite of being a woman in precarious health, probably a consumptive, she still wishes to be a homoeopathic
physician; Her courage, if not her prudence, is to be admired.

A Meeting of the County Society. Gymnocladus.

I escorted Father Hering to a meeting of the County
Society this evening. Arm in arm we went. He was more
jolly than I had yet seen him. Nothing of great importance was transacted at the meeting. Dr. Guernsey arose
and said a few words in favor of the much discussed Fair,
thereby showing courage in the presence of opponents.

When I had brought back Dr. Hering, we took seats in
the back office where he talked to me for an hour before
retiring. He told me of a proving he had made of the pulp
of a bean from a tree in Washington Square, the *Gymnocladus canadensis.* In Kentucky the bean is used in the
making of a substitute for coffee. Hering, too, tried the
preparation, in company with some friends, but did not
admire the beverage. "The proving caused some fine symptoms, but no patient so far has been found with symptoms
to correspond. They have some similarity to those of
Belladonna. The pulp is used for a fly poison.

"The *Musca domestica* is called *Fliege* in Northern
Germany and *Muecke* in Southern Germany. In the North
the mosquito is called *Muecke.* The Pennsylvania Germans owe a large part of their dialect to South Germany."

Plants. Provings. Williamson. Jeanes. Bute.

"In reference to provings to be made from plants, Williamson favors a distinction to be made between provings
from the plant itself and those made from its active

principle. They should be thrown together. Our Dr. Jeanes did a great deal of proving. Likewise Bute, who introduced *Daphne indica* and *Mezereum*. Jeanes made provings of the body-louse, the lady apple, the *Dolichos pruriens* and *Kino gummi*.

"Jeanes was satisfied to get one good symptom from a proving, on which he could prescribe. Guernsey admits that he got his idea of practising by the keynote system, from Jeanes.

"We should always have three characteristic symptoms to a remedy before we prescribe it. There are to be considered: 1. Time. 2. Space. 3. Locality. The third refers to right and left side, front and back, up and down, etc. The first belongs to modality. Jeanes had a medicine for almost every spot on the body! He classified headaches under the various regions assigned by phrenology."

Clinical Cases.

Dr. Raue began his studies by reading all of the cases reported in Medical Journals, by which he soon acquired knowledge useful in prescribing.

College Journal. Clinical Cases.

Dr. Hering still thinks Martin, co-editor of the College Journal, should submit copy of clinical matter to him before going to press. The June number is filled with cases which Hering has not had an opportunity to approve. Hering has in mind writing a book for young practitioners, but says he must first have a collection of a thousand cases for analysis.

Remedies—Their Origin. Arum Triphyllum. Hamamelis.

"I got the *Arum triphyllum* (Jack-in-the-Pulpit) from an up-country Pennsylvania German who had it from an old woman. It became a valuable remedy for scarlet fever in its worst form. I was called to see three children located in a basement on Cherry Street. The eldest child was in the last stage of the sickness, evidently dying. The second was in the second stage and very sick. The third had just begun to sicken. I thought of the Pennsylvania German's remedy, the *Arum triphyllum*, which I administered to each of the three children, in the sixth dilution. All three recovered.

"The chief indications for the remedy are *soreness of the mouth, cracked lips and salivation*. I tried the remedy again soon after; this time getting an aggravation, probably due to the use of a low potency; higher ones were made use of later.

"*Hamamelis* (witch hazel) was suggested to me by a consumptive at the point of death, who controlled his hemorrhages with a quack medicine, which he himself had introduced, and which made him rich, but which he kept a secret. A substance which can stop hemorrhages from a lung almost gone, must be a good remedy, I thought. The consumptive had a daughter who impressed me. She revealed to me the formula.

"Her father had planted acres with the witch hazel, had built a distillery by which to extract the sap from the bush during the month of February, when it is strongest, just before the flowering season, when all plants are strongest in sap. If it had not been for the daughter, I would not have had any time for a man who discovered a healing remedy and guarded its secret for material gain."

The Hering Family.

Hering has one brother, Karl, and a sister living. One brother, Julius, died young. He says he must look up the living ones, if he again goes to Europe. If respectable, he says, he will recognize them. If not, he won't concern himself about them. His brother, Karl, is a renowned musician, whom Mendelssohn pronounced the greatest contrapuntist in Germany.

The Young Woman Who Desires a Diploma.

This would-be-doctress spoke to Dr. Farrington and myself at the College this morning. She is desperate. She says she will get a degree if she has to go to France, or Germany for it. She says she has been thrice cured by homoeopathy.

May 17. 1869.

Signatura. Cranberries.

"Cranberry poultice, recommended for *erysipelas*, comes under the head of *signatura*, a very ancient doctrine, which has much to recommend it on the grounds of *Similia*."

The Lizard With the Broken Tail. Nature's Mistake.

"A lizard which had broken its tail and afterwards, for want of surgical aid grew two tails, was to be sent to a museum in Germany. It was intended to represent the old school notion of a *Vis medicatrix naturae*. A satire on Schiller's expression, 'Suesse heilige Natur, fuehre mich auf deiner spur' (Sweet and holy nature, lead me in thy ways). The specimen did not reach the museum, at least I did not find it there. Nature needs both wisdom and art to guide it."

Governor Pollock and the Poor Man.

A German by the name of Taxis, a simple hearted, honest man, lost his position as janitor at the United States Mint, when Governor Pollock became director of that institution. A son of Taxis, employed in the Union Bank, wrote a filial letter to Dr. Hering in behalf of his father, asking him to use his influence to get his father restored to his position, as on their combined salaries depended the sustenance of the family.

Unthinkingly and ill-advisedly I undertook to call on the newly elected Governor at his church, where he instructed a Bible Class, early on a Sunday morning. Pollock said: "I am sorry that you came on such a mission on a Sunday; I cannot break the Sabbath!"

Next day I visited the Governor at his office, with a letter signed by Dr. Hering. The letter set forth, in flattering terms, the philanthropy, as well as the politics of the Governor, but it failed to move his honor, who said that he was overwhelmed with applications, three thousand of which had already come in, three hundred of them being from women for whom he had only ten vacancies,

Widows, he said, come here with their children, weep, and
moan, and sigh, enough to take the heart out of a man.

A politician, I thought, with a heart; a *rara avis!* He
further said that he was not in favor of men appointed under Johnson's administration, all of whom he had discharged and that he intended to appoint his own men. He
thought there had been too many superfluous appoint-
ments. All of which boded ill for reinstatement of poor
Taxis, and I went away feeling that my visit had proved a
failure. Next day the son came to Dr. Hering with a
twenty dollar bill, intended as a present for the Governor,
but was told that probably a man as pious as the Governor
would reject such a gift. I had my first lesson in politics.

First Patient.

Today, when Dr. Hering was standing in the doorway
of the College, a lady passed. He said: "That lady was
my first patient when I came to Philadelphia."

Betts.

This afternoon we had a visit from Dr. Betts, one of the
younger men graduated from the College, who has just
returned from Europe, where he spent some time in travel
and some in making the acquaintance of homoeopathic
physicians abroad. Dr. Betts, who could not speak the
language a year ago, now speaks good German. He
brought the news that Fleischmann, a homoeopath in
Vienna, had died; that Eidherr is ill with lung-disease,
and that Haussman is not very old.

Dr. Hering says: "Haussman is the only man who
could bring me back over the ocean again." Betts showed
pictures of German professors at Vienna; Skoda and Roki-
tansky. Dr. Hering offers to tender him a reception.

Hering Family. Sons of the Third Wife.

As soon as his children were born Dr. Hering predicted
what profession they would enter when grown up. When
Rudolph, the eldest, was born his father said: "This one
will be an engineer." The next son, Walter, he said, "will
be a printer." Both of these predictions were fulfilled.

The third son, Carl, was born with a caul, which is considered lucky. The mother asked: "Why don't you say something for this one's future?" The father said: "This one is to be a physician." In this case he erred. Carl became an electrical engineer.

When the last of the sons, born to the father at the advanced age of sixty-three came into the world, he was named Hermann Siegfried, and his father said: "This one, too, will be a physician, but the one before him, Carl, will be a surgeon."

Rudolph, the oldest, became prominent as a Sanitary Engineer, a builder of bridges and designer of plans for city drainage. All of the sons rose to eminence in their professions, efficient and honored for their attainments. Hermann, the youngest, at first a teacher, joined the ranks of Christian Scientists, in which he gained eminence as a practitioner, and at present is a lecturer of world fame. He is one of the directors in Mrs. Eddy's Church.

Hepar Sulph.

Hering introduced *Hepar sulph. calc.* for the treatment of suppurations, as early as 1827, while in South America. About the same time Hartmann, in Germany, introduced *Mercurius.*

Korndoerfer.

Hering predicts that Dr. Korndoerfer will some day become co-editor of the College Journal, also a member of the Faculty, which prophecy was not fulfilled though Korndoerfer was one of our leading homoeopathic physicians, extremely active for the cause and helpful to Hering in his literary work.

The Murder of Mrs. Rademacher. Finger-Prints.

Rademacher, who lived on Arch Street, was one of the early homoeopaths in Philadelphia. His wife was murdered in her room. Dr. Hering secured a piece of wood from a post on which was left the bloody imprint of the murderer's hand. He placed this under a microscope and found that the hand, a delicate one, had left particles of shoe-maker's wax in the impress. He said the murderer is a shoe-maker. The murderer, Langenfeld by name, was tried, found guilty and executed.

While the criminal was in prison awaiting his execution, Hering suggested that his finger-prints be taken, but this was denied him. After the execution, Hering and some other physicians, were permitted to view the corpse. It was Dr. Hering's intention to take an impression from the hands, in wax, for comparison with the specimens obtained under the microscope; but the hands of the cadaver were found cut and multilated beyond recognition. This piece of vandalism had been committed by an eclectic who was jealous of a homoeopath's triumph in a matter of science.

Another murderer was discovered through the imprint of a bare foot on the floor of a mill, where some flour had been dropped. The murderer had the reputation of being an honest and godfearing man. Jealousy over a woman had been the incentive to the murder.

The Bertillon method was but little practised at the time of these occurrences. Now we know that the lines in the human hand are singular and never duplicated.

———————

May 20, 1869.
Trinks.

Trinks, a German claiming to be a homoeopath, was a promoter of literature; of books which others had written for him, one of which with the silly title, *Das Handbuch auf dem Standpunkt*, (The Handbook on a Standpoint) was a frequent mark for Dr. Hering's ridicule. Trinks, in ugliness and disposition, resembled the animal Gnu, and was so named by Hering on account of his irascible temper; a sobriquet which stuck to him.

Examination Before the Faculty of the University of Wuerzburg.

"First of all I had to pass a written examination. I was known to be a homoeopath, for which reason I met with great opposition which I had to overcome. I was made a butt for ridicule among my fellow-students. The faculty did not allow students to grow moustaches. I defied the custom and appeared before the faculty unshaven. I wished to show my independence, as a homoeopath, to the fullest, a dangerous thing to do, a thing which I would not advise a student of the present day to venture to do.

"A week before the regular examination the students were required to call upon their respective teachers to advise them of their intended appearance for examination.

"I first went before Texter, noted surgeon, who was terribly opposed to all homoeopaths. He looked extremely angry, and said: 'What is your wish?' 'Professor I have come for examination.' 'For examination?' said he very gruffly; 'How, and in what manner do you ever expect to make your way in the world?' I replied: 'Professor, I wish to go to Holland, and become a surgeon on board ship, in the navy.' He then asked in what subject I felt myself most interested. I told him, 'In the treatment of the peculiar wounds made by the splintering of wood on board ship.'

"On examination day we had to go to a large, dark hall. On the table stood an urn in which the professors deposited questions, written on slips of paper, which the students were required to draw and answer. The hall had an imposing appearance with its columns and dim walls. I sat down to one of the small tables and wrote my answer to the first question, which was followed by other questions and answers, promptly gathered by the janitor in charge. To me the janitor remarked: 'What! already finished?' Next came the oral examination. I first appeared before the botanist, who sat in one of the window niches; in a second niche sat another professor with his victim before him. The botanist was a mild, pleasant old gentleman. He had a small herbarium in his hand which he showed me and said: 'Can you tell me, maybe, what this plant is called?' I made the correct answer. He then handed me the herbarium and asked me to tell him the names of all the plants in it with which I was familiar. I picked up one plant after another, laid them carefully to one side, after the manner of botanists, mentioning the name of each one after the other. I came to a strange plant in the collection which made me hesitate. The professor said: 'What is the name of that one?' 'Oh! That,' said I, 'is a new plant, discovered lately. I saw a picture of it in one of your works, professor.' I then named the plants according to the order to which they belonged. Other professors were within hearing distance and no doubt thought, 'How can we manage to let this fellow fall through; a homoeopath should not be allowed to graduate from our institution.'

"I next went before the physiologist. After him again came Texter, the surgeon. He pitched right into me with, 'What's this? What's the answer to that?' and asked me as a test question: 'What are the various causes of cataract?' I named the ordinary conditions; eye-strain and traumatism as the most common, which, however, did not seem wholly to satisfy the professor, who said: 'What other cause is there for cataract?' Schoenlein, who did not sit far off, overheard the question and said: 'I, myself, know of no other cause.' All were silent! Texter said 'Old age is a cause of cataract!' Schoenlein turned about in his chair and laughed in his sleeve!

"The obstetrician on the faculty being absent, Texter examined me in that branch also. He questioned me in regard to the various positions and operations of childbirth. I explained these in the order of the three stages of parturition, which surprised the professor, but he wished to know if I could remember another. 'I do not.' 'Neither do I,' said he, with a smile. Then came the veterinary, whose examination I passed without any difficulty. Finally I came before Schoenlein, the man whose great knowledge of pathology had lured me to Wuerzburg. Knowing my leaning to homoeopathy he questioned me on the Hahnemannian treatment of scarlet fever. Here I was at home and passed the examination satisfactorily. In fact, I graduated with highest honours in all the departments. My nine months of study at Wuerzburg had enabled me to do this. Yet if Schoenlein had wished to be inimical to the young homoeopath he could have flunked me."

A Woman-Hater.

"The death of my second wife, Marianna Husmann, the mother of Max and Odelia, whom I loved dearly, affected my mind to such a degree that for a long time I felt a strange antipathy to all womankind. On the day of my wife's funeral I was in an exalted state of mind, which made me talk inordinately, without being aware of what was happening. My dislike of women became so extreme that I no longer wished to have them come to consult me. Such was the extent of my disaffection that I would have been seriously injured in my practice thereby.

"Fortunately I was cured in a way corresponding to the law of *Similia*. Fanny Ellsler, famous German dancer of that period, had arrived at New York. One of my friends coming from there to see me, spoke highly of the great art displayed by this woman, who, from patriotic reasons, had refused to be advertised as a French danseuse. 'I am a German,' she said, 'and will appear before the public as such.' This fealty to her nationality inspired me, and when she came to dance in Philadelphia, I went, together with my friend, Professor Knorr, to the Academy of Music to witness the ballet. The subject of this was a fairy tale in which a goddess descends to earth, takes on the form of a mortal, and falls in love with a man, whom she marries. Her husband clips her wings, treats her cruelly, and she dies. Angels descend from heaven and take her up on a sunny cloud.

"This beautiful exhibition of woman's tenderness and devotion, so often unappreciated by ordinary husbands, who too late discover the worth of those who have loved and cherished them when on earth, now left to grieve and wonder why they could have been so cruel, with only the hope left them of a reunion in a better world, which should lead every man toward heaven, all of which made a deep impression upon my sick mind.

"It was Fanny Ellsler, the woman, faithful to her

nationality, the charming talented artist, who, with her inimitable interpretation of the fairy tale, brought back health and reason to me, the bereaved physician. In earlier days I had disapproved of the ballet; could see neither art nor reason in its artificiality as I then considered it."

In his youth Hering had seen dancing in Amsterdam which affected him adversely. He wrote about this in a letter before departing for South America. It was six years after the loss of Marianna, who was his second wife, before he could make up his mind to marry again, a third time, Therese Bucheim, daughter of an old school physician, in Germany.

Religion. Gaertner. Creed.

"What would this great work of the Creator be if there were no hereafter? I do not know what will become of my children if I should die, but I know there is a God who will take care of them. I cannot see how men can be unbelievers. My friend, Carl Gaertner, musician, does not believe. I try to help him to believe and already he begins to think there might be a heaven.

"My simple creed is short and to the point—To love the truth because it is true, the good because it is good, and to shun evil because it is evil. Christianity consists in leading useful lives, for the good of the race, and from unselfish motives. In spite of there being natural laws, to man is given a free will to act according to the dictates of his conscience."

The following statement, "A Confession of Faith," written in German and addressed to his sons, was but lately discovered by me among Hering's papers, translated and printed for distribution among friends. It is a record in brief of a practical belief, to which no one can take exception:

It is great good fortune for a man to believe in a God. Fervently, with all his heart, with all his mind, with all his soul, constantly and enduringly. It should be quite impossible for him to think that this great truth could be an error; he knows it to be true. All of us have come forth from God. He cares for us all. He does not care more for one than for another. He cares for all alike. He gives to everyone as much, or as little, as he is willing to receive. He will show to everyone his vay according to his understanding. He always gives the right, always the best, and always what is most beneficial.

In spite of the many unaccountable happenings, shortcomings, and undeniable incongruities, also the very many follies man has committed, and the mistakes he diligently continues to make, the world still remains a pleasant place to live in. Aside from the circumstance that after all we have to take the world as it is, we must acknowledge the ingenious arrangement, as it might be called, by which everyone is given full freedom to act, and to choose, according to his lights.

May 21, 1869.

Pow-Wowing.

"We should not condemn pow-wowing, for we have no reason for so doing; we must neither accept nor condemn a thing without a reason."

Physiology. Nerve Currents.

"I believe, with Swedenborg, that the nerves contain a gaseous substance which circulates from the periphery to the centre, through the sensory nerves, and from the centre to the periphery through the motor nerves. In sleep this current is reversed. Medicines placed upon the tongue are there changed to a nerve-gas which is transmitted to diseased parts."

Would this explain the lightning-like cures as mentioned by P. P. Wells (See Eulogies,) also observed by others. Hering wonders if the metals contained in a battery are dissolved, disintegrated and thus pass on through the wires and says: "Now we have only the effects from copper and zinc. Other metals might come into use."

May 22, 1869.

Ice and Ice-Water. Charcoal.

"Americans cannot realize their rapid progress as a

nation. They will not readily believe that it is only a
short time since such a thing as ice was introduced. Ice
came into general use in 1833. I had a patient by the
name of Geisse, a lay homoeopath (who had sat at the
table with Hahnemann), at whose house I met a Frenchman by the name of Moliere, who spoke about introducing
ice into Philadelphia. He secured a farm near the Schuylkill River, on which he built a tank the size of a city block
into which he led the water from a spring and allowed it
to freeze, cut the ice and built an ice-house, the first on the
American continent. This was in 1833-34."

Hering tells how his first glass of ice-water made him
ill and how Carbo vegetabilis cured him. Hence the
characteristic "bad effects from cold drinks," so often
since verified in practice.

Caster Oil After Childbirth.

Hering was the first to condemn the giving of castor oil
on the third day after childbirth, which was almost universally done to produce a bowel movement with the lying-
in. Hering claims that the seventh day after childbirth is
the natural time for a passage; if it does not come then,
give a dose of *Bryonia,* or *Nux vomica.* The old practice
of purging has been largely abandoned and in consequence, together with better sanitary methods of delivery,
there has been far less of puerpural fever and its fatal
consequences.

Suriname. Climate.

"In Suriname the heat is more supportable than here.
There are the breezes from the sea. People live near the
coast. None in the interior. Between noon and four p. m.
the people are in their houses and sleep. At four they
dress and go out of doors."

Biography. Peppich. Lachesis.

"I was teacher in an institution in Dresden, under Blochmann, whence I was sent to Suriname, by way of Cayenne,
for the purpose of making zoological and botanical researches, and collections for the museum of the King of

Saxony. About the same time a man by the name of
Peppich was sent there, on a similar errand, by some rich
men from Philadelphia. Peppich was bitten by the
serpent *Lachesis trigonocephaltus*, but was saved by applying radiate heat from a heated gold coin. We both remained in Suriname for six years. I made collections,
with the help of Weigel the botanist, for one year, then
devoted myself to the practice of homoeopathy. Peppich
made collections in all of that time."

May 24, 1869.

A Boa Constrictor. Weigel.

"My friend, Weigel, the botanist, went one day into the
jungle with his gun. He trod on a large boa-constrictor
which lay concealed in the grass. He felt the huge snake
moving under his feet. He bounded across it but left his
gun behind him. He heard a fearful hissing. Growing
faint he leaned against a neighboring tree where he imagined himself safe from the monster. The hissing became
louder and louder. He saw the snake drag its length
through the grass, finally its tail. She was drawing herself into a coil ready for a spring. Although a courageous
man, who had faced shot and shell, now his courage failed
him, he grew faint. He rallied, and with a desperate
bound he reached his gun. He now had a means of defense. The hissing ceased. Weigel thought discretion the
better part of valor and made tracks for home. He arrived
weak and faint, became ill, and had to keep his bed for
seven days.

"We went to the place where the snake had been seen
and found a place as large as an ordinary sized room
where the grass had been beaten down. I tied a live kid
to a tree, hoping that the snake would swallow the bait,
become helpless and so be dragged in by a rope, but
though I kept watch for a long time, the python did not
again appear. I think the kid was eaten by the natives.

"When a boa sees her prey she fastens her tail to a fixed
point, a stake or a small tree, from which she can shoot
out her coils to envelope the animal and strangle it, which

she could not accomplish otherwise. While she is preparing to attack she rapidly turns her head from side to side, keenly watching for the moment when her victim comes within reach. She opens wide her mouth; with her tail fastened to the tree, she darts her length forward and with her poisonless fangs fastened into the animal, her muscles contracting, she pulls it to the ground, where she wraps her coils around it, tightens them until the victim's bones are crushed in her powerful strangle-hold. As soon as she thinks she has vanquished her prey, she glides her head forward to the mouth of the animal and listens. If she hears another gasp or breath, she tightens her coils like lightning and gives another squeeze to finish the victim, after which she opens her mouth wide to give one loud blowing sound, an expiration by which she completely empties her lung, a single sac, the other lung having become atrophied to leave room for the one which extends almost through the entire length of her body. When she has completely emptied the air she closes her mouth and begins to refill her single lung with fresh air. The air enters her nostrils and fills her mouth. When the mouth is full she gives a gulp and swallows the air. This process is continued until the lung is filled. She does this because in the act of swallowing her prey, there is a pressure on her larynx which prevents more air from entering.

"She now proceeds to swallow the animal, but does not cover it with saliva before the act of swallowing. The saliva runs freely as she swallows. With the aid of her coils, still wrapped about the animal's body, she pushes it down her throat. When this is accomplished the huge serpent is helpless and may be carried away. The only possible danger, negroes say, is from receiving a blow from her powerful tail, which they say could kill a man."

Hering was eyewitness to what is here related of the boa-constrictor, which inhabits the jungles about Suriname. He kept a young of the species as a pet. He trained it by feeding it as often as it grew hungry. He sometimes allowed her to wrap herself around his neck; once, he says, she squeezed a little too tight, and sometimes licked his nose and mouth, which he did not like.

Ole Bull, Violinist.

With Dr. Hering's niece, Bertha, I attended a farewell concert given to Ole Bull before his departure for Europe. The aged virtuoso glides on to the stage like a ghost. He has grey hair and wrinkles. He keeps his eyes fixed upon his old brown instrument, from which, with astonishing virtuosity, he draws the most perfect sounds. He favored the audience with our national airs *The Star Spangled Banner, Hail Columbia* and *Yankee Doodle,* also *Home Sweet Home,* with which he made great effect. There is a trifle of the charlatan about him; for instance, a trick of keeping his ear close to the violin, while his bow, with a diamond set in the end of it, is kept moving for some time after the last faint tone has become audible.

———

May 26, 1869.

Liebig. Chemist. Lord Bacon.

Hering asks Dr. Neidhard, who is about to sail for Europe, when he goes to Munich and visits Liebig, who is on friendly terms with Neidhard's relatives, to tell him that there are three things about Liebig Dr. Hering always speaks of in his lectures to his students.

"1—That Liebig was a school-mate of a certain man who told the story to Hering. It happened on examination day at the High School. Each student was asked, by the professor, what occupation he had chosen for his life-work. When the turn came to Liebig, the boy was silent. 'Well, Liebig, what are you going to be?' Liebig stood up and said: 'I am going to be a chemist.' At first all in the room were silent, then came a burst of loud laughter.

"2—Liebig went to Paris to a famous chemist, for whom he offered to make explosives—compounds with gold— the cyanides. The French professor was aghast. 'So you would risk your life,' he said to the young man. 'Yes! professor, if you will have a small shack built for me out-of-doors, on the edge of the moat, for experimentation, I will.' Liebig made the experiments and was successful.

"3—Because Liebig had the courage to attack Lord Bacon's philosophy."

May 27, 1869.

A Benefit for the Hospital.

An evening entertainment was given in the home for the benefit of the Homoeopathic Hospital.

Dr. Farrington appeared in a tableau as a simple Dutchman making love. Also as the "Veiled Prophet" in Lallah Rook. Dr. Rembaugh, with a long beard, appeared in the *Music Lesson*, in which Dad is discovered peeping out from behind the curtain; also as the Magician in the *Magic Mirror*, and in the last tableau as a Courtier. The costumes were of the richest, from Van Horn, at six dollars a piece. Expenses amounted to half of the proceeds!

Doctor Mondschein, a fat German homoeopath, who gives "zee little pills and zee mighty potencies," was played deliciously by Will Burnham, a son of the locomotive manufacturer. Miss Barrett, daughter of the Swedenborgian minister, played the languid lady, Mrs. Backbay, whose husband says "When I turn in, my wife turns out; both in white!"

Loelkes.

Dr. Loelkes, for a short time assistant to Dr. Hering, had come to Newark from Germany, where he had an uncle. He was introduced to Hering as "an orphan with only a grandmother, living in Germany." He came recommended: "A giant in strength, a child in disposition." Dr. Hering took him on trial, Mrs. Hering playing the motherly part. Loelkes soon fell out with the daughters and in with the office girl. Love is potent. Emma left the house, saying that it was not honest to remain. Courtship had been going on on the sly. Loelkes borrowed money and left for Belleville, Illinois, there to set up a practice. Emma soon followed him and they were married, against the wishes of the uncle, who had intended that his nephew should settle in Newark. Later much trouble came to the family, wife sick, no money, etc.

Dr. Hering thinks it is well for a young doctor to have a wife, as it will aid him in his practice, but he ought not to marry until he can support a wife.

Fair.

A physician from Cincinnati brought the news that the Hospital Fair, held in that city, realized about ten thousand dollars.

June 1, 1869.

Martin. Gregg.

Dr. Martin, Professor of Clinical Medicine at the College and co-editor of the Journal, related to me incidents from his life and his conversion to homoeopathy. When a boy of sixteen, while rummaging among his father's things, he discovered some human bones which he articulated and fell in love with the skeleton. He studied it and hung it up in his closet, to the consternation of his boy-companions. He was thought to be an eccentric lad. Some moonlight nights he would go to the graveyard, sit or lie down on a flat tombstone and meditate. When a few years older he visited an allopathic doctor, who took him to the clinics for Eye and Skin diseases. He occupied himself with putting up nauseous prescriptions in his father's store. Later he came to Buffalo, where he took a position as clerk, and again engaged in reading medical books.

Martin had been reading but a short time when, one day, his uncle came to his office and offered him a position with a certain business firm, dealers in iron, in partnership with two other men. He accepted this offer, began to make money rapidly, and soon had accumulated twenty thousand dollars. Later a hundred thousand was sunk in the same business, a part of which sum he owes to the present day, but does not think himself obligated to pay. He says he entered the business with the intention of doing right, tried to do so, was unfortunate, now does not feel willing, or able, to repay the large sum.

After the failure, which came in 1857, he joined the army as a private, reached the rank of first lieutenant, but had to return home on account of camp fever. While in the army he had occasion to witness many surgical operations. He came under the treatment of an allopathic doctor, but grew worse, and finally sent for a homoeopath, one who was crude in his methods of practice. He failed to recover; his friends urged him to abandon homoeopathy and return to the old school. This he refused to do because he was stubborn, he says, all his life. Dr. Gregg, a prominent homoeopathic physician, in Buffalo, was called, examined the patient minutely, and there being spasmodic symptoms, prescribed *Belladonna* in the 200th potency. The first dose helped him and he was speedily cured.

From this time Martin was converted to homoeopathy, though not at once to the higher potencies. He afterwards joined Dr. Gregg, as a student, who cured him of a lung-affection thought to be consumption. Dr. Gregg had made many remarkable cures of tuberculous patients. He had remedies for special spots and localities in the lungs and had plates, or pictures made to show his pulmonary regional method of prescribing.

Dr. Martin next attended a course of lectures in an allopathic institution. He was in the habit of talking homoeopathy to the other boys, between hours, and gave medicines to some of them. They asked him many questions.

One day, in the street, he was attacked with *cholera morbus*, went to a hotel; had vomiting and diarrhoea. When he got home his wife gave him a single dose of *Veratrum album*. He applied a mustard plaster to his stomach; got well promptly, but ascribed his recovery to the mustard plaster! This was before his complete conversion to homoeopathy, which happened before he came to Philadelphia to attend lectures on homoeopathy, to graduate, and finally to be given the chair of Clinical Medicine in the College, and Co-Editor with Hering on the Journal of Homoeopathic Clinics.

Hering. Thomas.

Dr. Hering is unwell; suffering from diarrhoea and a cold affecting the larynx. Dr. Thomas is getting better slowly. The abscess is expected to break.

A Letter From Hahnemann.

"At one time I received a letter from Hahnemann through Dr. Haynel, in Dresden, in whose care it was sent. Haynel was to have married Hahnemann's daughter, Lotta. They were engaged to be married, but the mother, the first Mrs. Hahnemann, objected to the union. Hahnemann called Haynel 'my son'."

Sunday Dispensary.

My request for permission to keep the College Dispensary, in Filbert Street, open on Sundays was granted.

Fair.

Oak wood obtained from the wreckage of the historical Lutheran Church at Fourth and Cherry Streets, has been cut and made ready to be used for objects to be sold at the Fair. Two saws have been broken in the process! Watson, the College janitor, is going to have extra canes made from the wood, one for Hering and another for Raue.

Nomenclature in Botany and Pathology.

Hering says the long and difficult names in botany and pathology were invented by the French. He would like to see plates made showing characteristics and structural differences in plants, which would greatly simplify the study of botany. Every plant has certain characteristics which distinguish it from all others.

———————

June 3, 1869.

*Oken. Medical Associations. American Institute
                of Homoeopathy.*

"Oken, the great German naturalist, came to Goettingen to attend a convention at which were exhibited some rare specimens. Among these was a snail which I had examined and studied in South America. The snail, which is many-coloured, lays eggs as large as those from sparrows, with a hard shell.

"Oken, then a young student, who looked more like a tailor's apprentice, walked up and down before the exhibits and noticed that this snail was placed among water-snails, while it actually belonged to a variety of land snails, and he so expressed himself. Blumemfeldt, and a few other scientific men, who overheard the remark, also the Duke who was present, challenged the young man's assertion, saying: 'Do you not see the tiny bivalve attached to the shell of the snail?' 'Certainly; but the snail must have fallen into the water,' the young naturalist said. They laughed him to scorn.

"Oken said nothing more, went home, where a few weeks later he was visited by the Duke, who first asked his name, then why he had contradicted the learned men at the exposition. 'My name is Ludwig Oken. My reason for saying that the snail is a land-snail is because a water snail breathes through a pair of small horns which, if they had dropped off from the specimen, would have left depressions.' The Duke was astonished at the young man's knowledge.

"Four weeks later he was given a professorship in one of the universities and shortly after he was married to the daughter of a prominent man. Oken was the first to start regular meetings, conventions of naturalists and other learned men. At first these were sparsely attended, but later crowded."

Dr. Hering led, in this country, by helping to organize the first medical association: the American Institute of Homoeopathy, of which he was the first president; later the allopaths followed suit, and there are now more conventions of every kind than you can shake a stick at, including men and women of all denominations.

The city of Boston has devoted twenty-five hundred dollars for the entertainment of members of the American Institute at its next meeting, to be held there in the coming week, which is the first public recognition of the kind our cause has received.

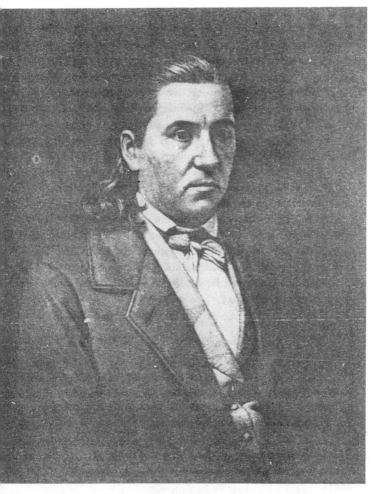

CONSTANTINE HERING.
PORTRAIT COPIED FROM AN ENGRAVING BY SARTAIN
AFTER A DAGUERREOTYPE BY G. H. WEEKS, MADE
SHORTLY AFTER HERING'S ARRIVAL IN PHILADELPHIA.

Special Form of Type (Organschrift).

"I began work on this while still in Suriname. The invention consists of signs to delineate form and position of mouth and tongue while pronouncing letters. Vowels are modifications of a circle. These must be very correct. The advantage of such a method would be its brevity, for as much as is ordinarily printed on a single page in our books could be printed in one line. The lines run from top to bottom of the page. The making of the type would not be difficult. There are certain signs, f.i., to express Schla, Schli, Schlo, Schlu. It was my desire that the students at the Allentown Academy should learn stenography to take notes of symptoms in shorthand."

This led me to make mention of my keeping tablets under the table for longhand notation. Hering said: "That you need not do; keep them on the table." It is this method I am pursuing, of making jottings in long hand, as rapidly as possible, with pencil on paper, which afterwards I copy, with pen and ink, into my diary. Fortunately the ink has preserved its quality in all the years; now more than half a century.

Lingen.

"One of my former assistants, Dr. Lingen, who died last July, left a fortune of about $200,000. He was a great speculator."

Sunday Dispensary.

Today I dispensed medicine for the first time from the Sunday dispensary. I had two women patients, of respectable appearance, who offered pay, which was not accepted. I hope the dispensary service will prove a blessing to the needy who are prevented from coming during working hours.

June 7, 1869.

Ignorance.

"I no longer have any sympathy for the ignorant. I once attended a family in which there was a daughter who steadily disobeyed my instructions, and sneered at homoeopathy. Her father compelled her to take the treatment. She had had a fall in which she hurt her knee. I treated her for the injury and she got better, but when her father died she returned to allopathic treatment. In a few months her leg was amputated above the knee. Her brother brought the severed limb to my office for inspection. I never saw a healthier appearing knee joint. The limb, which I should have kept, was buried. The victim is now limping about on an artificial leg. One of the leading allopaths pronounced the operation one of malpractice."

Allentown Academy.

"When the Academy was started the sum of seven thousand dollars was raised in one day. Four acres of land were bought and two handsome buildings put up. A dishonest local banker finally wrecked the institution. He died a miserable death."

Helfrich. Wesselhoeft.

"My friend, John Helfrich, a country clergyman, was a man of courage and indomitable character, with a well-grounded knowledge of homoeopathic therapeutics. On Sundays the farmers round about came to him in numbers to be treated. Dr. Wesselhoeft from Bath, Pa., visited him every four weeks, on Sundays, driving a horse and buggy, from Northampton to Maxatawney in the adjoining county, a distance of about twenty-five miles."

This clergyman was my great uncle. Following his example there were nine or more young men, including myself, who became homoeopathic practitioners.

June 11, 1869.

Hahnemann's Birthday, April 10th, 1755.
Hahnemann's Father.

In the German journal *Zeitschrift fuer Homoeopathische Klinik*, Feb. 1, 1855, No. 3, is found the following notice: "The one hundredth anniversary of Hahnemann's birth is to be celebrated, at Meissen. The committee is to

get information from city councils in regard to Hahnemann's earlier life. A bust of Hahnemann is to be placed
in the hall of the Public School."

Among documents, presented by Professor Peters, is the
following record of Hahnemann's birth: "Christian Friederich Samuel Hahnemann was born on April 11, 1755, and
christened on April 13 of the same year by M. Junghanns.
His father was Christian Gottfried Hahnemann, his
mother Johanna Christiana, nee Spiess. The names of the
sponsors are omitted from the church records; a space for
them is left blank."

It would appear as if Hahnemann was born under the
sign of Venus. The number eleven is plainly written and
admits of no doubt as to the date of his birth. From the
register of the Latin school, in Meissen, we obtain the
following: "No 20. Christian Gottfried Samuel Hahnemann, son of the porcelain painter, age 12. Class 11,
January 20th, 1767." Corroborated by Gottlob Ehren-
fried Dietrich, Rector of Public Schools in Meissen.
Friederich August Buerger was rector of the school which
Hahnemann entered, and M. Johann August Mueller, who
later became active as Tertius, Conrector and Rector in
the Public School.

From accounts in the ledgers of the public school we
have the following: "Christian Friederich Samuel Hahnemann visited the *Fuerstenschule* (college for the sons of
nobility) up to Easter 1775. The name first appears in
the account of Easter, 1771, which corresponds with the
signature in the album for Nov. 29th, 1770. Hahnemann
was also Extraner (day pupil) in the house of the Three
Colleagues, under M. Mueller, who is said to have been a
splendid instructor. He was given the position of *Famulus*
(amenuensis) to Mueller. On April 24th, 1775, Hahnemann and his fellow-student, Karl Friederich Lehman,
from Dresden, delivered valedictory addresses in public
which were responded to by Karl August Funke."

The above extracts are pronounced authenic by Professor Dr. Peters. The reason for Hahnemann's name being registered as born on the 11th of April, is that it was

a custom to bring newly-born infants to church for baptism a couple of days after birth. Nurses, to gain a day, sometimes gave the date of the child's birth a day later than its actual occurrence. It was so in Hahnemann's case; also with Schiller, who was born on the tenth of the month, but registered on the eleventh, which confirms a duplicature of events in history.

"A Professor Fluegel told me that he had been informed by one of the older workers in the Porcelain factory of Meissen that Hahnemann's father was in the habit of locking-in his young son when leaving for the factory, after having given him a difficult problem to solve, or to think about, until his return; thus striving to make him a thinker."

Botany.

"In my boyhood days I became interested in the study of botany. On my excursions into the neighboring hills, and through the country, I stopped by the wayside, in Inns and Kneipen (saloons) to assort and press my plants. Here, when a boy, I heard and learned the popular phrases and expressions of the people, which I had never heard at home. My father, who was very strict, did not allow us to make use of any vulgar expressions. One time when walking along the road I met a farmer who asked me if I knew what the word *Standpunkt* (Standpoint) meant; saying that his minister was preaching all the time about standpoint, and to him, the farmer, it seemed to be a most ridiculous thing to talk about, a thing without a meaning. In the evening I repeated this conversation to my father, and several older gentlemen, who were present. They all laughed heartily and said it was nonsense to use such unmeaning language, especially when speaking to the illiterate."

Cruelty to Animals. Pedigree.

"A nobleman had a horse which angered him by becoming balky on the road. The owner of the horse, wishing to take revenge upon the beast, decided to imprison it within stone walls, so that the horse would die of hunger.

For air was left a small window near the top of the prison,
through which kind neighbors passed provisions to the
animal to keep it alive. When the nobleman found this
out he ordered the aperture to be closed. The neighbors
muttered, revolted and formed a mob threatening the
nobleman with violence. One of the men present, of
humble birth, indignantly stepped forward and said: 'I
too was born in the regular way, not dropped by the road-
side, but had a natural origin, the same as this nobleman.
Let him take care!' "

Militia.

"The military system of Prussia, the formation of a
militia for state protection, had its origin with General
Washington. Papers containing his plans were found by
some one in Washington, who afterwards went abroad and
there introduced the system; the same as planned and
made popular by Washington in this Country."

Liszt. Coal Mines. Railroads.

"A man by the name of Liszt came to this country from
Germany and opened coal-mines here. To him we are indebted for the use of coal for heating our houses and fac-
tories. He went back to Europe, poor as he had come. He
there initiated the railroad system. He built the first railroad running from Leipzig to Dresden. Liszt was a great
mechanic.

"I am thinking of our Henry Carey (political economist,
in Philadelphia) as being to Liszt what I am trying to be
to Hahnemann, a promoter of his doctrines. Liszt was a
brother-in-law to our Dr. Neidhard."

Bricks.

"When the first fire happened in Pittsburg, and while it
was still raging, an enterprising young man went about
making contracts to furnish bricks for rebuilding. He
secured such workers as were homeless, and out of employ,
and in a short time made an incalculable number of bricks,
the sale of which made him a millionaire."

Thomas. Abscess.

Professor Thomas had his abscess opened by Doctors Macfarlan and Morgan. No pus was found. Hering says the so-called abscess should not have been tampered with. The surgeons were disappointed and at a loss for a diagnosis. The case has assumed a threatening aspect. Hering devoutly says: "Our only hope is that Heaven will look kindly upon us and save him for us." Dr. Thomas desired the operation, hoping that a discharge of pus would relieve him. Doctors Raue and Hering both disapproved, thinking that well-chosen remedies would have done better, especially if given in higher potency.

Bute.

"My friend and former student, Dr. George Bute, who practised in Nazareth, Pa., had been sold, upon his arrival from Germany, to a man who paid his passage money on board ship. A Catholic priest, who accompanied Bute on the voyage, had promised to pay his fare, but vanished immediately upon their arrival to parts unknown. The man who took the stranded passenger into his service was named Pratt, a Philadelphian, who made him a gardener.

"By another man Bute was brought free from Pratt, came among the Moravians at Bethlehem, Pa., and was thence sent as missionary to the Moravian Colony in Suriname, South America. There he made my acquaintance and I took him as a student and for eighteen months taught him anatomy, physiology and *materia medica*. It had been Bute's intention to practise allopathy, but the Moravians, who had been under my care, said, 'We are homoeopaths.' Before he came to be a student of homoeopathy he had been sick. He recovered and was thereby converted to the cause. He later became dissatisfied with life in the tropics and came North, to Philadelphia, where, in one of the hospitals, he distinguished himself by curing the cholera, which raged there epidemically with frightful mortality. He, sometime later, while the cholera was still raging, urged me to come North and help him to cope with it."

Croup. Belladonna. Arsenicum.

"In five years I have not given either *Hepar* or *Spongia*, considered favorite remedies in croup. Generally *Belladonna* for the spamodic variety, and *Arsenicum* where there is great weakness, or a suppressed *urticaria*, as sometimes happens."

Hydrocephalus.

"My first death this year is a case of *hydrocephalus* which I treated in consultation with Dr. Martin. A puny child, born at seven months. The remedies given were: *Rheum, Acon., Ipecac. and Sepia.* None was of any avail. This morning when I arrived the ominous white ribbon was on the door. The parents seemed to be glad, rather than otherwise; particularly the father."

Martin.

"Dr. Martin returned from a visit to Boston, where he was hospitably received at a meeting of the Institute. There was a brilliant reception. Council had donated twenty-five hundred dollars for a grand levee; this, in spite of the mayor, an allopathic physician. There was also a banquet given by the Massachusetts Homoeopathic Medical Society.

Dr. Ludlam of Chicago was president of the meeting. At the banquet toasts were proposed to the city, the Cause, the President of the U. S., the Legal profession, and the Military, all of which were responded to by men of prominence in these branches. A toast to our College was responded to by Martin. Dr. Gause also made a speech. The programme included sight seeing to places of interest for visiting physicians."

The next meeting is to be held in Chicago. Hering says: "Then Philadelphia must return the compliment, with a grand concert, a promenade, a collation and a hop, and the usual banquet."

College.

"Our College has promise of a glorious future. Doctors Carroll Dunham and Timothy F. Allen, of New York, have offered to give one lecture each a week, gratis, in our next winter course. The New York Homoeopathic College is about to break up, which will probably increase the number of our students in Philadelphia."

Martin proposes that Dunham should lecture on Institutes. He still thinks that Morgan, for want of discretion, is the one member of the faculty who is likely to injure the cause.

Fair.

Our friends in Boston are taking an interest in the Fair. They propose having a Boston table, sponsored by Doctors Payne, Wesselhoeft, etc.

The Infected Hand. Arsenicum.

"The following is a translation from a letter, by me, printed in a German journal, Vol. 3, No. 15, August, 1860, edited by F. A. Guenther, in Langensalsa. The heading is *Homoeopathy is dead!* I had left Leipzig. After another year had passed, homoeopathy was still living, although I myself had nearly died, from an infected hand, received when making a dissection; an accident which has carried off many a young physician by a horrible death. The dissection was made upon the exhumed body of a suicide, a job side-stepped by others, and over which I lingered a bit too long, while dabbling among the entrails with a partly healed cut on the forefinger of the right hand, thinly covered by a scab.

"Before making the post mortem I washed my hands in hot soapy water which left the cut uncovered. A man from Jena had asked for a dissection of the kidneys, with ureters and bladder, and all that belonged to the specimen, which I promised to make for him.

"After several days my finger began to show signs of infection. I was given an opportunity to observe, on myself, that malady against which leeches, calomel and hellstone (nitrate of silver) had proved powerless in allopathic hands. I refused amputation, because with a crippled hand I would have had but little show of becoming an obstetrician or a surgeon. I preferred death to

this. I was, at the time, still deeply sunk in that superstitious belief that external diseases could not be reached
by internal remedies, least of all when given in small
doses.

"I was saved by one of Hahnemann's earliest students
who persuaded me to try *Arsenic*, in ridiculously small
doses. When, after taking a few doses of the remedy on
my tongue, a sense of relief from the horrible affliction
began to pervade my body, the last obstruction that had
made me blind to the rising sun of the new healing art
vanished before my eyes.

"I still have the finger; it is the same with which I write
this, and more than all I have devoted my entire hand,
body and soul, to the cause which Hahnemann gave to
suffering humanity. His teachings had not only restored
my bodily health but gave me a new purpose in life.

"And it was to me they told: 'Homoeopathy is dead!'
Many times since, 'The dead have buried their dead.' Progress goes on. The world is moving."

June 15, 1869.

Fair.

I assisted all day at a Strawberry Festival to raise money
for the Fair. Grand decorations. Beautiful flowers.
Baskets, bouquets and wreaths. Cakes, ices and straw-
berries in profusion. Between three and four hundred
people in attendance in the afternoon. In the evening
the hall was crowded to overflowing. A grand success.
People enthusiastic. Hosts of beautiful young ladies.
Flower-selling girls. Rebecca at the well selling lemon-
ade. Auctioning off of cakes. Dancing. A great adver-
tisement for the coming Fair.

June 16, 1869.

In the evening while sitting at the table cutting slips for
an index to Kafka's book, Hering says: "In Germany
when a new book appears the students will say, 'Have you
read So-and-so's new book?' 'No? Then you have read
nothing!'"

Wine.

There is wine on the table. The doctor quotes the old German saying, *Drei Maenner Wein* (Three men wine). Two men must hold the third until he finishes drinking the sour wine.

A Satire. Homoeopathy vs. Allopathy. A Will. Ridicule.

"I wrote a satire, 'Allopathy vs. Homoeopathy.' In it I pictured a man who dies and leaves a will. The day for reading the will is appointed. The doctors meet. They make Death president. A homoeopath, from America, is present who can work miracles. They ask him what he can do. He informs them that Spirits enable him to call up the dead. They ask for Hippocrates. The magician says the books must be at hand, and must be produced. They place them on the table. Hippocrates is invoked, appears and speaks. They next ask for Galen. His books are produced. Galen appears but talks about nothing but making money. They wish him dismissed. The magician, who is a homoeopath, whispers the word 'cholera' into the ghost's ear. The spectre vanishes. They next ask for Paracelsus, whose books are available. He speaks for homoeopathy. They now wish to see Hahnemann. He cannot be invoked because they have failed to produce his books.

"The meeting adjourns. All disperse excepting the American who alone remains to hear a codicil read, which decrees that the money is to be divided among those who remain last at the conference. He is the only one left to hear the last of the will. The money which amounts to a sum well advanced on the road to a million cannot be inherited by the American because a division among one is not possible. There were prior bequests in the will, made void by the last codicil. One of these favored any college that had not made any changes in its faculty in a certain number of years."

Some so-called homoeopaths did not escape well-merited castigation in this satire, one of many, which Dr. Hering wrote in defense of the cause. He gave it as his

opinion that when a thing is due for annihilation nothing
will prove so effectual as killing it with ridicule.

_____

June 18, 1869.

A Clinical Case. Warts on the Vocal Cords.

"A patient, a young girl of thirteen, came to me today
with a rasping, almost constant, distressing cough which
makes the listener nervous. I sent her to Macfarlan for a
laryngoscopic examination. He found a great many warts,
like fig-warts growing on the vocal cords, almost ob-
structing the passage. The cough is caused by constant
irritation of the pneumogastric nerve. If the warts could
be cured the cough would cease. On account of a sycotic
dyscrasia, and the warts, the patient received *Thuja*, in a
high dilution."

Hering does not expect the case to recover, without an
operation. Foreign bodies in the larynx, or trachea, he
says, cause hepatization of the lungs.

A Clinical Case. A Foreign Body in the Larynx. Ethics.

"A very bad, stubborn boy played with a metallic pencil-case which he accidentally swallowed. The metal tube
had separated into three sections at one end, by which it
was held fast in the larynx. There were no immediate
bad effects and nothing could be done with him at the
moment. He would not admit having swallowed the
pencil-case. Next day there was a slight cough, which
grew worse on the following day. On the third day the
cough had increased to a harsh bellowing sound. The
family now called in two doctors who diagnosed croup,
and gave the patient *Phosphorus*. Both were low potency
prescribers. The patient not improving, I was again
called. The mother asked if it was croup. I hesitated.
She saw my hesitation and said: 'Doctor, is it a foreign
body; could my son after all have swallowed the pencil-
case?' 'Yes, I said, that is it.'

"It was too late then to perform an operation; the boy
was already dying. Next morning I asked that a post
mortem be made. Dr. W. carefully removed the larynx.

I sent a member of the family from the room to procure a sponge. Dr. W. pocketed the specimen, which, afterwards, on being opened disclosed the metallic pencil-case. When the mother learned the truth she fainted, overcome by the thought that her child had died from neglect, when an operation might have saved his life.

"I told the mother that the operation should have been done on the first day, which greatly angered W. who, for a long time remained my enemy. but later became friendly.

"Some time after this episode Dr. Lippe and myself were called to attend Dr. Gosewisch, in Wilmington. We had to run to get the train. In my absence a Mr. Johnson, a rich type-founder, came to my office to ask me to call on his wife who was very sick. Not finding me he called on Dr. W. and informed him that Dr. Hering, who was his family doctor, was out of town, would he please come to see his wife. The doctor strutted about his office and said: 'It is about time that I stopped playing second fiddle to Dr. Hering!' And he refused to go.

"Mr. Johnson went away with a heavy heart, but remembered that Dr. Kitchen did not live far away. He called on him. He had scarcely mentioned the sick wife and the name of Hering when Kitchen had his hat on, ready to make the visit. I turned the family over to him.

"W. had come to Philadelphia an allopath. It was with great difficulty that he was persuaded to abandon the practice of giving castor-oil to women after childbirth. He was an obstetrician. I sent him many families, in fact set him up in practice.

"On the day following the postmortem on the body of the boy who had swallowed the pencil W. took the specimen with him to his lecture room to show it to the students. He told them that on the previous day he had been in consultation with Doctors Hering and Neidhard, on the case, that both of them had diagnosed croup, that he alone had pronounced it a case of a foreign body lodged in the larynx.

"Dr. W. has done a great deal for homoeopathy; neither could we have done without Lippe. It is only when men go too far, so as to injure the cause, that they must be checked."

Foreign Body in the Windpipe.

"I had heard of the case of a young man who, in rough play with his sweetheart, took a ring off her finger with his mouth. The ring lodged in his windpipe where it remained for some time, just above the bronchial bifurcation. It frequently moved from one side to the other. He died, probably from inflammation and hepatization of the lungs; a martyr to his amorous playfulness."

Nemesis.

"Retribution follows the misdeeds of people. It is not for us to judge, nor to malign. We should never quarrel with, or defame others, for personal reasons. Nor be jealous of them. My daughter Odelia often got angry when she thought others had stolen my thunder. I replied: Let them steal the thunder as long as I am left the lightning."

Rev. Brobst, of Allentown.

"I once asked Brobst to correct me if I had made a misstatement as to his ancestry, in which I declared that it was his great, great, great grandfather who had come over from Germany. That is the exact truth, said Brobst. The name originally was written with P, Propst, meaning provost."

History.

"Particular events, as they happen, count most in making history. *Einzelheiten in der Geschichte sind die Hauptsache.*"

Silly Phrases.

Hering is frequently annoyed by such. As for example the German word, *Leider,* meaning alas, or unhappily. Another, frequently used, is: *Eine Rolle spielen,* (to play a part, as in a drama). Also the word standpoint *(Standpunkt)* is objectionable to him when missapplied.

The First Homoeopath.

"St. Paul was the first homoeopath; for in Acts, Chap. 14, verse 15, he says: 'We are *homoeopatois*,' a Greek word signifying of like passions; in German *aehnlich leidende*, of like suffering."

Hering laughs and says that is something the old man (meaning Hahnemann) did not know.

Wine. Hahnemann. Carey.

"Hahnemann drank his wine in thimblefuls. A strong German wine. Henry Carey, Political Economist, did the same, and treated his guests in the same way."

June 20, 1869.

An Adventure. The Inebriated College Trustee.

A note came to Dr. Hering asking him to go to the stationhouse, at 15th and Locust Streets, to see a Mr. Norton, one of the trustees of our College; that he had been picked up intoxicated on Chestnut Street the night before. We were amazed, but thought if it were Mr. Norton, the President of our College, he must have been ill and found unconscious. Hering did not feel like going, and no official person being available I volunteered to go.

It was not our President whom I found at the stationhouse, in a cell, where a man had been confined all night without anything to eat, but one of our talented trustees, a portrait-painter, who had been picked up by an officer and brought in the night before.

The painter's story was the following: "I was on my way out of town to paint a portrait and got in with some friends who persuaded me to go with them to Harmer's Cornucopia, where I got tight, and in going up Chestnut Street, I was arrested and brought here. I was robbed of the last two dollars I had in my pocket, also of my spectacles, from which only the case was left me and I have had nothing to eat since yesterday."

He had mentioned the name of Mr. Norton to the turn-key as being one of his friends, which led to the misunderstanding, implicating our abstemious and worthy president. I gave the complainant a single dose of *Nux vomica* to sober him, went to the nearest magistrate to obtain a release for the unlucky trustee, which cost $4.50, and gave him carfare with which to return home.

The painter's wife is actively engaged in working for our Fair, and the artist is painting a portrait of Hering to be exhibited there. Hering said the bibulous artist when appointed had been a member of the former College, as trustee, so he could not well have been dropped from the board. A good man, but like many, weak in resisting liquor.

Thomas. Hepar Sulph. in Suppuration.

Dr. Thomas is improving. In Morgan's absence he received the indicated remedy, *Hepar sulph.*, from the hands of Doctors Koch and Macfarlan; which remedy he should have had much earlier, and before the unsuccessful operation was attempted.

Morgan had pinned his hopes on the hypo-phosphites-of-lime, given empirically. After the stage in which suppuration cannot be prevented by the prescribed remedy, it is proper that it should be encouraged, therefore *Hepar* is given in a higher potency. Pus is now discharged copiously from the abscess and the patient is on the road to recovery. Morgan felt a bit hurt at what had transpired in his absence.

After all, we may say, that Dr. Hering should have the credit for giving the *Hepar*, since it was he who had first proposed the remedy.

Inimical Remedies.

"Certain remedies are inimical and should not be allowed to follow one another closely, as for instance: *Phosphorus* and *Causticum;* also *Rhus tox* and *Apis;* likewise *Nux vom.* and *Ignatia.* Only one of them can be properly indicated and if a wrong one is given it will do harm.

"Always a bridge can be built from one to the other remedy by giving a complementary medicine, such as *Belladonna,* after *Rhus tox., Pulsatilla* after *Nux vom.,* etc., etc."

See Chapter 48, Guiding Symptoms: Relationship of Drugs.

Diet. Coffee, Etc.

"Coffee, and all roasted substances, aggravate catarrhal complaints, sore throat, coryza, etc."

A German Picnic.

On last Saturday a picnic was arranged. The party included Mrs. Hering, Hering's niece Bertha; three of the boys, Walter, Carl and Herman; Ernestine (a niece of Dr. Raue); a Miss Froehlich, lately arrived from Germany, and Mrs. Seiler, a singing teacher, and myself. In a beautiful retreat by the Schuylkill River, the company enjoyed some beer and wine; also a favorite drink with German people in hot weather, called *Bierkaltschaale,* composed of beer, water, sugar and crumbs of ryebread. There were crackers and cherries. German songs were sung, the boys played ball, and when evening came we went home in a crowded street car drawn by horses, which was not quite as pleasant as had been the journey up the river by boat. German *gemuethlichkeit* dominated the party, and everybody had a good time. These outings were of frequent occurrence with the Hering family.

Bayard.

"I once made a visit to Dr. Edward Bayard, in New York. As I entered the parlor, there, on the mantlepiece I saw an image of the *Chevalier sans peur et sans reproche,* in bronze, the French Knight of the Middle Ages, dubbed: 'without fear and without reproach.' The figure, to all appearances, was a likeness of my friend Bayard, to the wart on his face. The Knight was mounted on his horse, ready to join the Crusaders. I marvelled, could a sensible man like my friend Edward, a descendant from the Bayards, have sent his portrait to Paris to have it reproduced in this form? This could hardly have been the case.

"Mrs. Bayard came into the room to receive me and saw that I was puzzled while regarding the effigy. She told me that she, and her mother, when travelling by themselves in Europe—the doctor having been too busy to leave home—had, while in Paris, entered a jeweller's shop, where, to their amazement, they beheld this bronze figure, mounted on a clock. Both of them observed at once that the image bore the very likeness of Dr. Bayard, even to the wart on his face. They decided to buy it and bring it home. The picture of the Knight 'without fear and without reproach' of more than a thousand years ago was the image of the man of today. So much for family likeness by heredity."

June 21, 1869.

Doctor's Fees. Macfarlan.

Dr. Macfarlan is subpoenaed to go to court as a witness in the case of a College dispensary patient, by which he will lose both time and money. Not long ago he reduced a strangulated hernia for a shopkeeper, who thought a fee of ten dollars too much for the service; the regular fee being thirty. The usual case of the ungrateful patient. Hering says we must not expect gratitude, and we will not be disappointed.

Malpractice.

"Cases of malpractice occur in the same ratio in which suits for the same are brought against physicians. The patient has no right to take a bungler for his doctor, hence should not have the right to sue.

"If a man loses a child which has been poisoned by the prescription of a drunken physician, the man has erred in having employed the services of an inebriate for his sick child.

"I remember a case in which an applicant came to me asking to be taught homoeopathy. As there was then no college of our own I advised him to go to an allopathic institution, for at least two years. He refused to do this and I would not take him as my student. He went to a doctor by the name of Schmoele, who advised him to hang out a shingle and practice on his own hook; saying that he had done the same way.

"The young man opened an office on Front Street. A lady who had previously consulted me went to the new doctor, who gave her a heavy dose of strychnia, from which she died in convulsions. The husband came to me threatening to sue the ignorant practitioner for malpractice. I said: 'You will only make yourself and your wife ridiculous for having employed such a quack. You are to blame and should bear the censure.'

"I say to all: Cursed be he who defends the bringing of suits against physicians for malpractice!"

Music. First Piano.

We had a visit, this evening, from Mr. Himmelsbach, a musician who came to say goodbye before leaving for Germany. Hering told him that he would not stay long over there; that no American, nor any German who had lived here for long could exist there. That this is the land of progress and Philadelphia the place from which all important things eminate. As for instance: the first Maennerchor (Male Singing Society), the first Library, College, etc., etc. Pianos were first sold here, from the store of a man by the name of Wittig, who had the first music store in America.

Wittig sold his first piano to a Jersey farmer. After three weeks the farmer came back to town with the instrument on his wagon, drove up in front of the store, went in and said to the proprietor: "For heaven's sake, take this thing off my hands, or I will be ruined! Get what you can for it and give me the money." "But why? What is the trouble?" "Trouble?" said the farmer, "nothing else but. My house is made a pandemonium. My daughter plays fairly well on the thing, but in consequence all the sons and daughters of my neighbors, for miles around, come and fill my parlor, drum on the instrument, dance and raise Cain in general. The young country fellows bring their horses to be stabled and fed. I see ruin staring me in the face. Even my daughter consents to be rid of the nuisance. Take it for what you can get for it!"

At the present time (1869) there are over six thousand pianos in Philadelphia. You will find them in back streets and everywhere.

Music. Allentown.

"At Allentown, in 1835, one evening a couple of German students raised a German song: *Ich geh an's Bruennele, trink awwer net,* (I go to the well but do not drink), popular among people in Germany. The singers were soon joined by others, by myself also, and we passed around the Academy on the way to a nearby place to drink beer, and to sing some more. We made a sensation."

Wine.

"In a few more years we will have banquets with ladies present, and there will be wine too."

Gartenlaube. Homoeopathy.

"The editors of the German magazine, *Die Gartenlaube,* are opposed to homoeopathy and will print everything against it, but nothing in favor of it."

Hausmann.

"The great book, just issued by Hausmann, will only be fully understood two or three centuries from now. It will be the great basis for homoeopathy. Hausmann proceeds from the study of elements or metals which form crystals in the tissues of the body. In places and organs, where found they will perform cures. Copper traced to its destination in the tissues will be creative of the diseases located there.

"Hausmann, who apparently knows everything, is not so well at home in botany as in other branches of science. I intend to write a book to make him intelligible to the students."

The book, for want of time devoted to *Materia medica,* was never printed. There are a few prefatory notes.

June 27, 1869.

Hahnemann's Son, Frederick.   Humphreys.

Hering speaking to Dr. H. M. Smith, from New York:
"The first opponent to Hahnemann was Hecker. A bad
fellow; malicious, feared, hated and despised. Hahnemann took no notice of him. Hecker was crazy because
Hahnemann printed the *Organon*. Wished to see him
dead. Hecker had a son.

Hahnemann's son, Frederick, was injured, had his back
broken, when the wagon upset with the family in one of
the many movings from one place to another; the daughters were unhurt. Frederick, a hunchback, became a painful sight in the eyes of his father, which the son sensed.
He wanted more money than the father had to give him,
so he left home, and with what money he had saved bought
an apothecary-shop somewhere in Saxony.

"The father had no great luck with his children. He
was a strict man, a bit pedantic. Being a friend of liberty,
he hated Napoleon.

"The son began to thrive, had a good run of customers
from the better classes. The market-place, in front of his
apothecary-shop, was regularly lined with carriages. He
cured a girl who had been blind from birth. He asked
the girl to look straight into the sun until she could see.
She saw the sun and later her father. Frederick was a
low dilutionist. He used *Mercurius* and *Sulphur* in the
first, second and third dilutions, but went up to the sixth
and twelfth because he got symptoms from the lower preparations.

"The multitude hurrahed and hosanned. I know this
from an eye witness. He did not sell drugs; only had the
right to dispense; apothecary rights. A law had been
passed taking from doctors the privilege of keeping an
apothecary shop. Suit was brought and there was the case
of the State against Frederick Hahnemann. Friends wrote
to his father to come and defend his disorderly son. The
son said: 'Let them go to the devil,' or words to that
effect, made his personal property over to his wife, left his
shop to the state, and departed for Scotland. Orders had

been issued to arrest him for contempt of court. Hahne-mann said: 'Poor Frederick, he will go insane.' These were the last words he ever again spoke of his son. While in Scotland there was a bust made of Frederick which I tried to recover, but it had been lost or broken. He had left Scotland for parts unknown. It is almost certain that he came to America. For this I had the word of my old friend, William Wesselhoeft.

"Frederick Hahnemann had been traced to some mines in the far West. He may have been here, in the East. A farmer, somewhere near the Jersey border, described him so accurately that there could scarcely have been left a doubt. A small man, a hunchback, little pills, very pre-cise in making his prescriptions, forbidding things that are injurious to homoeopathic treatment, saying: 'If you don't do so-and-so, as I tell you, I will not come near you again.' Gruffly spoken. It must have been Frederick Hahnemann.

"Again, I read somewhere, that while the cholera was raging in the Mississippi valley, a man dressed in a long Turkish garment, such as Frederick was known to wear, came out of a lead-mine, put a few small globules from a small vial, on people's tongues and cured many of the cholera. To those who offered to pay he told them not to give money but to follow him to help nurse and cure the afflicted. He was reported as being small, with a hump on his back, and a long beard, such as he had dared to wear when it was against the custom in Germany, and on ac-count of which his father had not allowed him to appear before him. He had a habit of spitting, almost continu-ally, which, on account of his short stature, and by having to raise his face to people when speaking to them, made him a nuisance.

"Humphreys, whom I disliked on account of his quack-ery and morals, also had heard of Frederick Hahnemann from speaking with a man who had described him to a T. Humphreys also knew about his having been in Scotland, and of the words of the father: 'Poor Frederick will go crazy,' and that he had ceased to speak of his son."

Sharks. Jurisprudence.

"While I lived in Paramaribo, Surinam, a human head was washed ashore. It had been torn from the body and its muscles and ligaments were terribly lacerated. A coroner's inquest was held, to which I was invited to make a post mortem examination. I was asked to give my opinion in court. My evidence was somewhat tantalizing for I mentioned all sorts of possibilities that might have happened. Could the man have been killed and his body thrown overboard? There were no signs of a deadly instrument having been used. Could the victim have been caught in the wheels of machinery? Unlikely, judging from the appearance of the head. Could this, or any other fatality have occurred? The answer was always, No. The head showed several wounds, similar to those made by sharp teeth. The pupils were dilated.

"I concluded that the man had fallen overboard from some vessel, perhaps while intoxicated, and that sharks had mangled him as soon as he had struck the water; that the head had been severed from the trunk and washed ashore while the body of the man had been swallowed piece-meal by the hungry sharks. The animal with several rows of sharp teeth pointing inward, forming a saw, has a small gullet no wider than an ordinary teacup at its widest end; consequently he could not make away with the head.

"The shark, with belly turned up, attacks his prey by shaking it sideways, to and fro, with incredible rapidity, until it is sufficiently mangled to be swallowed.

"It is dangerous to bathe in tropical waters. White men take negroes with them to ward off the sharks. The negroes are stationed out, in advance of the bathers, as guards. As soon as a shark approaches and stares at the negro, with small but terrible eyes, the negro, quick as lightning, strikes the water a resounding blow with the flat of his hand. This frightens the cowardly marauder who turns and darts away. The negro makes for the shore. He knows that the shark prefers dark meat; which statement I have heard corroborated.

"The shark not only turns on his back to do his deadly work, but the negroes say he revolves so rapidly as to complete a circle at each turn, all done quick as lightning, which deceives the eye. I have observed the black men when they go out in a boat to feed the sharks, which come up to snatch the bait and disappear like a flash.

"The case here related belongs in a book on Medical Jurisprudence, but has been steadily refused as 'evidence coming from a homoeopath!' The incident marked a great triumph for me in Paramaribo. A set of saw-teeth from a shark was brought into court and fitted to the wounds on the mutilated head. The man who lent the specimens brought an armful of them."

Balling. Portrait.

Balling, a portrait painter from New York, a friend of Dr. Fincke, came to Philadelphia on a commission to paint some portraits, and while here as a guest, offered to paint Hering's portrait. The result was a rather bricky-looking sketch which was relegated to the garret, whence later it disappeared. It had been intended for the Fair, where better pictures of Hering were exhibited. Balling played on the cello. He had made a sketch of a log cabin, which for a time hung on the wall in the office. This also disappeared.

Portrait of Hahnemann, Painted by Madame Hahnemann.

The history of this splendid portrait of the father of homoeopathy which hung on the wall of the doctor's reception room, and is now in my possession, is told by Dr. Hering:

"Dr. Wesselhoeft of Boston, had for a patient an artist by the name of Miller. Being unable to pay for his treatment the artist offered to do something for his benefactor. He was about to leave for Paris. Wesselhoeft said: 'Bring me back a portrait of Hahnemann.' Miller promised faithfully, and soon after he arrived in Paris, sought the house of Hahnemann. He there met Madame Hahnemann to whom he made his request. She said her husband could not be put to the trouble of a sitting. Miller said: 'But I

have promised to bring back a portrait of him to my
physician, and I must keep my promise.' Madame Hahnemann, herself an artist of great ability, showed him a
portrait she had painted of her good 'papa' as she called
him. Miller said: 'Why the little black cap on his head?'
'That,' said the lady: 'is intended to hide the high forehead which draws everyone's attention away from his
kindly face.' She must have possessed both talent and
genius. The painting is the best of all known portraits
of Hahnemann.

"On condition that the painter would follow her idea
she permitted him to see Hahnemann, and paint his picture
with the little black velvet cap on the forehead as suggested
by Madame, which impresses all who look at the portrait.
When Miller had finished the painting and was about to
send it on its journey to America, the thought came to
him—what if the picture should be lost on the way? I
must paint a duplicate. So he made a second copy from
the original and sent one of the portraits by way of England, the other direct to Boston. The one sent direct got
there first; soon after, the second one arrived. Wesselhoeft was puzzled. He said: 'Is the man gone crazy?'

"He had already ordered a costly frame for the first
picture, and expressed his great delight with the painting.
The second picture, presumably a copy of the first, he
thought, might, after all, have been the original. His
friends could not decide which of the two had the greater
merit. In order to help make a decision he had the second
picture framed, like the first, and for comparison placed
both portraits, side by side in their frames. Still he could
not come to a decision.

"In desperation Wesselhoeft told his man to pack one
of the pictures, either one, and send it to his friend Hering
in Philadelphia. So I received one of the fine portraits,
for a gift, whether the original or the copy, I never knew."

This portrait is one of the valued possessions of the
writer, together with the marble statuette of the master
by the sculptor Rauenthaler, and also a marvelous portrait
of Jenichen, representing him in the act of potentizing, by

hand, *Pulsatilla* to the 16,000th potency. In addition there is a bronze medallion of Hahnemann in profile, by the celebrated French artist David, besides other interesting relics, including a small picture showing the statue of Hahnemann in Leipzig, and a portrait of the youthful Hering painted on ivory. Besides these treasures there are letters both from Hahnemann and from his widow. The latter contain fervid invitations to Hering, none too delicately veiled, to come to Paris and become the successor of Hahnemann. The doctor declined, in words not any too friendly, as it would appear from his replies to Madame Hahnemann. He was a widower at the time with two children, Max and Odelia, whom he says he did not wish to be made French, but remain Americans.

Hom. Dispensatory. Henry M. Smith.

Henry M. Smith, from New York, came to consult Hering about publishing a Homoeopathic Dispensatory. Hering suggested, as part of the plan, to have microscopic cross-sections made from the roots and other parts of plants, for the purpose of diagnosis and identification. Smith favored the idea and promised that it should be carried out, but this was not accomplished.

Wine.

"Blackberry wine can hardly be distinguished from Port."

Fireflies.

"In Surinam, in the tropics, thousands of fireflies illuminate the landscape at night; myriads of them sparkle at the same time."

June 28, 1869.

Von Tagen.

Hering has a visit from Dr. Von Tagen, from Harrisburg, who comes to consult him about his little girl, ill with diptheria. Von Tagen promises a Harrisburg Table for the Fair.

Hering said, in conversation with the visitor, "If you get wives and children for patients, husbands, if worth having, will follow; but sometimes the men think if they join our ranks, they will have to give up alcoholic drinks."

July 1, 1869.

Balling. Cathedral of Cologne. Banquet. Prophecy.

In the evening, at the supper table. Balling, the painter. prepared to make a sketch of Hering. The doctor said: "So you are about to steal something?"

The conversation turns upon a favorite topic, the Cathedral of Cologne. "My friend Weigel and I, one morning found ourselves floating down the Rhine to Cologne. I said I wish to see the Cathedral. Weigel said: 'You are foolish, we cannot afford the delay.' We were on our way to Amsterdam to set sail for South America. We stopped off in Cologne and put up in a boarding-house, temporarily, while visiting that marvel of architecture, the dome. We saw the unfinished edifice with a crane on top of it, and deep mud in the streets all around it, an enormous pile of masonry resembling a grand ruin.

"We had a meal at our boarding-house, and later were invited to a banquet given by the King of Saxony, who was present at the dinner. On the table stood a huge piece of meat like a small mountain, from which the King, with a sharp pointed knife, carved a coneshaped section from which he cut smaller slices, dripping with blood. Weigel claimed that he saw his portion still twitching on his plate. A gravy was served with the meat, the best, I thought, I had ever tasted.

"I remarked to the guests that we had come to see the Cathedral. At that time the people on the Rhine preferred to be French rather than German. Some one at the table expressed himself in regard to the dome: 'Only fools could imagine that anything could be made out of these ruins!' I stood up and said: 'I am of that opinion.' Ho! Ho! Ho!; loud laughter followed this speech.

"Toasts were in order. I proposed the toast: 'The dome of Cologne will be finished!' More loud laughter. A celebrated architect, present at the table, said: 'I have examined the foundations of the structure and have found them thoroughly rotten, and decayed.'

"I remarked that I had read a different account, and again rose to propose a second toast: 'The dome of Cologne will be completed as surely as Germany will become united.' Greater laughter than before greeted this proposition. The architect came over to me and said: 'I now know whom I have before me. A great satirist!' I replied: 'When I again return to Germany, the Dome at Cologne will be finished and Germany will be united.' The answer came: 'Permit us to laugh.' This was in 1826."

In later years, when Hering returned to visit his fatherland, both of his early prophecies had been fulfilled. The Cathedral, with both spires, stood completed, and Germany, under Bismarck, had become united.

Hering, deeply interested in the famous Gothic structure at Cologne, had collected numerous pictures and views of the Cathedral, one of them so large that to be seen in its entirety, it had to be hung out of a second story window into the garden. The large picture of the Dome is made from an original plan drawn by the architect 800 years ago. It is thirteen feet in length. Catholics in this country show no interest in the Cathedral in Cologne. They are devoted to the one in Rome which houses the Pope.

History. Laws.

"The French have a saying, *Jusque a la mer* (all the way to the sea), meaning that they would like to have possession of the Rhine to its outlet into the sea, on both sides. Nemesis will overtake them. Hollanders cannot abide Belgians. World history will run its course. Many have already seen certain laws of history come to fruition. With an understanding of these laws, one can make quite wonderful predictions. Events in history are polarized, have a duality. They strike a balance. Aristotle and Plato came after each other. Prophecies are nothing but logical conclusions. When we observe certain symptoms we expect others to follow, and a prognosis is possible."

Following the above conversation, Hering remarked to

Balling, still busy with his sketch: "What gave you this idea? You would do better to play on your cello. May I take a pinch of snuff?" "Two if you like." "One will do!" "I have made a preparatory sketch for a portrait of you, Dr. Hering, if I have the courage to go on with it."

The result was as described on a previous page.

College Days. Expositions.

"At school there were three of us, in particular. from whom ideas originated. Meyer, whom we named the 'Rose-red,' Boehme. and myself, to whom was given the nickname of 'Buffalo.' Hard studying was called buffaloing at school. Boehme was tall as a sapling, slim and dry. My specialty was medicine; his, Greek philosophy. 'Rose-red' became secretary to Prince Albert of England, to whom he gave the idea of opening a World Exposition. Another student, Schambrok by name, was knighted for his discovery of the *Victoria Regia*, a tropical plant so large that a house had to be built to receive it, the blossom alone being the size of this table (over ten feet long and four feet wide). Seeing this building in London gave 'Rose-red' his idea for an Exposition.

"The Exposition in Paris exceeded, in size, five times the one in London. I am proposing permanent expositions, with kitchens and houses made of iron. Waitresses from all nations, such as were serving beer at the Paris Exposition, are to be excluded as something that mixes up art with things natural. There should be medallions, of gold, for special distribution, as rewards."

Soldiers. Napoleon.

"It should be the care of the Latin nation to improve the souls of its soldiers. 'Back of the bayonets are heads, back of the heads, human wills,' said Napoleon."

July 5, 1869.

Fourth of July. A Fire. Paintings.

The fourth of July, which came on a Sunday, was celebrated on the fifth. On the evening of the third some fire-crackers were set off in Hering's garden, including a penny rocket, which lit on the house of Dr. Koch, two doors away, and started a blaze on the roof. This was done by one of the boys, Walter. We ran next door thinking the fire was there. In the meantime a man from Cherry Street, close by, saw the blaze, came and put it out with a bucketful of water. Suspicion fell upon this man's boys. As yet no revelation has been made.

On Monday evening the family, including everyone from the youngest to the doctor himself, stationed himself on the roof to observe the display of fireworks against a background of dark sky. When it was over we descended to the parlor where there was music, on the cello by Balling, the painter, and some duets on the piano by Rudolph and Bertha. There was wine, and conversation from Father Hering, who told us the history of two paintings in his parlor, which were done by two artists, named Koch and Gruenewald. One of the pictures represents a shepherd driving home his flock of sheep through a blinding storm; the other shows the shepherd of another flock which has been brought safely under cover in a cave sheltered from the storm, illustrated by the German proverb: *Er hat seine Schaefchen ins trockene gebracht* (His lambs are safely housed), meaning that his undertakings have been crowned with success.

July 6, 1869.

The Magnetic Telegraph. Morse.

"The idea of the magnetic telegraph was given to Morse by a Frenchman on board ship. My friend, General Hubbell, a Philadelphian, had the honour of finding this out. Morse, who was stupid, took out a patent with the help of a man by the name of Campbell. The first test was made over a wire from Boston to Washington. As if a distance of a few miles, or a million, could have made any difference in the result of the experiment! Others, who disputed the right of taking out a patent on a principle, began to make better instruments. I thought Morse should have received a premium for his share in the invention. Some were in agreement with this, others were not. I was told that I did not know our people. I replied: 'Nor do I know the devil's grandmother, for that matter, since I have never seen her!' There should not be any patents. A fair reward should be given to the inventor; not a million, but a sum proportionate to the value of his discovery."

Inventions. Malleable Glass. Varnish. Platinum. Stapf.

"There was a king in ancient Syracuse to whom came a man saying: 'Your Majesty, I have made this beautiful glass goblet. Take it and cast it upon the floor.' 'No!' said the king, 'It is too beautiful to be destroyed;' But he threw it down, and it was not broken by the fall, only bent out of shape. The man took a hammer and hammered it back to its original shape. The king gave orders to have the fellow hanged."

A fairy tale now come true through the discovery of malleable and nonshatterable glass.

"Dr. Zumbrook, my chemist, has made an accidental discovery of a wonderful varnish in a combination of sugar, saltpeter and sulphuric acid, under a freezing process. When applied to paper, or to an engraving, it refracted light as brilliantly as a diamond. It would have been a valuable varnish to use on oil paintings. The discovery might have made Zumbrook rich, but he could not reproduce the article. The varnish did not have the quality to resist alcohol. Peterhofer discovered a method by which to restore oil paintings.

"Platinum was discovered in Mexico. A shipload of it was to be sent to Spain. The Spanish government had the ship scuttled and sunk. The first platinum was smuggled into England. A nugget of it, a rare gift, was sent to Carl August.

"A certain German duke owned a museum which contained a large collection of minerals, among which were some valuable specimens of Platinum. Some one remarked that these could be of no use to the world.

"There was an apothecary, in a certain small town, by the name of Doebereiner, whose genius Goethe discovered, and helped him to secure a professorship in chemistry at the University of Jena. Doebereiner, of a retiring disposition, hesitated a while but finally accepted the position. The students were slow to accept him but he began to lecture and to make experiments which soon aroused enthusiasm for chemistry in the classes.

"The duke sent his specimens of Platinum to Doebereiner and asked him to put them to some use. Doebereiner wept for joy, like a child, when he saw what he had received. He examined the Platinum and found out its properties. The English went into a jealous rage, as they always do when a German makes a discovery. Doebereiner made public his findings. Later, Wollaston, of England, discovered the ductile properties of the metal.

"A retort was manufactured in which Sulphuric acid, the basis of the newer chemistry, was distilled. Doebereiner obtained a precipitate from the metal, of a spongelike character, which resembled tiny trees or mosses. He brought various gases in contact with these without any apparent result, until he tried nitrogen gas which caused them to burn like tinder. When the flame went out, the little sponge remained unchanged. He allowed the gas to pass through this which caused it to glow. He had brought the heaviest substance in contact with the lightest—the result was a flame. He next invented a lighter, for lighting cigars. He informed Goethe of his discovery. Goethe wrote: 'I will come at once to see you.'

"In Berlin were made the first medallions from Platinum. Stapf, the first to follow Hahnemann, was my intimate friend. Hahnemann had proved the metals silver, gold and zinc. Stapf undertook to prove Platinum. With considerable difficulty he obtained a trituration from the spongy metallic substance and made a proving of it. He had a hard time to induce Doebereiner to let him have even a small quantity of the valuable metal. The chemist said he must first ask the Duke's permission. 'All I need,' said Stapf, 'is a single gramme.' The chemist laughed heartily and said: 'You are welcome to that much. Take it and dissolve the tiny sponges in nitromuriatic acid.' Stapf at first tried to make a triturate but did not succeed. After some reflection he made the solution, suspended small bars of steel in it, which attracted the dust particles, thus obtaining a precipitate from which he made his provings. With the potentized *Platina* he cured three or four ladies at the ducal court, which later won him the title of *Medicinalrath*, (Medical adviser at court). It was a case of 'cast your bread upon the waters.' All honour and glory to Stapf!

"I have made mention of these occurrences in American Drug Provings. What was there printed was read daily to Stapf after he had gone blind. He had written to me: 'Hering, stay in America. It is the land for homoeopathy'."

Inventors. A Cannon. Petchke. Secrets.

Next to Hering, at table, sat one Petchke, a German, nicknamed "Canonicus" because he had invented a cannon which he called the Pacificator, which would not explode and could hit the mark at ten miles. Hering said ironically: "I would hang every single inventor!" "But doctor," said the inventor of the big gun, "that would be a bit too severe." "No!" said Hering, "I would not do that to inventors, but I would propose a government reward. I would hang them only for keeping their discoveries a secret!"

Eclipses.

"Eclipses of the sun and moon are occasions which I would like to see observed as national holidays."

———

July 8, 1869.

The Jenichen Potencies. Lippe. Hofrath. Ridicule.
          Phrases. Secrets.

A number of the *Allgemeine Zeitung*, the principal German Homoeopathic Journal, arrived this morning. It contained an article, by Hofrath, in Prague, entitled *Again the High Potencies.*

There had been a letter from Lippe, to Hofrath or maybe to the Journal, accusing Hering of conspiring with Jenichen to keep his method of potentizing a secret. The letter charges commercialism and secrecy *(Geheimnisskraemerei)*. Lippe, writing at a midnight hour, disclaims that he is trying to injure Hering by laying blame upon him; and calls this *Scheuslichkeiten in die Schuhe schieben* (shoving abominable things into men's shoes). He expresses regret that the homoeopaths, in Germany, fail to acknowledge work done here; notably that they have avoided making a translation of his article in the *Hahnemannian Monthly*, in which he scolds Fincke, whom he calls before a tribunal to answer for putting the seal of secrecy upon his method of potentizing; more *Geheimnisskraemerei.*

Further Hofrath says that he has always regarded Hering, as by nature, an honourable man, who would not have anything to do with secret-mongers, and hopes that this blot, which blackens homoeopathy, will soon be obliterated. He winds up with the hope that Dr. Hering will tell!

Hering read the scurrilous article quite coolly and laughed. I myself was furious; at Lippe, at Hofrath, at their unfair imputations. I believe, I swore for the first time since my early days on the farm. I said Lippe ought to be shot! Dr. Hering still laughed. Now arrived our Lion, Raue, who stormed and said: "Dr. Hering must reply at once!" Hering said: "No! I have already violated my rule not to read anything that appears against me in print."

At luncheon Dr. Hering told the following: "It was Jenichen's intention to leave his fortune to me with which to erect a hospital in this country, in which only his potencies were to be used. He had made this bequest through the President of the United States; I think it was Fillmore, to be carried out in case of my death. I had a long correspondence with Jenichen during this period. In his letters he made known to me the method by which he made his potencies, viz: he first of all triturates his drugs, adds the alcohol, gives the preparation a thorough shaking, and then allows it to evaporate before continuing the process of dynamization.

"Copies of his letters, made by my secretary, I have sent to my brother-in-law, Hartlaub, in Germany. On a sudden Jenichen changed his mind and willed his money to any physician living in a small town in Germany, who will be willing to make use of his potencies in treating the poor.

"It was Rentsch who accepted this proposition, but he began to place the Jenichen potencies on the market, in fact, wrote to me and asked me to sell them in America, which I refused to do. The great secret of the whole business is that Jenichen allowed his drugs to evaporate before adding alcohol and shaking them, by hand, in the regular way. Fincke did not shake his potencies; said it was not necessary.

"Jenichen was a powerfully built man, with a strong arm (as shown in his portrait). At one time, on the street, he forcibly held a team of runaway horses harnessed to a carriage in which the Duke and Duchess were riding. For this service he was knighted and given the title of Master of Horse.

"The heavy succussion, of which his mighty arms were capable shook the framework of his house, on the second floor of which he did his work. The constant armwork he practised seemed to divert his vitality from other parts of his body; he became dropsical, melancholic, partly in consequence of the death, by scarlet fever, of a girl he was about to marry, and he ended his life by his own hand.

"I am minded to try to find out the secret of Fincke's method, by experimentation. It will make him terribly angry, but I cannot help it."

As for the scurrilous article, suggested by Lippe, and published in the *Allgemeine Homoeopatische Zeitung*, over Hofrath's name, Hering at first chose to ignore it, then to treat it with a certain amount of ridicule. He came to this conclusion one day after returning from his round of visits. He proceeded to finish his article on a meeting of the American Institute, held at Boston, to which he appended some remarks, in a humourous vein, relative to the libellous criticism. "Shoving abominable things into men's shoes, at the midnight hour," became a household word, and a part of Dr. Hering's collection of silly phrases. It was his opinion that to make a thing ridiculous is the nearest way to killing it. The laugh must not be loud and uproarious, at once, but begin with a chuckle, under the diaphragm, gradually growing to a sidesplitting guffaw.

In this wise he purposed to answer his slanderers, in their own palaver. He had no patience with empty phrases such as had been coined by some of his opponents, in Germany.

Pennsylvania German Hospitality. The Tramp and the Flies.

"The Pennsylvania German people have always been noted for their hospitality. This subjected them to frequent visits from loafers and beggars. A young fellow once started out from Philadelphia to beg his way to Pittsburgh. Finding begging a rather unprofitable business he began to meditate and finally hit upon the following plan: When stopping at a farmhouse he asked the farmer's wife, 'Do you have any trouble with flies, on your table, at meal time?' 'Oh yes,' she said, 'we are badly bothered with them.' Then: 'Do any of the flies ever fall into the butter?' 'Oh yes,' said the farmer's wife, 'it is there that they are most annoying.' The young man said: 'I can tell you how to prevent flies from falling into the butter.' 'All right, then, come in and take supper with us, we are ready to sit down as soon as my husband and the boys come in from washing at the water trough.'

"The young man did not refuse, but sat down with the family and ate like a woodchopper. By and by the flies began to settle upon the butter. 'Now,' said the farmer's wife, 'is the time to try your skill.' The young magician took two crusts of rye-bread, fastened them together in the form of a cross which he planted upright into the centre of the butter. Not a fly touched the butter. The farmer and his family were astonished and extremely delighted with the result of the experiment. They asked the tramp to stay the night with them, prepared him a good lodging, a breakfast in the morning, and gave him a lift in their wagon to the next farm, where he sold his secret for a dollar. It is a well known fact that flies avoid settling where their feet are apt to be caught, as long as there is a drier perch to light upon."

College Journal. Editorship. Martin.

Hering threatens to resign. Is dissatisfied with Martin. On July 10, 1869, Dr. Hering wrote a letter to Martin in which he declared his intention to withdraw from the editorship of the College Journal. The August number was to be the last one to bear his name upon its cover. This letter Dr. Hering handed to me, for perusal, at the same time declaring that he would have nothing more to do with Martin; that he was careless, arrogant, his work full of mistakes, unpardonably negligent, and that he could no longer continue to co-operate with him. That he would undertake to publish extra volumes of his *Materia medica,* independently of the Journal, in which parts of his work had appeared as an appendix.

Hering had promise of a liberal contribution which would materially assist the project. I begged the doctor to reconsider. Asked him not to send the letter; but to speak to Martin, and keep on good terms, without quarrelling. That if he wished to withdraw he could do so amicably. I pictured to him the probable results of his withdrawal. Would it not injure the College? He thought not. He was bound to give up; he could no longer work with Martin. He could not stand for such gross negligence, carelessness and ignorance.

When Raue made his usual morning visit, before he went up to the study, I told him about the letter. He too, thought it should not be sent; that Hering should not give up his part of the work on the Journal. The letter was not sent.

July 12, 1869.

Anecdote. Adventure Among the Indians in South
America. Victoria Regia.

"On an expedition in the tropics we travelled up a river
to hunt a certain mysterious animal which the natives said
inhabited a house of stone, built by the Great Spirit. That
the monster devoured people, but only if they were sleeping in hammocks. My party consisted of myself and a
band of negroes who served me. I unfortunately had given
orders to one of them to dig up for me the skeleton of an
Arrowackian Indian. He unfortunately dug up the remains of an old grandmother, belonging to one of the
tribes of Caribs, who were of a mixture with negroes.

"The act was discovered by the Indians. I had to fly
for my life as quickly as possible. They placed the blame
upon me, not the negroes, who were not considered to be
human beings, therefore it was I who must die. I took
to the boat. The pursuit began at once. I gathered my
firearms about me. The negroes were cowardly and refused to row. I threatened that I would shoot them. They
insisted that I must sit up on top of the cabin of the boat,
in my white suit, trousers, vest and straw hat, a mark for
the enraged Indians who ran along the banks of the
stream, shooting at me with their arrows. Otherwise the
cowardly blacks were going to drop their oars, and hide
below. It was dark and I was the only object visible in the
gloom. I kept on discharging my double-barrelled rifle,
two shots in succession, as fast as the blacks below could
reload. Double shooting scares the wild men; they cannot understand how a gun can go off twice at the same
moment. As the river widened we grew momentarily
safer. We landed exhausted and laid ourselves down to
sleep. I slept like a rat for seven hours.

"Among the Indians I had a Madi, a blood brother,
with whom I had exchanged blood, he drinking mine, I
his. If he were alive today he would give his life for me.
Directly after the episode related I met with this friend on
one of the plantations. The natives here were somewhat
under restraint from the government. But they thirsted

for my blood, and would have killed me. I had to mount a cask, at the foot of which sat my friend. I made a speech to the natives. I said: 'My friends, how can you believe the words of a negro, who you say is not a human being, and not believe me who am your friend. I am speaking to you as a friend. Will you still believe the negro? A creature without a soul. You would not believe a monkey. Believe me.'

"One of the natives stepped forward and said: 'We will believe you, but you must give us whiskey to drink!' My bloodfriend said: 'They will kill both of us if you give them the firewater!' I spoke to my blacks and told them to get into the boat to leave the place at a moment's notice. I had the whiskey jugs filled with water in the meantime; gave them a small quantity of whiskey to taste and hurried to the boat, which, by hard rowing, soon brought us to the nearest town where I was safe.

"If it had been my fortune to follow the stream further, on which we were travelling, I would have discovered the Victoria Regia, which in that case, would have gone to Dresden instead of to England. Fate willed it otherwise."

Children.

"Every seventh day children will learn something new."

Menstruation. Indian Squaws.

"Every healthy woman menstruates either at full, or at new moon. Indian squaws do not tell when their periods are due, nor mention them in conversation. Their husbands do. Negroes are less reserved on the subject."

A Big Fish Story. The Ray.

"When I was in Suriname the negroes, and others, spoke of a huge fish, big as a house, that could swallow anything that came in its way, but could never be caught. I asked the Indians to make me a strong rope of palmetto and attach thereto a triple hook of iron.

"Together with a number of blacks and some white fishermen, we went out to the sea. We planted a windlass

on shore and tied to that the powerful rope. For bait I
fastened a chicken to the hook and tossed it into the sea.
It had scarcely touched the water when we had a strike.
I ordered the negroes to pull slowly, very slowly, until
the heavy object came nearer.

"All at once I beheld, in the water, close to the shore,
a monstrous thing, the size of a barn door. I ordered
the negroes to get into a boat, with an axe, and strike the
gigantic object a blow on the head. The blow landed but
the quarry shot out into the sea quick as lightning, taking
all of the heavy rope with it, windlass and fixtures. The
boat upset with the blacks who were pulled under water;
some of them were entangled in the rope. I stood on the
shore anxiously waiting for one after another of them to
come to the surface and swim ashore.

"Everyone of the men, if they had been drowned, would
have cost me a large sum of money. The fish was the
Ray. A full grown one was never caught, only smaller
specimens, supposedly the young of this remarkable fish."

Conversion To Homoeopathy.

"When a student, I was writing a book against homoeopathy. My first question had been: What is the meaning
of similar? A painter has painted a portrait. Some one
looks at it and says: 'How great the resemblance!' Another person says: 'It is not at all like him!' Now then,
what can it mean for one thing to be similar to another?
I then began to study the Materia medica. Under every
remedy I found vertigo; in German *Schwindel*. I almost
came to the conclusion that the whole business was nothing
but a swindle!

"I explored further and it seemed to me as if the devil
was at the bottom of the whole thing by the way it all
came out. Everything agreeing.

"I am very glad that my book was never printed. My
old friend, the apothecary, who was happy when I began
to write against homoeopathy, was always ready to secure
for me anything I might need to carry on the work. One
day I came to ask him for a good tincture of Peruvian bark,

unadulterated. This was a drug in common use, at the time, against malarial fevers, which were prevalent. I saw a change come over the face of the druggist, who sensed my purpose. He knew that this drug had paved the way for Hahnemann to make his discovery. 'That, my young friend, is very dangerous,' remarked the druggist. 'Have no fear,' said I. 'I have studied mathematics and am able to tell the true from what is not true.'

"In a fortnight I was forbidden his house and lost my stipend. I came near starving. No one gave me any help. My friends avoided me. One of them said: 'Hering is going crazy!' Another, a friend, offered to play sick so that he might have an excuse for paying me a fee for attending him.

"I was mad to discover the boundaries between the true and the false in homoeopathy. I was persuaded to call upon a certain boarding-house mistress who they said wished to try homoeopathic treatment. I called. She said: 'I have no time at the moment. Sit down, and eat.' I ate like a woodchopper. The woman said: 'Come again tomorrow, at one, then I will have time.' One o'clock was mealtime. Again I was asked to sit down at table and satisfy my hunger.

"I began to barter medical treatment for food, and once more regained my strength, which I devoted to further study of Hahnemann's books. It was a year and a half later when my finger, and with it my life were saved. A few drops of medicine (a preparation of *Arsenic*) had sufficed for a cure. I had shown my ignorance by demanding that the drug should be applied outwardly. Lord! How stupid one can be!

"My enthusiasm grew. I became a fanatic. I went about the country, visited Inns, where I got up on tables and benches to harangue whoever might be present to listen to my enthusiastic speeches on homoeopathy. I told the people that they were in the hands of cut-throats and murderers. I made many cures. Success came everywhere. I almost thought I could raise the dead.

"I wrote an essay. I wrote in a spirit of prophecy. I thought what a tremendous influence my writing will have on medicine. I sent the essay to Stapf. I wrote about things that might come true in a hundred years. Things to benefit suffering humanity. Stapf wrote about me to his friend Gross. Stapf, Gross, Hartmann, and Moritz Mueller had already joined the ranks of homoeopaths.

"One morning, a woman who served me with milk, reminded me that she had not received any pay for a long time, that she could not continue to go on in this way, because she had to buy the milk which she sold to her customers.

"On the same day a messenger came to ask me to go to Dr. Hartlaub, a brother to the homoeopathic physician who had married my sister Clara.

"After having suffered from starvation, for almost a year, I went to a farm nearby, where I found plenty to eat. The owner of the farm was a distant relative who had deprived a branch of my family from their property-rights, and I felt justified in squaring myself with him in this manner. Of this family but two members remain at the present time, the rest of my people being scattered.

"When I came to the farm I had a lean and hungry appearance, my clothes were full of rents; but I was very proud. It would not have been well for anyone to have made remarks about my shabby condition.

"I left the farm, although my cousin Reuslitz had asked me to remain, and went back to town. At one of the banks where I went to collect my monthly stipend of five dollars, which I had not drawn for three months, I was met with a notice from one of the clerks asking me to interview one of the higher officials.

"I was confronted with a short, stout, husky, pompous person, who said to me: 'I hear that you are occupying yourself with experiments in homoeopathy. This I must beg you to discontinue. Here is the money for your last payments. I cannot permit the money placed in my charge to salvage a homoeopath.' I replied: 'By what right do you address me in this insulting manner?' and threw his silver on the counter. 'Not a penny will I take of it'!"

Never at any time did I see the good doctor so excited as at this moment, when he struck the table with his fist, pushed back his chair, sawed the air, his eyes full of fire, and his blood seeming to boil. One of the daughters looked across the table at her cousin, in surprise. She afterwards said she had never seen her father so excited.

"This man, who had insulted the poor student, in later life himself became a homoeopath. He offered to return my money but I would not accept it, nor would I again go near him. From the moment in which I had thrown the money at his feet I never had occasion to go hungry; nor at any time since during my long life. When I returned home from my visit to the bank, there was a call from a patient waiting for me.

"I had to work hard for Hartlaub while I was his assistant; harder than my old scribe has to work for me. But two groschen a day were enough to make me happy. I was not legally entitled to practice, for as yet I had no diploma, but I was sure that I knew more than my employer. I devoted an entire year to the study of Materia medica. In the following winter came the episode of the injured hand. In the summer that followed, I travelled. It was my fanatical summer. I assisted some farmers to break into, and rob a storehouse with grain, to help keep them from starving.

"Every day new and favorable things turned up for me. One of these was a brilliant offer of a position, as private tutor in a wealthy family in Russia. I went to my brother Ewald. While there, there came two letters which the carrier refused to deliver because there was an unpaid charge for postage. My brother paid this for me. One of the letters was from Hahnemann giving me information on the subject of iron; it was short. The other was from Jean Paul Richter, the poet, who asked me for some vials.

"My brother said: 'You will not go to Luefland. A man who gets letters from two of the greatest men of the age must not go to Russia. You will remain here.'

"There were things to be forgiven my brother. He had taken the books belonging to my father, taken them to Leipzig and sold them. It was a saying of Jean Paul: 'That all events happen in doubles.' On the same afternoon I declared that I was not going to Luefland, where a brilliant position awaited me, not at all to my taste. I was never made to serve royalty and would have made a poor lackey."

Jean Paul Richter.

"Jean Paul Friederich Richter, the novelist, was a great man. He had always reverenced Rousseau until he learned that he had sent his children to an institution for foundlings.

"Jean Paul was very witty. His conversation was full of humour. Once he said to me: 'You young folks have it easy; you can get along on two feet while I require a dozen.' I said: 'Then you must have two horses, a coachman and your own two feet, which make a dozen!' He was much pleased with my ready remark.

"Jean Paul was an atheist. One day when sitting by him, on a sofa, he said: 'I cannot understand how people can be so ignorant as to place Christ, although the most perfect human being upon earth, on an equality with God.'

"I replied: 'If you will permit me to say so: "The square is equal to the circle'."

"He sprang from his seat and rushed about the room wildly, saying: 'No! No! No! That's not it! It cannot be so explained! It cannot be!' He did not, however, seem to be displeased with me.

"Jean Paul had two daughters; one named Emma, the other, Ottilia. Emma was the more intellectual of the two. Ottilia was of a more humble and retiring disposition. Emma was a trifle slack. But she was learned; so much so that I was afraid she might know more than I which made me stand in awe of her. Her father said: 'Emma, you could finish all of my writings, if this should become necessary.' 'But papa,' said she, 'that would not be at all to my taste; I would rather make my living at

darning stockings.' 'But, my dear' said her father, 'I did
not say that you *should*, but that you *could*.' Ottilia was
the more sociable of the two *(gemuethlich)*. It was rum-
oured that I was to marry Emma. I had observed, that,
from visit to visit, a rent in her apron remained unrepaired,
which annoyed me. Also the family was not homoeopathic,
consequently I had no desire that way. Emma was married to a nobleman, Ottilia, to an officer in the army."

Dr. Ameise. A Fairy Tale.

"To cure myself of a passion to travel in foreign countries I wrote a fairy tale which I named Dr. Ameise (Dr.
Ant).

"A young doctor leaves home to travel in foreign parts.
He comes to a mountain where dwells a fairy who changes
him to an ant. He comes down from the mountain and
sees an ant hill in the valley. He stops and gazes at the
turmoil which goes on before his eyes. Hither and thither,
in all directions, rush the busy creatures as if their lives
depended on getting their work done, as do inhabitants in
the streets of a big city during business hours.

"He did not like the turmoil, wished himself back in his
home with his sweetheart. Early one morning he climbs
a stalk on which hangs a drop of dew, sparkling in the
sunlight. In the dewdrop is mirrored the image of his
beloved. He experiences tearful regrets at having wandered away from home.

"He returns there and marries the girl of his choice,
and I suppose they lived happily ever after. When I read
the fairy tale to Emma Richter she was delighted. Went
into ecstacies over it. 'But,' I said: 'I must first find out
if the story of the dewdrop is true to nature.' 'By no
means,' said she, 'The tale must remain as it is told.' By
this I saw that after all her mind did not tend toward strict
scientific investigation."

Peter Merten. A Fairy Tale.

"Peter Merten, a young goatherd, went to the Queen of
the Clouds to complain about her many weeping maidens,
who brought too much rain, which caused the rocks to roll

down from the mountain side. 'I am afraid that I cannot stop them,' said the Queen of the Clouds. 'You must go to the King of the Winds and ask him to stop blowing so hard in this direction, then I will no longer have to drift over your mountain.'

"Peter went to the King of the Winds. The King flew into a rage, and began to swear horribly. 'Thunder and lightning,' said he, 'Don't you see that I *must* blow? Don't you see that the sun is burning like mad, and everything on earth would sizzle and go up in flames if I stopped blowing? Can't you smell the smoking Sahara down there? Go to the Queen of the Sun and ask her to cool off a bit.'

" 'Well and good,' said Peter, 'but how will I get there?' Then the Wind King's soldiers—he had a regiment of them cursing and fuming, loaded him into one of their cannons and shot him to the Sun. When he arrived there he asked for the Sun Queen and soon was in her presence. She lost no time in telling him that if she granted his request, nothing would grow here he came from, and his goats would perish for want of something to eat, and all other creatures upon earth with them.

"She gave him this advice: 'Plant shrubbery on the side of your mountain to keep the rocks from rolling down to the valley.' This appealed to Peter who promised to follow the advice of the Sun Queen. 'But,' said he: 'How will I get down from here?' 'Observe my maidens,' said the Queen, 'who are drawing water at this hour' (It was just before sundown.) 'See how they climb up the sunbeams, which they use for ladders, to fill their buckets from the clouds and slide down again to earth upon them just before dark. They will carry you down on their hands and leave you at your home on the mountainside.' The maidens accomplished their task with many a giggle and roguish glance at the handsome herder.

"When he had come down, he was an old man whose children were married and had children of their own. Where had stood his hut there was a small town, and, most remarkable of all, the inhabitants had planted shrubbery to keep the rocks from rolling. Peter was elected to a public office and lived happily ever after.

"The moral of the tale. It was my intention to write a satire against the *Tolle causam* (remove the cause) so often mentioned in the books of the allopaths. Peter Merten could not remove the cause. The Sun Queen had taught him that all was wisely planned, that evil consequences must be removed by useful remedies. Of course Peter was an old fogy, and behind the times, but his descendents were progressive.

"My daughter Odelia has the fairy tale in her possession. It was elaborated pretty thoroughly by me, but should be abbreviated, as much as possible. When completed we will ask Balling to make the illustrations."

The Grey Donkey. A Fairy Tale.

"The story of 'The Grey Donkey' belonged to my friend, the Rev. John Helfrich who had it from his father, and he from his father. Wesselhoeft made a joke of it. Helfrich told it to a party of us when on a ride to the Blue Mountains.

"We assembled at Bath, near Allentown. Wesselhoeft drove us in his large wagon to which was harnessed his big sorrel horse, in the direction of Helfrich's home, and beyond. The trip lasted two days.

"In the party was a foreigner by the name of Fehrentheil, a political refugee from Germany. It was Wesselhoeft's intention to get him to study homoeopathy at the Allentown Academy, for which purpose we were to contribute the money. Fehrentheil was a maker of plans, a promoter. He had discovered a lake, broad as the Schuylkill River, and shaped like a horseshoe, with a waterfall at one end, forming an outlet. The property could be bought for a song. Fehrentheil wished us to buy the land, he would engineer the job, blast ten or twelve feet away from the rocks at the top of the waterfall, completely draining the lake thereby and gaining from ten to thirty acres of meadowland on which to pasture and raise oxen.

"All about us, where we stood, reaching into the valley

far below, was a wide expanse of red from the blossoms of the mountain laurel *(Kalmia latifolia)* then in full bloom, delighting the eye. The beautiful lake was to have been made small, the waterfall destroyed in order to secure an income of five thousand per year from pasture lands.

"Like Peter Mertens, in the fairy tale, the promoter's expectations ran too high and nothing came of the plan."

A Caterpillar. Dolichos Pruriens.

One day a hairy caterpillar crept up Mrs. Hering's arm and left its bristles in her flesh. On the following day, another of the same description, got on the doctor's leg. Rubbing had aggravated the condition. Hundreds of the sharp hairs had entered the skin and set up a violent irritation.

Early next morning I was called to his bedside—he slept on a couch in his studio—and asked to perform the operation of removing the offending foreign bodies which had caused the irritation. Armed with a magnifying glass and a small forceps, with which to pick out corked vials from boxes of Jenichen's potencies, the venerable Aesculapius in his night gown, placed in a rather uncomfortable position on a parlor chair, I proceeded with great care, and as much delicacy as possible, to extract the tiny bristles which came out, one at a time, or in small bunches.

While thus employed Hering related to Balling, the artist, who was busy making a pencil sketch of the picture, an experience he had in the tropics when accidentally getting his arm in contact with a specimen of the *Dolichos pruriens,* a tropical climbing plant, named Cowhage or Cowitch, which bears a seed pod about three inches long, covered with bristles. The plant was proved by Jeanes and is a remedy recommended for *Herpes zoster,* and the neuralgic condition supervening. It also helps inflammation of the gums (See *Dolichos,* Guiding Symptoms, vol. 5.) By advice of natives Dr. Hering removed the irritating bristles from his arm by applying pure oil to the skin and passing a sharp razor blade over the surface.

September 18, 1870.
Anniversaries.

"On the occasion of a Fiftieth Anniversary it is expected of one to write a dissertation. I desire no celebration for myself. Not even a serenade. I am going away. Such occasions do not make a good impression on the children; though wives enjoy seeing their husbands honoured.

"I had proved as many as a hundred remedies at that time (fifty years ago). Watzke, then notorious with his 'Leider, Leider,' (Alas, alas!) is dead.

"Trinks bragged about his correspondence with Hahnemann concerning a disease he had picked up in Paris. If I should be given an honorary degree in the form of a diploma, I will send it back as a thing for which I have no use whatever."

Sanitation. Atmosphere.

"The air between partitions and in walls of houses, as likewise the air in churches, becomes stagnant and thus poisonous and is the frequent cause of sickness in children."

Dyspepsia. Causes of Disease.

"The causes of sickness are usually internal; occasionally external. More often the blame is laid to the climate. Quack medicines are frequently the cause. Hot foods and drinks. These cause Southern dyspepsia. Hot cakes and hot coffee cause callosities. One might as well swallow molten lead. Such cases usually require three years of treatment.

"Northern dyspepsia is caused by cold things; ice water and ice cream, which are more dangerous than hot things. Water, to drink, should be of the medium temperature of a place. Five minutes for dinner, with insufficient chewing, is another cause. An hour should be allowed for a meal. A walk of twenty squares, there, and twenty back, before dinner, is advisable. I had in mind to write a book on the Causes of Disease but at the time no one wished to publish it."

Wesselhoeft.

"William and I had but one quarrel. Oh! How mad we were! He said he owed me a hundred dollars. I said No! I owe *you* a hundred!

"Later I found my note of hand, but he said, 'Forget it; and don't say another word about it!' It was paid. We used to sit up and talk late at night and then lie down on the floor and sleep until morning when we would drink a cup of coffee to the honor of Hahnemann. He wished me to move to Boston, which I could not do because he expected to play second fiddle to me! Later, when ill, he wished me to come and see him, which I had to refuse because we then thought differently about certain things."

Hahnemann.

"When Hahnemann died it affected me dreadfully. Three days after his death I took a ride to Fairmount Park to a place where no one could see me and cried like a child. People thought I would get sick. As a rule things do not affect me deeply at first, but grow and grow until they become almost unbearable; especially things pertaining to Homoeopathy.

"Hahnemann always thought to try to explain thé *Why* of things. Here he was in the wrong. Before his death came he had ceased to believe in his theories. He thought more of me than of any of his followers. Called me his John."

Hering had the courage to express himself frankly, both in writing and in speech in opposition to some of Hahnemann's theories, but was in perfect accord with him on the soundness of his Practical rules, and so remained to the end of his life.

To Dr. Ray Barton from Philadelphia, a friendly allopath, who visited Hahnemann, the latter said in allusion to Hering's criticisms:—"They made me—made me—well, I don't know, made me feel afraid that I was not right; it stopped me, checked, chilled me for a while!" He then asked, "How much has Hering written about this, and how has it been received?" Finally he said, "Well, no matter!"

September 20, 1870.

Grauvogl.

"Grauvogl appeared in military trappings, as staff physician, at a medical meeting. He opened the meeting abruptly, in business style, pulled out his watch and disappeared, not to return."

Hausmann.

"Another great man whose work appeared from the hands of a publisher who also printed an allopathic journal. Homoeopathy is not mentioned in his book. He quotes Drysdale's provings but does not refer to the British Quarterly. He evidently thought of making a grand impression upon the Old School.

"I devoted a Summer course to lecturing on Hausmann, explaining him to the students as far as I understood him. I wrote and asked him for the titles of books of which he had made use in his studies, but received no reply. Probably because I am a German, and he took sides with the French."

Business. At Table.

"Question: What is honesty in business?
Answer: Honesty in business is where
both sides gain proportionately."

Diet. Nutrition.

"Certain tissues require certain condiments. There remains muscular weakness from all sickness. In such cases a diet of mushrooms will be beneficial. They contain potash and phosphoric acid in a high percentage, which restore muscular tissue. For travellers on foot, rowers, and mountain climbers, they prove a restorative of wasted muscular tissue. *Potash* restores muscle; *Ferrum,* the blood globules; *Arsenic,* the aponeuroses; *Rhus tox.,* the joints; *Wine,* the brain; *Okra,* the abdominal organs; *Lentils, Beans* and *Peas,* the bones.

"Condiments are important; peas require pepper; beans, herbs; beef, onions; and mutton, garlic."

Grauvogl.

"A remarkable person, and an expert fencer in logic. He says he makes daily use of Hausmann's book, which means work. I have made an arrangement of the different kinds of pain mentioned in the book."

Potencies.

"Our potencies are explained by the molecular theory. Molecules are widely spaced and move with more than planetary rapidity."

Leprosy.

"To my ginger plantation in South America there came a boat bringing a girl from Holland who had leprosy. I was asked to treat her. I was given a horse and carriage and no objections were raised as to my right to practice. After six months I had 200 patients. The ginger farm was forgotten. Indians provided me with all my needs, while I practiced.

"Sometime later it was borne in upon me that I needed a relief from the tropics; that according to a German saying, 'Wine needs a winter,' and I left for Philadelphia where I was rushed into a practice. Here I saw for the first time the future mother of my son Max and my daughter Odelia, who was washing the marble steps in a small street. I shall never forget how she looked when she turned around and I saw her for the first time. She was blonde with blue eyes and a fair complexion. She had made her home here after coming from abroad with people who had no servant, so she did the housework for them."

October 15, 1870. To C, Wesselhoeft.

Recreation.

"Rest comes when one engages in amusements that have a mental stimulus."

Satires. Marx.

"My Introductory address as Professor of Homoeopathy in Strasburg. Shall I send it to Germany? A nation must have a conscience. Marx, that divine fellow (Goettinger Anzeiger) has written in vain."

Provings. Jeanes.

"Jeanes makes his provings and gets some symptoms. A man with peculiar symptoms comes to him and receives a few drops in a glass of water, then swallows the contents of another glass of water, and the glass is washed. The patient's old symptoms return."

Potentizing.

"About grafting of potencies. They act. How or why they do passes our small stock of comprehension."

Provings.

"He who makes provings of the higher potencies remains in good health, and lives to a ripe old age."

Physiology.

"C. W. makes physiologic gymnastics."

Phrenology.

"When young I made a collection of animal skulls in reference to this subject. My friend, the forester, gave me those of rare animals. I helped him with his trout fisheries."

Nov. 2, 1870. To Dr. Hills.

"Someone told me: 'You will make friends but you cannot keep them; you will make money but cannot keep it.' So it has been. Scarcely a year has passed without my losing a friend."

Money was spent, as fast as made, for useful purposes; it never accumulated.

Bath Houses.

"When I came to Philadelphia I wanted a bath house. They laughed at me! I had a tent built over the garden hydrant. When I rented another house I carried the tent with me. My friends said, 'Don't talk about this; you will be laughed at'!"

Houses. Graperies.

"I call a double house, a plain simple house. Do you call a man double because he has a right side and a left side? In Philadelphia, at the present time, a house will not easily sell, or be rented, unless it has a grapery."

Diatetics.

"What does B . . . know about the subject? Only the observations of physicians can furnish rules for this branch of medicine."

Typhoid Fever. Graperies.

"A man with typhoid fever might get well alone by sleeping in a grapery."

Bedsores.

"May be prevented by placing a tub of water under the bed."

Spirals. Lightning. Snails.

"I was probably the first man in the world to say lightning is in the form of a spiral. One can only observe it when the lightning is opposite to one. Formation of water is the cause of lightning, thunder as well as rain.

"All planetary motion appears in a right spiral direction when observed from the outside. The snails I saw in Surinam all turned to the right. I made this observation together with my wife, the mother of John. When I mechanically turned the snails to the left, they, after going on a while, came to a standstill and then again turned right. This gave me a flood of new ideas."

Guns.

"A South American Indian, who for the first time saw a gun fired, said: 'You men are friends of God who has given you a Book, and you can make thunder and lightning.' He saw the lightning, then the thunder and that something was struck by the gun. I said to the whites, who laughed at the Indian, 'You are greater fools than he with your ideas of thunder and lightning. You say that the lightning, makes thunder, while both are caused by something else.' Lightning is electricity caused by condensation of steam into water. Clouds are formed from bubbles of water, in immense numbers, forming a large surface. The drops bring electricity and ozone down with them. The vacuum which is left by condensation is rapidly filled with air which causes the report. Soap bubbles will rise, but fall as soon as they burst."

Platina.

"When I first read the provings of *Platina* (by Stapf) when a student, I felt like Balboa when he discovered the Pacific Ocean. It is now nearly fifty years ago. Materia medica will now become a science, I said. *Palladium* stands nearest *Platina*. I saw clearly that a new period had arrived with Hahnemann."

Hering speaks of Doebereiner, and the Preface dedicated to Stapf.

_____

Nov. 3, 1870. To Dr. Hills.

Paracelsus.

"That mean, malicious, shocking, horrible, awful scamp who slandered Paracelsus! There is nothing I despise more, in a physician, than the keeping of a remedy secret. If F. had killed his children and eaten them, he would not have done so great a crime as to make a secret of his discovery. A man who keeps a secret of what might benefit the race is infamous."

Domestic Practice. Home Remedies.
    Domestic Physician.

"When making the first boxes for the Domestic Physician I thought it best to use numbers, in place of names, for the medicines. This was done because I thought, for instance, the name of *Ipecac.* might suggest vomiting, and that of *Ferrum*, weakness. The medicines at first were put up in quills, for we had neither vials nor corks. Lingen's advice was to put up the medicines myself, and sell them to make money. I said: 'Sooner than do that, I wish that the whole world might go to nothing'!"

Jenichen.

"Jenichen was a powerful man, who could break a horseshoe with his hand, like a cracker. He once came to a blacksmith together with some other young noblemen and asked him if he could make a good horseshoe. The answer was 'Yes.' When the shoe was made Jenichen took it and broke it with his hands. 'You must be a devil,' said the blacksmith; 'no human being could do such a thing.' Jenichen laughed, paid for the shoe and left. He could roll a silver fork, or plate, into a scroll.

"Jenichen was in love. When, after a long absence from his sweetheart, he rode to her home, to a village at some distance, where the people he met looked serious, he was informed that his bride to be had died on the previous night from scarlet fever. He turned his horse's head and rode away. He never married. To me he wrote, 'You could never have loved your wife, or you never would have married again.'

"Jenichen now gave his love to homoeopathy, which he said would have saved his bride, and some of it to horses. One time when he wished to give *Veratrum* to a sick horse, he found the vial empty. Thinking that some of the remedy must still cling to the glass, and the cork, he put some globules into the vial and gave those to the sick animal."

Potentization. My Multiplication Scale.

"I made triturations 1 to 10, in a much quicker way. I made 1 to 100, 1 to 1000, to see what the difference might be. I had provers make provings of the billionth and the decillionth, in three different ways. I found, by the aid of the microscope, that any medicine could be triturated in fifteen minutes. To begin a proving I always swallowed first the rinsings from a mortar, after making a trituration. A prover may have a return of symptoms after a year. Observe Rhus poisoning. We again arrive in the same position to the planets. He, Jenichen, said he washed a bottle then allowed it to evaporate; he then added alcohol to the drug and shook. He did not count it a shake unless he heard a ring.

"Pehrson who knew him, wrote books in Latin, and thought himself inspired. He prayed for his patients and thought the Lord would show him the remedy. He called everything an inflammation. He was cracked!"

Fevers.

"While practicing in Surinam I was never left more than five days without a case of putrid fever, and never lost a case unless my orders were disobeyed."

Practice.

"We should be governed by symptoms; not by a single one either. Three highly characteristic ones are necessary —like a chair which will stand firmly on three legs."

Voting.

"I think every one who has the right to vote should do so from a sense of duty."

Paracelsus.

"The saying *Mundus vult decipe* (the world wishes to be deceived) has, for years, been attributed to Paracelsus. He said: 'Apothecaries think that wisdom comes flying in to them through the window,' and of Jews he said that they claim knowledge of great secrets from their Talmud and Cabala, also that since the world asks to be deceived, it is just as well that the deceiving be done by both Jews and Christians!"

Nov. 9, 1870. *Studio.*

"Let some one turn a somersault! Here is what I call a cure! Gosewisch's case of pterygium. Old woman and nettles! The *Urtica urens* contains formicic acid."

Aegidi.

"Aegidi successfully prescribed *Angustura* for my daughter Hildegard's necrosed foot. At the same time that it was helping her, Aegidi's life was saved by my

Benzoic acid! I had refused my consent to an amputation of my child's foot just as I had refused the removal of my infected hand, in early life. Aegidi is opposed to Boenninghausen. B. was a layman; Aegidi, a thoroughly educated physician. So it was between Lippe and myself."

Wesselhoeft.

"The old doctor was a man of high ideals. If he is not in the very first heaven I would not care to go there. Albeit he could say some awful swear words!"

Frederick Hahnemann.

Hering says: "If you can get me the books of Frederick Hahnemann when you go to Edinburgh, I will give a feast. Frederick was very talented, but a hunchback and a freak. Went about in oriental costume, allowed his beard to grow untrimmed and was always spitting. I knew that he had lived for a time in Scotland. At one time mention was made of a portrait bust of Hahnemann. Soon after it was declared to be the bust of Frederick, the son. He must have ended in some Western lead mines, in Missouri, where he had gone to treat patients in an epidemic of cholera. He was a misanthrope.

"I wonder if one could learn something about him from places in Missouri? I had written something about the man for a journal signed "Ostner" which was flatly contradicted by Hartmann, who said that Frederick Hahnemann had disappeared while in Scotland. A hunchback seldom lives to the age of eighty; they die young. In Hahnemann's last letter he wrote to me: 'My poor Frederick will become insane.' This made me feel very sad."

Plumbum.

"Hahnemann wrote, in a letter to Stapf, that he did not wish to have *Plumbum* proved. This fact made me decide to have it done. In spite of the unreasonable respect for Hahnemann with which I had been charged, I made the proving. Probably Hahnemann may have given it without result. Hartlaub then opened his *Materia Medica* with it. I did not send my proving to Stapf fearing that, from strong feelings of reverence, he might refuse to print it. Nenning's wife kept a dressmaking establishment, in which many girls were employed, who were set to making provings of the *Plumbum*."

Dec. 2, 1870.

Naturalist.

"At the age of nine to ten I had found the caterpillar *Sphynx Atropos* on my father's grapevine, which was the beginning of my studies in natural history. Later came the *Lachesis*, and finally *Clotho*, third of the three Fates, who are supposed to sway the lives of men; thus coming into my life in reverse order."

Dec. 4, 1870.

Knorr.

"There came the news that my once intimate friend, Professor Knorr, teacher of German, had mysteriously disappeared, two days ago. Knorr, who resided in a section of the city close to the river, where prowled suspicious characters, called the Schuylkill rangers, had left his house at twilight, to get an order for coal placed before the office closed. He was never seen again. He must have been assaulted and foully murdered. We had a falling out over some disparaging remarks the latter had made about German workers, which, for some time, kept us apart. If I should meet my friend now, or at some future time on the street, I would embrace him and say all is forgotten."

The disappearance of Professor Knorr has remained one of the many unsolved mysteries in the annals of crime.

Dec. 26, 1872.

After the interval, covered by my absence abroad, these notes were resumed, and added to, from time to time, until Hering's death, in July of 1880.

Surinam. Servants.

"I kept a footboy who always slept in front of my door at night, a female slave who had nothing to do but attend to the laundry, a boy who had to cut grass for the horse, another to take care of the animal, and a third to hitch him to the carriage."

Dec. 30, 1872.

Fatherland.

"With every breath I take I cherish the memory of my fatherland. Never have I forgotten it, for a moment. No one knows what he loses when he leaves the land of his birth, a stranger in a strange land! I bore it all for the sake of homoeopathy. This, now, is the country of my children."

Jan. 6, 1873.

Practice. Death of a valued patient. Mrs. Babcock.

"It is so terrible for me to stand and look on where I cannot help, particularly where it concerns a person for whom I have entertained feelings of affection and respect."

Records.

Gideon Leeds was the name of a patient who on a certain date, long past, had hemorrhages, which returned later, at a time when Dr. Hering was absent in Europe. His assistant, Dr. Husmann, consulted the books and found there recorded *Conium.* The remedy was again prescribed, successfully. A similar instance happened to me when a Mr. Daniel Smith sent a request for a remedy he had received fourteen years previously. The name of this medicine was *Clematis,* which again helped as before. So much for accurate book keeping and preserving records indefinitely.

Wens. The case of Mrs. Benton.

"An old lady patient had wens on her head. She had a son, a politician, who may have been in the senate. One time she had a fall and broke a leg. McClellan, a prominent surgeon in Philadelphia, was called to attend her.

The doctor happened to see the wens and said: 'They must be cut out.' The patient said: 'My doctor does not approve of an operation.' 'Who is your doctor?' 'Dr. Hering,' she said. 'Ha! Ha! These homoeopaths, what do they know?' The surgeon removed the wens. Some time after, the patient developed dropsy, sent for me and said: 'Doctor, do you remember my wens? I know I shall die!' It happened, some time later, that I was summoned to attend the postmortem. The allopathic doctors who officiated found nothing pathologic in any of the many cavities that were opened and were ready to desist from further examination, when I said to them; 'Have you looked at the kidneys?' If a bomb had fallen in their midst they could not have been worse scared. They removed the kidneys and there were the wens, in the form of ulcers, which had brought about the dropsy and which had caused the patient's death. Again the 'damned Dutch' had scored, and the allopaths had to take the blame!"

Jan. 11, 1873.

The Missing Muffler.

"Today, when I came downstairs to get into my carriage I put on my hat but could not find my woolen scarf. It was cold out of doors. I knew that I had not left it in the carriage, the day before. I adjusted my glasses, looked down, and there, under my feet, like a small heap of misery lay the missing scarf! The children have gone to see Dum Dum (Tom Thumb)."

The Saxon speaks the T as a D, and *vice versa.*

Haynel. Typhoid Fever.

"Rice came to my house on Vine Street, Philadelphia, and said, 'Don't get frightened but they will bring a dying man here on a stretcher, and you must take him into your house. Do not be frightened, the man is dead.' On the stretcher lay a man who looked like a species of Don Quixote. It was Dr. Haynel, from Baltimore, who had sickened with typhoid fever, and just before losing consciousness, had expressed a wish to be taken to Dr. Hering, in Philadelphia. A back room was prepared to receive him, and I had him on my hands. In his delirium, he, like a general, commanded soldiers about to take Constantinople. He had a nurse who wished to boss the patient, became hysterical at first, wept, then screamed.

"When he had sufficiently improved, in plain language we were ready to be rid of him, particularly since the nurse had made herself impossible. I pondered over the situation. I gave the patient some of my very best old Rhine wine, dispensed it to him in small bottles, as medicine. By chance I had left two full bottles, from which the labels had been removed, on a table beside his bed. When he awoke and saw the bottles he thought they were filled with fluid medicines. When I came into the room he said: 'Dr. Hering, I hope that you have not given me tinctures; rather than you had fallen so low I would have died!' When I laughed and showed him that the bottles contained wine, he humbly said: 'Forgive me. I am a sick man, and irritable and thought that you had turned into a dispenser of tinctures!' When he heard that his Lotta (Hahnemann's daughter) had died, he turned more sour than ever."

Teacher. Hahnemann. Jenichen.

"I believe that after I die I will sooner ask to meet my teacher Rudolph than Hahnemann. I do not think that I could get along as well with Hahnemann, nor with Jenichen."

Hahnemann.

"All of what Hahnemann had left undetermined, or vaguely said, I ground to a finer edge, or made more pointed. 'We do not heal diseases but sick individuals' was a great observation. We may say of all who lived before or after him, that there was not one who, in the least, could compare with him. Not a thought of it! Hahnemann could easily be made very angry. But he allowed both of his wives to domineer him; not in matters of principles or affairs, but in a general way."

Convalescents. Greeting.

"Now you are again risen from the dead!" was the Doctor's greeting to those who returned to the table after a spell of sickness.

Jan. 18, 1873.

De Kalb.

"John De Kalb was a German soldier who came to America with Lafayette, and served under Washington. Politicians wished to exhume his bones, and save them from obscurity by burying them with pomp, to make propaganda. As a German of some prominence, I undertook to make a speech in which I referred to the man's remains as 'De Kalb's bones,' which cast so much ridicule upon the project that it fell through."

A Wounded General.

"A general, from New Jersey, died from what was reported to have been a shot in the back of the neck. McClellan, the surgeon who had extracted the ball, reported a fractured coccyx. The general happened to have received the wound when raising himself in the saddle when giving a command. The surgeon gave out that the man had been wounded in the abdomen and had died from gangrene."

Jan. 23, 1873. To Dr. Tafel.

An Invitation.

"I am sorry that I cannot accept your invitation, with a good conscience. I must confess that I bungled the matter and am not satisfied with what I have done. Homoeopathy in Germany is on the wane."

Faith.

"My faith in the Trinity has been wanting all my life."

Strauss. History.

"Strauss wrote a book to prove that Christ had never lived. Afterwards an Englishman wrote a satire in which he claimed that Napoleon had never existed."

Logic. Proof.

"Proof is nothing more than the acceptation of an axiom. There must, however, be two persons to agree upon the truth of the axiom."

Providence.

"Providence permits of no boundaries."

Man, As a Whole.

"Man is a whole; an entirety. In my student days I challenged my fellows to quote me something better."

Bible. Greek Poetry.

"The scene in Maccabeus where the mother exhorts the youngest and last of her sons, has much more of spiritual beauty, than the Greek Niobe, whose children are shot by Apollo from revenge. The Bible excels in beauty all of the poetry of the Greeks."

Palestine. Providence. Fairy Tales.

"It was the custom, at one time, to make journeys to the Holy land. Some one, Noack by name, wrote a book, in which he said that all of the localities mentioned are falsely stated, and supports his statement by reference to contradictions. He claims that all that is written about places there is authentic, but did not happen in the places which people visit.

"In the manner in which we tell our children fairy tales, such as stories about the stork, of Snow White and the Seven Dwarfs, Providence takes the same course with us larger children. And why not?"

Jan. 29, 1873.

Diet.

"The following three combinations have become as pillars in my dietetics: 1. Rice and Raisins; 2. Oatmeal and currants; 3. Barley and prunes."

Feb. 2, 1873.

Dreams. In the studio, on Sunday morning.

"I had a very vivid dream toward morning. I had a look into the spirit world. All things there seemed small to me; everything, people and objects, were diminutive. I saw children at play, and people walking about and conversing. It then appeared to me as if I heard a voice saying: 'If thou wilt, this world may be opened to you.' I said: 'No! I do not wish it,' and awoke.

"In Surinam too I had a remarkable dream. I saw in my dream a young girl with blonde hair and blue eyes, offspring from a negress and a German father, to whom I was to be married, as it seemed in my dream. This happened after John's mother had died. On the evening before my dream, I had in my mind the young girl answering to this description, a Miss B. In my dream I heard a loud 'No!' When, on the following morning, I had a hurried visit to make to a servant at the girl's house, I made a quick entrance by the back door instead of at the front, as usual. I had scarcely come into the house when I saw the girl of my dream rushing toward me, with uplifted hands, like a fury, in pursuit of a female slave whom she intended to strike. Her face turned purple, like that of a turkey cock. She was also dressed in a disorderly manner, not in the way I was accustomed to be met when visiting at the house. Later she apologised and made the excuse that the slave had become so abusive that she had lost her temper; that it would not happen again. I was disillusioned. She was no longer the girl of my dreams! The girl's brother had studied at Goettingen and spoke good German. The girl too was interesting."

Surinam. At Parting.

"It was very hard for me to make up my mind to leave Surinam to come North. The following incident determined my decision. I had at one time met a German farmer who complained that his grapevines were not producing as they should. On questioning him why he felt so, he answered 'Because they will not blossom.' 'Why won't they blossom?' 'Because the wine must have a winter.' The wine must have a winter, I thought, and said to myself: 'And so must you after living six years in a winterless country!'

"The Moravians, my friends and patients, were decidedly averse to my leaving. Among them was a baker, of whom I thought a great deal, for he was as honest as the day is long, though once arrested for a shortage in size of his bread, which almost grieved him to death.

"This man preached to me: 'God is to be found everywhere, and here you can foster the natural sciences and make your patients well.' I replied, 'The wine must have a winter!'

"They brought out their lottery-machine, provided with acorns cut in half, on which were printed numbers which referred to Bible verses. According to the reading of these was to depend the outcome. I submitted to the ruling of this game of chance, particularly because I had already postponed my going for a whole year; mainly because I did not have the means. One is only paid at the beginning of the year for one's services. Consequently I agreed to suffer myself to be led by the Bible verses. Amid the most solemn surroundings I drew a number. I believe it was the number 113. As soon as the man saw the number, he exclaimed: 'Oh! Doctor, we will have to let you go!' The verse read: 'Depart in peace, good and faithful servant, thou hast been faithful over little and shall be placed over much.' All of them consented to let me depart in peace. The women began at once to make shirts for me, and to get everything ready for the journey."

Family. First Marriage. First Child.

I asked the Doctor about the death of his first wife, and of what sickness she had died. He took a pinch of snuff, was quiet for a moment, then said: "She died shortly after the birth of John." I asked: "In childbed, then I suppose?" "No," he said, "she was taken to the country directly after her confinement, against my wishes. I had objected to employing a negress for a wet nurse. The mother thought she was too young to nurse her child; that doing so would make her prematurely old and ugly. She was taken from me, to the country, by her mother, where she was given herbs to suppress her milk, from which she sickened, coughed up milk, and before I had received timely notice, she was beyond help and died on the following day. I vowed never to be married again to a wife who had a mother. Some mothers-in-law can do great mischief, are apt to come between husband and wife and cause much wretchedness in the family. The wife is always in a dilemma between mother and husband.

"My wife's family name was Van Kemper. They kept my son in their care for some years, later lost their money, and I brought the boy North at an age when he needed schooling."

Feb. 10, 1873. Sunday afternoon in the back office. Present Dr. Opelt and Dr. Boericke.

Apples. Pocket Cases.

Opelt presents some apples to Hering who, standing between the two visitors, says: "Here I approach immortality through the kingdom of apples! But what becomes of the honour due me for the invention of the first pocket cases?"

Maybe this was intended for a mild rebuke to Boericke, who had appropriated the invention!

A Quack.

"Peter Frank, in Vienna, had a student who had failed repeatedly to pass examinations, but finally got his diploma on condition that he would leave the country to practice elsewhere. After a year or two he returned and managed to acquire one of the largest practices in Vienna. After bungling a case badly he called his preceptor in consultation. Dr. Frank did not speak to the family about the terrible blunder that had been made. The former student expressed his appreciation of the kindness shown him. He called Dr. Frank to the window to look out upon the street and the many passers by. He asked the older man: 'How many of the people that pass are wise, how many fools?' 'Oh,' the answer, came, 'Nearly all are fools!' 'Well,' said the quack, 'The fools want doctoring as well as the wise'!"

Providence.

"Nothing should ever be done without the thought: 'Thy kingdom come'."

"It was my friend Kummer who advised *Arsenicum.* I did not wish to lose my right hand, which I needed for drawing, writing and anatomical work, and for future use as a surgeon. I could not see the sense in taking the *Arsenic* inwardly. Kummer made me give him my left hand, the well one, and solemnly swear that I would take the medicine, as directed, which I did and in three days I was out of danger. For some time my finger remained weak. Once a certain person scoffed at homoeopathy and called me a fool. I went to the window, opened it and held my finger out long enough to see it turn blue. then was ready to challenge the man to fight a duel. I became an enthusiast for the cause, a true fanatic. I mounted tables in public places from which to harangue the people, and barely escaped arrest. Gradually I returned to a calmer state of mind and said to myself: After all there is provision made which keeps trees from growing into heaven."

Feb. 17, 1873.

Family.

"From the location of the battle field of Sadowa can be seen the castle in which dwelt my ancestor who was put to the torture. He told his three sons to depart from there and follow the river Elbe until they came to Saxony. It was after the battle of Sadowa that the German army formed a semicircle and sang, 'Nun danket alle Gott' (Now thanks be given to God)."

Feb. 19, 1873.

Life.

"All stages in my life were sharply marked. The first sign I had of growing old was when I noticed that I could not turn the leaves of a book with the accustomed ease and

celerity. I always had considerable facility in the use
of my fingers, which came mainly from making drawings."

Feb. 27, 1873. To Dr. Farrington.
History.

"Let Providence rule. We cannot make history. We
must work. Our little bit of wisdom is but like motes
in the sun, no more."

Practice.

"I will not grumble about the low dilutionists. They
are the bark to the tree. We, the splint, are protected by
the bark."

Jahr. Mental Symptoms. Boenninghausen.

"Jahr murdered the mental symptoms; Boenninghausen
neglected them."

Natural History. To Mrs. Pope, Sr.

"It was a specimen of the Sphynx Atropos which put
its head out of the ground, and made a squeaking noise,
that brought me, then a mere boy, to the study of natural
history. I went to the woods and collected all sorts of
insects. When I had learned to distinguish these I turned
my attention to botany and mineralogy. I now think
that to be able to cure a man with toothache is worth
more than all the animals in creation."

Hydrophobia.

"A man came to my office and said: 'I am crazy. I
know it. I am rich and have no cause for complaint. I
walk the floor every night until my wife comes, with tears
in her eyes, and implores me to lie down. I fear that I
shall die with hydrophobia. I have read all the books on
the subject and know I shall die from the disease. It is
very clear to me. Why don't you promise to cure me?'
'Well,' I said: 'We do cure horses, and they do not imagine things.' 'You *do* cure horses?' 'Yes.' 'Well, have you
had any cases to treat like mine?' 'Yes, similar ones.
We will try.' He promised to take the medicine and I
gave him a single dose in a high potency, of *Hydrophobin
(Lyssin).* Later he returned once more to say that he had

not missed a night of sleep, but thought that imagination
had made him well.

"The case brought me one dollar in fees, at fifty cents
each, but I would not have missed the cure for a thousand!

"My son Max was bitten by a mad dog. He took the
Lyssin and no bad consequences followed the bite."

The treatment has been verified many times since in
cases of dog bite, with or without rabies.

"The mad dog from which I took the saliva belonged
to a baker, here in Philadelphia. I put the saliva in alcohol, potentized it, and at once began the proving. I had
to desist when I had become almost crazy with mental
forebodings and anxiety. A chemical substance in the
saliva gives it its poisonous quality. After evaporating
this substance on a watch glass I could observe tiny
crystals. *Sulpho cyanic acid* is a normal constituent in
the human saliva. The test is made by adding *muriatic
acid* which reddens the saliva of persons in health. Sheep
always have it. Something similar must be contained
in the saliva of the snake which kills by causing fermentation in the blood. I have always reasoned from analogy,
and experimented mathematically and philosophically.
In Surinam dogs are not subject to rabies. In smallpox
the *sulpho cyanides* leave the saliva and are found in the
pustules."

Smallpox. Sulpho Cyanates.

"A black man came to me, here in Philadelphia, saying
that he had dyspepsia. I had frequently tested the saliva
of dyspeptics. I examined this man's saliva and found
the *sulpho cyanates* absent. Next day he had a fever and
on the day following, smallpox developed. Dr. Raue
who took charge of the patient, applied the muriatic test
to the contents of the pustules and found the *sulpho
cyanogen* had migrated there."

See *Sinapis nigra*, (black mustard) as a remedy in
Smallpox.

Psorinum.

"When in Surinam, I examined a strong, healthy look-

ing negro with the itch, a tailor by trade. I looked for
the *acarus* but could not find it. I know that the bug
accompanies the disease, but it may be a product caused
by disease, and there may be itch without the *acarus*.
I took the pus and poured alcohol over it. It coagulated.
I put some of it on a watch glass where crystals formed.
I swallowed the potentized preparation. If I ever was sick
in my life it was then. The effect was shocking.

"We homoeopaths are called pariahs, but we are a
hundred years ahead of the times. I dislike making experiments upon patients, but myself am willing to prove
any substance, when in health. We could find out by
the use of the spectroscope what chemical elements are
produced by the salivary glands."

A Nostrum.   Calcarea Phosphorica.

"Soon after the English took possession in the East
Indies there appeared there a quack who made 'Dr. Jones'
Powders for Fevers,' which became an article of export.
The East India Company sent thousands of pounds sterling to the Indies for it. Jones made his recipe public.
Another Company worked a mine from which they got
a great quantity of Phosphate of Lime which enabled
them to put the powder on the market at half price. Because the article manufactured from this phosphate did
not have the same curative effect, the powders were sent
back, and a lawsuit for infringement of a patent was instituted against the ri...l company. English, French and
German chemists were consulted, all of whom stated that
the ingredients were ordinary *phosphate of lime*, with
crude *antimony*. There was a clever chap in New York,
publisher of an agricultural paper, who learned from this
trial that phosphate of lime, made from bones, is different; also that it makes a better fertilizer because being
animalized it is more readily absorbed by vegetable
organisms."

Sinapis Nigra.   Smallpox.

"*Sulfo cyanide* obtained from black mustard seed, being a natural product, was found to be a more effective

prophylactic, and remedy in smallpox than the chemical
preparation, although this, used in silverplating establishments during an epidemic of smallpox in Philadelphia had immunized the workers, and proved a useful dis-
infectant in the sickroom . I came to find out about the
healing virtues of mustard in a strange way. My friend
Raue came to congratulate me on a first of January, my
birthday, and called to mind the case of Gross who, when
ill and expecting to die, had bid farewell to his friends.
Remembering that mustard had cured paralysis of nerves.
the same as were affected in his case, he asked his wife to
give him the mustard, and got well. A Mrs. R., one of
my patients, failed to recover from a severe case of smallpox, accompanied by hemorrhages from the lungs, possibly caused, certainly aggravated by a sachet of *carbolic
acid* worn on her chest for a preventive. The patient had.
as I remembered, all the symptoms of mustard but I found
this out too late. Thereafter we began to use the potentized *Sinapis nigra*, both as a prophylactic and a curative
of smallpox, with excellent results.

"Certain normal constituents of the human body, during certain pathologic states, leave their habitat where
they have a function to perform and appear in places
where they do not belong and there act as irritants, which
is the case in scarlet fever, measles, smallpox, etc., etc.
The question is not yet solved."

A Sore Finger. Petroleum.

Hering has a sore on the first joint of the first finger
of the right hand, which gives him a great deal of trouble.
He cannot bear a bandage on it, licks it, blows it and
further irritates it by getting snuff on it. He thinks he
will have considerable trouble, and is very impatient
about it. He took *Petroleum* and the finger made a good
recovery.

Order.

"I will have to take a day off, stay at home and put
things to rights in my study. I made a beginning this

morning; no one else can see any change, but I know there is one."

Nativism.

"Must be eradicated in this country. This will be done by descendants from the German people."

Materia Medica.

"I am having my *Condensed Materia Medica* printed in four kinds of type, so that he who runs may read."

Viola Odorata.

"Compare it with *Zincum*. Violets, growing on zinc beds, were found to contain zinc in quantity."

Proverb.

"He who is born to ill luck will fall on his back, break his nose, and spoil his clothes. (Wer Unglueck soll haben der stolpert im Grase, faellt auf den Ruecken und bricht sich die Nase.)"

Philosophy.

"Things in nature are words and colour in form; a language which expresses itself to those who can read."

Erysipelas. Apis.

"An old woman, living in the hills of Saxony, was asked by me what she had used in treating facial erysipelas. She answered: 'You would not believe it anyhow!' When promised a Kronenthaler for the information she said: 'Take honey in which a bee has died and apply it to the spot.' What happens to a bee when she dies in this way? She relaxes, and the poison remains in the honey."

Animal Breathing.

"Crocodiles and snakes breathe through their noses. They have no diaphragms, so they suck in the air."

Pathologic, or Symptomatic Indications.

"It is according to these that we differ most in our School of Medicine, not according to high or low dilutions."

Critics.

"A man must serve his time to every trade save censure: critics are ready made."—*Byron.*

"No one has more suffering heaped upon him in this world than the poor pitiable critics. He may be working for pay in the service of some one, and do his work at command, or he may be sacrificing himself for humanity, or it may have become a habit with him like chewing tobacco. In any case he deserves our commiseration for having to 'chew the rag,' *ad nauseam.* The man who offers us something new, might, on occasions be allowed to err. A critic never. Otherwise he is no critic."—*Helbig.*

"One man cannot know everything."—*Oken.*

"Not one among us but will be willing, or should be, to admit that the things he undertakes to critizise may be criticised as well by a dozen, or maybe a hundred others, each from his own point of view. The result will be different in every case. Should not the reader himself be allowed to pass judgment? Which after all is a matter we cannot hinder. We have not the right to play the schoolmaster in matters of the kind.

"Nothing can be more stupid than to play critic without a reason for so doing. It is silly to find fault with an experiment not yet made, or which perhaps cannot be made.

" 'Kill the dog, he is a critic,' is a saying by Goethe, which may be a somewhat impolite way of expressing oneself, but the epithet may be justifiable if made in a measure not too forceful, and comparison be made with our canine friends and resemblances be pointed out, prominent among which are the cold nose with which the critic noses out his subject, and sprinkles it with acrid baptismal fluid as he pursues his devious ways. Odious as the comparison may seem, it is not intended for any but the professional fault finder who slams where he cannot boost. Where there are no grounds for honest criticism judicious silence should be maintained. Let not one donkey repeat what another jackass has said."

Gratitude. Shakespeare.

"The word gratitude is mentioned but four times in all of Shakespeare's works; ingratitude twenty-two times."

"Throw him out with wondrous potency."—Hamlet 3, 4.

"Stand all aloof and bark at him."—Henry VI, 2, 1.

"They bark at me."—Lear 2, 6.

History. Politics. Germany. A Good Answer.

"When little Thiers, the biographer of the great Napoleon Bonaparte, made his fiz-gig trip through Europe, after the surrender at Sedan, he lodged in the same hotel in Vienna. in which the world famous historian Ranke had taken rooms when on a visit to examine Austrian archives. Ranke politely invited Thiers to dinner, at which the latter, turning the conversation upon events of the day, expressed the idiotic view that the war had been a quarrel between two crowned heads and would have to cease with the surrender of either of the two. Taking a pinch of snuff Thiers added the question: 'With whom then do the Germans really fight now?' 'With Louis the XIVth,' said Ranke, thus silencing the Frenchman with a single word; which tells all. The Germans take back what was wrested from them while suffering from their Thirty Years' War for religious liberty, take again what was then snatched from them by the infamous acts of that king. They take only what belonged to them before the Thirty Years' War."

A Fairy Tale. The Devil's Bite. (Teufels Abbiss).

"Children of the present day are scarcely ever told the fairy stories of the olden days. The grandmother is growing scarce who was wont to tell of how the devil would bite off squarely the roots of certain healing plants, under the ground, so that they might no longer grow and be useful to people for their sicknesses. The devil thought he knew which part of the plant to destroy to keep it from growing again in the springtime.

"Learned school masters taught the children the tale, with a difference. They said, 'The plant has roots which drop off once a year when new shoots replace the old, which makes the roots look as if bitten, perhaps by said devil, but more likely in some other way.' The school-master wisely comments: 'Since we no longer believe in a devil we know that he cannot be blamed for what happens to the roots of the healing plant,' and the children smile with him at the curious tale. It pleases them to think that they belong to a wiser generation than those of the old days. We will let them think so, but will try to give to the fairy story a more useful interpretation. It is not quite fair to think ourselves wiser and better than the people who lived before us, who after all might not have been as stupid as we sometimes are willing to believe. One need not be overwise to observe that the plant we are telling about puts out a new root, or branch, to the old stock, grows a new stem, which flowers and bears seed in its season. Even though the devil might be blamed for biting off the best part of the plant, which after all might not have made good in all cases, or have done what was claimed for it, we must remember that while the ancient enemy is still going about in the world busy destroying what makes for good, plants still go on making roots, new shoots, blossoms and seeds which ripen for uses. It is so ordained. Hence we may find in this beautiful little tale a great general truth, a parable from which to draw a useful lesson. Everytime a new truth comes into the world, or a new discovery is made, the devil is at hand ready to bite off the best part of it. Evil, in the form of self love, self interest, meanness, jealousy or idleness, is ever ready to bite off the best part, to rob humanity of benefits. So we must content ourselves with what remains of good and wait for new roots to grow.

"It is so with Christianity, which had scarcely become established among the people before the enemy came to bite off its roots. It was so with Hahnemann's doctrines, which had scarcely been made known before they were assailed. Countless other instances could be cited of roots into which the devil was ready to sink his teeth. Nothing is suffered to go untouched or unbitten. It is the way of the world. We must wait for the All Pervading Spirit of the world to accomplish its ends, while, putting our hands to the plough, we look for Spring to come, as it always will, to grow new roots, new stems, blossoms and seeds with healing virtues to bring health to mankind. Let the devil nibble the old roots while newer ones bring forth fresh life and use. Fortunately his Infernal Majesty, the Prince of Darkness is stupid. He thinks he bites off the best pieces, but is doomed to help where he seeks to destroy. The better parts of the roots remain."

Philosophy. Truth. A Confession of Faith.

"All who live under the sweet illusion that men love truth are like children who while enjoying their piece of cake, kindly make motions to hand it out to others to take a bite, most of whom will make believe to bite, smile and say, 'Thank you.' The great multitude cares little for the truth; never has. If asked what most they wish for, the answer comes: 'Something for myself, something for number one; all I can get!'

"Every individual has a right to be what he desires to be, above all to be happy. Why is it that so few of us find happiness? Because we reach out for unessentials. There are so many wishes to be satisfied of which few are of moment. If the great desideratum is kept before us, which is to realize the importance of the general good to mankind, and work for this assiduously, with all our hearts and minds, happiness must be ours. Seek for the kingdom to come and all else will be added thereto."

Philosophy and Mathematics.

"Philosophy has not been without its uses. In the period when skepticism became the rule and the silliest incredulity prevailed among so-called thinkers who imagined that a doubting mind was in reason, seekers after truth learned, or at least should have learned what measure of truth is contained in the following formula:

"*It is against reason to deny or to pronounce false any affirmation without sufficient proof; it is intellectual weakness to be satisfied with weak proofs; it is plebeian to agree with public opinion when this is carried away by unreason and credulity; in short it is unscientific to declare anything to be false without having put it to the test of strictest experimentation.*

"In a second period, the opposite course prevailed. Many theories were advanced and postulated as truths in natural science, which were accepted and believed without sufficient investigation or guarantee that things were as represented. From this the following formula is proposed: *It is rational to accept as truths only such as have been subjected to the severest tests and strictest investigation the subject will allow.*

"In comparison with life, which is fluctuating, we have the swinging of the pendulum back and forth, in matters of science. The later proposition is the one which should be adopted by the masses. Both the microscope and chemistry have come to judgment, and rightly. There are, however, here as elsewhere, misleading possibilities, which an application of our first formula might prevent. Let us take time to think, and examine, before we take sides.

"There are still many among the admirers of the exact method of investigation who lean to the opposite side, which rejects new discoveries before these have had time to ripen and to be confirmed. These come under the head of our first proposition. The tendency to ignore new discoveries is often due to the air of importance men give themselves—the 'know it all' kind—who think it clever to reject anything not sired by themselves.

"The great progress made in the domain of the natural sciences we owe to the newer methods of observation, which have been more strict, exact, reliable and definite. All of this we owe to mathematics. Philosophy has often proved misleading, mathematics has never failed unless improperly applied. In philosophy one error has constantly taken the place of another, whereas in mathematics, correctly applied, error is impossible."

Materia Medica.

"A knowledge of drugs is an entirely different field from Physiology and Pathology. We can never cure diseases, only sick individuals, for we have nothing to do with abstract things, but solely with individuals. We must individualize cases as well as suffering individuals, likewise the drugs to be applied. Pathological phenomena have an altogether different value and importance in the scheme of posology (dosage) of our day, as also in *Materia Medica* as effects from drugs. Pathology may be of some use in the study of our *Materia Medica*, but less so than Physiology. Of paramount importance is that which we can neither explain nor understand under the terms of physiology or pathology, viz,: *Mental states and conditions.*"

Symptomatology.

"We have comparative arrangements of symptoms of each particular drug, called comparative *Materia Medica*. Essential symptoms. Differential symptoms. Characteristic symptoms and indications. Predominating symptoms. Verified and probable symptoms. Of prime importance are the mental symptoms."

Prophylactics. Curatives.

"1. Lemon juice intensifies the action of *Belladonna* and increases its curative effect.

"2. Charcoal will prevent yellow fever; given in potency it will cure it.

"3. *Tellurium* given chemically, in tolerable quantities, will destroy *trichinae.*

"4. Radiate heat will destroy the poison of serpents and rabies.

"5. *Cyanide of potassium*, a normal constituent of human saliva, is an antidote to smallpox. A mild solution of it is to be used on cloths hung in the sickroom. A remedy is *Sinapis nigra.*

"6. As a preventive, ozonized oil of turpentine is advised in African fevers (Malarial); a drop daily on a lump of sugar; also *Terebinth* as a remedy in potency.

"7. *Lac. Sulphur*, a pinch of it placed daily in each stocking will keep off cholera. *Sulphur*, in potency, is a remedy."

Memory.

"It has been observed that old people who have completely forgotten their mother tongue while using a foreign language exclusively through middle life. have recovered the use of their mother tongue, possibly a dialect. in extreme old age, while foreign languages have completely vanished from their memories."

Blindness. Psora.

"Might not many who are born blind or deaf, though in good health, or possibly tainted from suppressed psora have their sight and hearing restored by homoeopathic treatment? Observations of this kind, made by an intelligent physician, would be of great interest, not alone on account of the relief to be given, but the discovery of characteristic symptoms of the remedies employed."

Birthmarks.

"Has there ever been a case reported of a cure of a birthmark with an antipsoric remedy? (See *Guiding Symptoms, Fluoric acid* and *Calcarea fluorica*). I know an epileptic who has premonition of coming attacks by a change of color in a birthmark."

Lycopodium. Wine. Sulphur.

"*Lycopodium* is frequently used as an agent in the adulteration of wines. Probably the shaking of the bottles developes dynamic forces in the wine, as is the case with sulphur in alcohol. When wine, thus treated, is used as a common beverage, it would be useless to expect results from prescribing the *Lycopodium* in potency, and, in reverse order, when *Lycopodium* fails to act when indicated, the reason may be that wine so adulterated is being used by the patient.

"Vintners in all countries give their casks a yearly cleaning with sulphur. This cannot materially affect the wine if it is put through the process of fermentation a second time, for this will rid it of the medicinal effects of the sulphur, which might act injuriously in wine not so treated. Sulphur, if dissolved in water, will impart to it a medicinal quality. If sulphur be poured over a red hot iron into water it forms a precipitate containing iron, and the water will be strongly medicinal. This preparation will help serious cases of diarrhoea and dysenteries. I have made use of it, several times, with the best results in cases of the kind in animals."

Clinical Experience.

"An ideal homoeopathic cure, made according to rule, should exhibit the following characteristics:

"1. Limitation of the usual course of the disease to a shorter space of time.

"2. Perceptible moderation, or total prevention of pathological products, without arriving at what is usually understood by a crisis.

"3. Rapid recuperation of strength and bodily vigor: marked shortening of the period of convalescence.

"4. Removal of a tendency to recurrence of the disease. prophylaxis against relapses, even where exciting causes are unavoidable.

"5. Improvement in the mental condition of the patient, apparent to the skilled observer from the moment he enters the sick room, by the attitude and demeanor of his patient."

Music. Fairy Tales.

"In my younger days, I was passionately fond of music and the theatre, and wrote several opera texts and fairy stories. Among the former were *Der Arme Heinrich* (Poor Henry) which I submitted to the great musician Spohr with whom, however, I could not come to an agreement over details. Also *Der Wassermann,* a grand opera text in three acts, elaborated according to Eichendorf, German poet, dramatist, and novelist. The hero is a water god, the heroine a peasant girl wooed by a young nobleman from a castle nearby. The chorus is composed of water-sprites and of fishermen living by the sea, one of whom falls in love with the beautiful peasant girl who comes to the beach to commune with her ideal lover, a young Neptune.

"Titles of fairy stories are *Peter Mertens*, a shepherd. who sees beautiful maidens descending from the clouds on a sunbeam with buckets to fill and carry aloft; the other *Doktor Ameise* (Doctor Ant) is a romantic story of a father, his daughter and a young enthusiastic lover who listens to the whisperings of angels."

Apparently the writings, though interesting, were too idealistic even for an age in which poetry of a senti- mental kind flourished. The writer had his reward in the pleasure it gave him to write as his fancy dictated. What he wrote came from a ready pen, in the best of German diction, and was read with loving interest by his family and intimate friends. Only one of his productions, a short novel, was printed, but, as he was wont to express himself in later life, "went for waste paper." While at this period of his life he had a strong inclination to adopt literature as a profession, he was providentially moved to vary his course and devote his talents to medical author- ship in the service of Hahnemann and homoeopathy.

Darwin. Cats. A Satire.

"A proposition declaring that raising clover seed de- pends upon old maids who keep cats, is thought by some to be very clever. Old maids keep cats, cats catch mice which destroy the nests of bumblebees, bumblebees fertil- ize the clover which enables the farmer to raise seed. All of which is nothing but a chain of stupidities supported by somersaults.

"A clever person can make a logical addition to every one of the statements mentioned. For instance this one, which is a variation on some Darwinistic propositions: viz, that increase of sturdy young men in Old England depends upon the number of old maids in that country. Old maids keep cats, cats kill mice, mice destroy bumble- bees, bumblebees fertilize clover, clover makes pasture for steers, steers furnish meat on which young men thrive and grow strong.

"On the other hand if the first crinoline originated in a struggle for the survival of the fittest, and thereby the

necessity to expand, or to spread oneself, to be in the
mode, later followed by the Grecian bend resembling the
rear of an ostrich, and still later the coming into fashion
of high heels which distorted the pelvis of growing young
women, another parallel may be found therein to the
chain of circumstances handed down by Darwinists. And
again, in this, we have a pretty good imitation from the
way naturalists introduce new and unnatural language in
words that require an apology for lack of thought (Woer-
ter die sich einstellen wo Begriffe fehlen). In such
manner useful discoveries in science are bedizened and
distorted."

A Doctor's Catechism.

"When patients discharge their physicians they seldom,
if ever, think it worth their while to give a reason for so
doing. Exceptions are rare. In a practice of fifty years
I can remember but one. A lady sent word that she was
compelled to change her physician because she could not
tolerate one who took snuff! She sent for me later when
it was too late to save her.

"What is a doctor? A thing that comes when you send
for it. Is the practice of medicine a business? It is, but
should not be. Why not? Because there are many differences between this and any other business.

"What is the main difference? In every other business
the person interested may advertise his services. Not so
the Physician. Not even when in dire need, but only
when others are in need.

"What other differences? The physician is always,
and the only one, who works against his own advantage,
unless a criminal. He must prevent sickness whereever
possible, cure his patients so that they may never have
to return for his services, or at least as far as this may be
made possible by strict homoeopathic treatment."

Napoleon. Lilienstein, a Fortress In Saxony.
Prophet Hering.

"In 1810 Napoleon ordered two of the cannons, called
the Twelve Apostles, to be moved to the fortress, on the

Elbe, to find out if the Koenigstein opposite, could be bombarded from there. The cannon balls fell short of the mark. The Austrians surprised Napoleon, who fled and left the two cannons in their possession. These are now located in one of the fortresses of Theresenstadt, in Bohemia."

See account of Prophet Hering who was named Shepherd Thomas. He predicted railroads, and that a certain bridge would be built over which horseless carriages would pass.

Science.

"Our position in the Universe is such that we appear to stand and to move upon a flat surface with the heavens above us. The area of ground under our feet, even when standing on highest mountain tops is very small compared to the wide canopy over our heads. In the course of time we have become acquainted with the three great kingdoms of our world: the minerals in the earth; the plants and animals on top of it; likewise with the wonders of the air, the moon and stars in their course about the sun.

"Science has taught us the composition and the uses in the wider of the three kingdoms—the mineral; the narrower, called the vegetable, and the still more limited, the animal kingdom; and finally, highest of all, that of man in their midst."

Remarks (to the author) by Saladin, A German
　　　Homoeopath in Berlin.

Allium sativa. The juice of garlic helps children in convulsions from teething.

Fever and Ague attacks are abated by the daily use of Chamomile tea.

Convulsions. Valerianate of Zinc.

Dropsy. *Chininum arsenicosum.*

Belladonna. When it fails to act try Sulphate of atropine.

Belladonna and *Glonoine* should not be given after each other.

Alum. Patient must not eat potatoes when taking it.

Arnica. Is to be given for eight days before confinement, and for eight days after it.

Calendula. Pyemia. From Jahr's *Clinical Experience.*

Hahnemann. A visit to Hahnemann's Oldest Daughter, Frau Moosdorf, in Coethen, in 1872.

Madame Moosdorf spoke bitterly of Melanie, the second wife. Said she kept Hahnemann in a back room on a mattress where he died, calling for help. That she reviled his mother whom she did not know and prevented Hahnemann from revisiting Germany, which he longed for. She made him wear wooden shoes. We made no claim upon any property belonging to father. She did not write to the family when he was ill. Did not admit his daughter. It was on a morning that he spoke his last words. Rain fell in torrents on the day of the funeral. The pall bearers scraped the wall which made her scold and stamp her feet. We had hopes of bringing father to his hundredth year.

"From 12 to 1 he smoked his little pipe. The serpent on a rod is carved from a single piece of wood. Steinhauser was here at the age of seventeen. Hartlaub was Hahnemann's favorite assistant. Lehman was strongly magnetic. Scoppe, from Berlin, painted a picture and delivered it when he came here through influence of the Duke in 1821. In 1835 father went away. In 1830 his mother had died. Melanie took him away secretly one morning. We wished to accompany him a distance and drove a long way by extra post. In the Crown Prince's palace, in Halle, we were assembled and wept at his going. We telegraphed from Leipzig and wrote every week. After two years Malchen wrote to Melanie: 'Why do you not write? What has become of our letters?' The answer came: 'I purposely hid them away that he might not get homesick;' This angered father. Melanie's mother died of the gout from grieving. Melanie spent two years at sea. At Paris she belonged to a Literary club, all men. She aimed to have Hahnemann made

President of a medical faculty. She made Doctor Roth very angry. She was a disgusting old coquette. She appeared, in 1821, as a very poor girl and in a few weeks was dressed in silk. She kept bringing *bon bons*. Father suddenly became estranged from us. They were married in father's front room, the bride wearing a wreath of myrtle. 'I am your servant,' said father. 'No, my son,' said she. He left nothing behind but diploma and relics.

"In 1862 Lotta died in this house. She had helped making potencies. I helped with writing. Melanie wore men's clothes, arrived at the hotel in a hunting suit. She was fond of playing cards and was said to be proficient in the black arts."

Hahnemann. Coethen. As related by Hartlaub to the author.

"Hahnemann did not go out to visit patients; they came to him in the forenoon up to 12 o'clock. The evenings he spent in his garden; he carried a lantern when dark, to go about among his flowers. His rooms were small. Against a wall stood a desk beside which was room for patients to sit. Hofrath Lehman occupied another corner with his patients. I was near by. Hahnemann was very frank, and surprised one by his kindly treatment. I was a favorite. Hahnemann attended to his correspondence in the afternoon, from two to six; supper was served at seven. He only ate bread and milk in the evening and liked to talk afterwards about homoeopathy and current events, before he went into his garden. Friends were invited in the evening. It was then that I occupied myself with studies of mesmerism. Lotta had a toothache. I touched her tooth and the pain was gone. The girls, Lotta and Frau Moosdorf, made sugar of milk powders, on a small table which was quickly covered when company came. Hahnemann, small of stature, stood erect and gestured with his hands, giving out magnetic force. His head was crowned with short white locks. He was always shaven clean. His pipe, which Lotta lit for him, never went out. On Sundays he rode to a farm, sometimes accompanied by myself and Lehman, where good grapes were to be found; the only place he visited.

"Steinhauser, a young sculptor from Berlin, came to model Hahnemann's bust in plaster. It is the best of all portrait busts of Hahnemann. Hirschfeldt, from Bremen, brought with him a phrenologist whose advice was asked on correcting contours of the head. The same wrote a small book on *Homoeopathy and Respiration*. Hahnemann received a letter asking about an infant that was to be vaccinated; he counselled that *Sulphur* should be given before and after the operation."

Frederick Hahnemann. Provings.

Hartlaub says Frederick made provings on insane persons so drastic as to endanger lives; no one else would have submitted to like experiments. When mention was made of the son, Hahnemann always became very sad.

A Visit to Aegidi. Cantharides. A Case of Dysentery. Remarks to the author.

"A child of five years had one hundred and fifty stools in one night; stools resembled chewed cherries; gave *Cantharides* from one of Hahnemann's pocket cases; the globules were yellowed with age. In five minutes the trouble was stopped."

Aegidi says that Burkhard maintains that medicated globules improve with age, and that alcoholic preparations degenerate. I always use globules, believing the alcohol to be injurious. I gave a single dose, to be dissolved in water, and taken night and morning for three days, to be followed by powders of sugar of milk. With certain temperaments homoeopathic remedies, high or low, will not take effect. Cases of Paralysis from spinal irritation were helped remarkably by *Plumbum* and by *Aesculus hippocastanum*.

Aegidi says of Hering's conversion: "A Saul who was converted into a Paul."

He continues: "Hering is the greatest authority. Boenninghausen comes next. Boenninghausen came from France; was consumptive and was converted to homoeopathy by Dr. Weihe."

Aegidi has a box of medicines from Jenichen, and a pen from Hahnemann. He made a visit to Madame Hahnemann. We talked of Grauvogl who is in Gastein, of Hausmann, and Aegidi's daughter-in-law, wife of his son, who is private secretary to Bismarck. There were wonderful trees from South America, about Aegidi's home and a pavilion, in marble, dedicated to Apollo. He suffers from gout. Regrets that he has no son-in-law to be a physician. All his effects are to be burned. Spoke of *Rubidium*. Calls Kafka a dog!

After luncheon and coffee, I left for Berlin, on the 3 o'clock train. Later I spent some happy hours with the son, Secretary Aegidi and his charming wife, in Berlin. I met there, at dinner, a daughter of Goethe's Bettina, an old Portuguese countess.

Aegidi is 78 years old. In a letter to Dr. Hering he wrote: "A hundred thousand thanks for Dr. Knerr." The son was wounded in the Franco-Prussian war, where he suffered the loss of his toes. Aegidi thinks that music, a divine art, has but few votaries excepting among the frivolous and gay.

The Declaration of Independence. An Oratorio.

"Since 1776 the Declaration of Independence has been read, publicly, every year, on the anniversary of the day on which it was signed. On its centenary anniversary it will be read once more, audibly, solemnly with appropriate ceremonies. This will be done, not alone here, in this great country grown to a world power, but in all parts of the earth where Americans are to be found, and in all places where there is love for liberty and independence.

"On all occasions where the heart overflows and seeks utterance there is no better medium than song. Music is the language of the heart and the emotions. To give full expression to the sentiments of the people, at the coming Jubilee of this great nation, instruments and voices should combine in giving expression to harmonies inspired by love for God and country. This could not be done more effectively than through the medium of an oratorio, the text of which would closely follow and embrace words from the Declaration of Independence, which would further be ennobled by the music from the soul of an inspired composer in this great land.

"The creation of a musical work, in the form of an oratorio, with which to celebrate fitly this great national event has been in my mind for many years. There can be no doubt that a work of this kind would receive applause and approbation from people throughout the country. Imagine the suspense in which an audience would await the performance of a stirring festival overture, from a full orchestra, under the leadership of a great director, to be followed by the combined voices of a well-trained massed chorus of men and women, giving utterance to the inspired words of the text in sounds rushing along like mighty waters. Imagine the forceful recitatives, the trios and quartettes sustained by an accompaniment from a well-trained orchestra, its volume gradually increasing, finally rising to an overpowering height of musical expression, ending in a burst of glory accompanied by waving of flags. Would not this stir an audience to an amazing pitch of excitement and admiration, seldom witnessed even under the influence of the highest patriotic fervor?"

Synopsis of the Oratorio.

Overture. Pilgrim fathers. Early settlers. Disturbances. Dissatisfaction. Mutterings, Resolve.

Introduction.   "When in the course of human events," etc.
Quartette.

"And to assume," etc.   Crescendo.

"Laws of nature and of nature's God." Climax.

Part First.

"We hold these truths."   Recitative.

"That all men are created equal,"   "

"That men are endowed with inalienable rights,"   "

"Life liberty and the pursuit, of happiness,"

"Deriving their power from the consent of the governed."

Repeated in Chorus.

"From prudence in deed, to tyranny over these states,"

Chorus in Crescendo, continually growing like the *Song of Tell* composed by Karl Hering.

Part Second.

Recitative.

1. "To prove this," etc. "We have, he has," 13 times. Followed by a storm of indignation. Sound of Kettle-drums and Oboes. Forte. Fortissimo. Grave.

2. "He has abdicated,"
   "He has plundered,"
   "He is at this time,"
   "He has crushed,"
   "He has excited." A women's chorus, for a beginning.
   "In every stage," etc.,　　　　Impressive trio.
   　　　　A Male chorus joins.

Part Third.

"Nor have we."

"We have"　　　　Alternating chorus. Dolce.

"We must therefore," etc.　　　　Great resolution.

Full chorus—Enemies in War, Friends in Peace.

"We pledge to each other our lives, our fortunes, our sacred honour."

　　　　Augmented Chorus in Brilliant Style.　　Finis.

Thoughts on Religion.

"The beginning of wisdom is the realization of God who is without end. God being infinite the realization of Him must be so likewise.

"God is eternal, therefore, true wisdom must be eternal and all science a state of growth. All things come from God and through Him; they have their origin and continuance in Him. God is the primary cause and the All.

the source and promoter of all things.

"The order of the Universe and the things in it, their progress under constant change, is governed by laws which have their foundation in God, are harmonious, concordant, analogous and inherently alike.

"We believe in God because we know that He is; this knowledge is in every human being. He who says he cannot believe, lies because he does not wish to believe, thereby putting himself beyond the pale, his mind unhinged, distorted, his thoughts twisted and his judgment warped.

"He who wishes to prove a God is foolish for he is without logic. He might as well deny the principles of mathematics and the axioms upon which this is founded. Denial declares him to be a traitor to human intelligence, to so-called philosophic reasoning."

PART II

A SEA VOYAGE
AND
LETTERS FROM THE TROPICS.

JOURNEY FROM SAXONY TO PARAMARIBO,
SOUTH AMERICA, IN 1827.
*(Written by Dr. Hering while waiting in Amsterdam for
the East Wind.)*

It was on Oct. 10th, at noon that Weigel and I entered
the stagecoach. The space about us was crammed with
people. We felt in our new surroundings as must feel a
peasant bride in her wedding outfit, scarcely knowing how
to move, yet compelled to do so constantly. The horses
pulled us along, indifferent to all but their load, which
concerned them far more than the burden that lay upon
our hearts and minds.

I stopped off in Oschatz for a painful parting with Luise
who would not listen to the word America, which, she
said, would shatter all her hopes. Even the word Amsterdam sounded harshly to her ears. I had to let the matter
rest there, although keeping silence pained me. Every
thing seemed to conspire to keep me in Oschatz. Many
things had to be done in Leipzig, where my companion,
Weigel (a botanist appointed by the crown) was chafing
at the delay. The passage money for the diligence had
been paid. I had to hire a private conveyance; no other
being available. There was sufficient time, when later
I arrived in Leipzig, to attend to my affairs and to deliver
a letter to Plass.

It is well, when at parting, the gray threads in the
fabric of care are shot through with the red of joyful
anticipation, as was the case with us who were leaving. It

is always those who remain behind that doubly feel the pain of separation. For us the burden was lighter; for our friends in Dresden, Oschatz and Leipzig it was heavier.

In the evening the leave taking in Leipzig was enlivened by a quarrel with the authorities over our firearms. There was plenty of room, for besides the main coach there were four extra wagons, nevertheless we were to be debarred from taking our rifles. The Prussian officer did not wish to shoulder the responsibility, and the matter had to be referred to his eminence, the Postmaster General of Saxony himself, who was willing to let us take our guns, but ruled that we must leave our dogs behind.

We started on our journey. We occupied first places in one of the extra coaches. There was a scramble among the passengers. Weigel and I were to be separated, because armed as we were, to the teeth, with four guns, numbering five barrels, and two swords, we were accounted unsafe, and no one was willing to share our conveyance, to which we did not object in the least. For a while we harbored a Prussian officer, a major, who had missed the coach ahead in the scramble for seats. He later gave a favorable report of us to the rest of the passengers. The caravan reminded one of a centipede, with a very rapid crawl. It had about fifty horses' feet with which to cover the road. Its segmented body was equipped, in front, with a yellow head and chest, and whips for antennae. Its entrails, with ramifications, were represented by the twenty-four or twenty-five passengers inside the coaches. As Parasites, on its sides, rode five outriders on horseback; that these were suckers was shown at every stop. In all the centipede numbered one hundred and ten legs, ten more than belong to the many jointed myriapod, commonly named hundred-legger. If at first we had a mathematical problem to solve, it was now a geographic one. Our journey took us through seven lordly domains. The second country we came to was Prussia, where, in Naumburg, where we had a longer stop, I received a warm welcome and godspeed.

Stapf, a mainstay of our school of medicine, who was

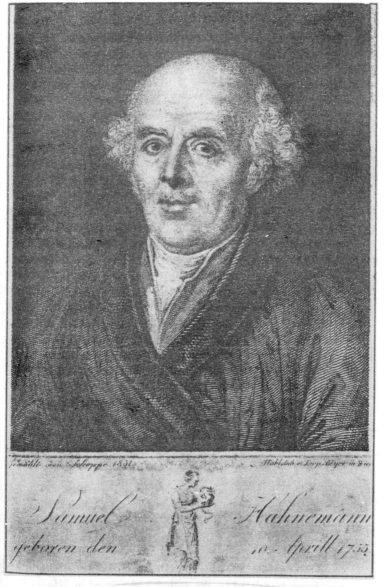

SAMUEL HAHNEMANN.
COPY OF STEEL ENGRAVING PRINTED IN GERMANY IN 1831.
(Over)

Facsimile of a Letter to Ernst Stapf by
Samuel Hahnemann.

Lieber Freund und College!
Diess ist das Conterfey des Mannes,
der Ihren Eifer für unsre wohlthätige
Heilkunst zu schätzen weiss und Sie liebt,
Coethen den 7. Febr. 1832. Ihr Samuel Hahnemann

(Translation)

Dear Friend and Colleague:

This is a picture of the man who knows how to value your zeal for our beneficent healing art, and who loves you.

Your Samuel Hahnemann.

Coethen, February 7, 1832.

Note: This picture and the accompanying message was sent by Hahnemann to his first student, Ernst Stapf, of Naumburg, Saxony, later Editor of "The Archives." The picture was received by Dr. Hering subsequent to Stapf's death together with a collection of 127 letters in German from Hahnemann, covering a period from 1813 to 1838, now being translated by the author and printed in "Hospital Tidings," a periodical of Hahnemann Medical College and Hospital of Philadelphia.

(Over)

expecting me, according to appointment, was waiting. Although in correspondence with him for a long time we had never met, and the time seemed all too short for this meeting, in the brief time allowed for the stopover. We had expected to arrive at midnight, but it was two o'clock when I alighted to look for my friend. I made out to see strangers, whom if I had known them I could not have recognized in the dark, there being no moon. My principal object in meeting Stapf was to obtain certain medicines which I needed to complete my outfit, and also to get his counsel about certain things to be done for our cause. Furthermore there were medicines to reach me at the local postoffice, and possibly a letter. Anxiety gripped me; for rather than be without my Hahnemannian medicines I would go without coat and pants. Nothing at the postoffice! Furiously I demanded to see the postmaster, who was asleep. A postillion standing nearby asked: "What is the matter? Why the hurry? Here is a package from Dr. Stapf for a traveller who is to come through. This must be the party," he said, pointing his finger at me. He had observed me with my cap off, my mantle over my ears, under it gun and hunting knife, a terrifying object. At this moment a man slightly stooped, simply dressed, of scholarly appearance, with a box under his arm, stepped forward saying: "Surely you must be Dr. Hering?" "That I am; and you, Dr. Stapf." "My dear friend," said he "What a solemn first meeting with so soon a parting! What an enormous undertaking, this journey, what gain, very great gain, and what danger in a thousand ways! But come; come quickly."

As we walked through the dark streets, our voices made us acquainted, our faces being revealed but in shadowy outlines. At his home my friend provided me with the medicines I had asked for in my letter, with several more, all genuine and of the best preparations, carefully packed and ready for the long journey. All I had to give in return was promises, thanks and some observations for his advice. Doubtful things were cleared up. Uncertain matters corroborated. But more of this for a later page.

With all the worries and anxieties the prospect of leaving home had caused me, my heart was made glad by meeting face to face a great man, like Stapf, whom I had thus far only been able to admire from a distance. To me this was the crowning point: that words such as he spoke would illuminate whatever of darkest night might come over me.

It was granted me, at the last moment before leaving, to receive a greeting from another, from Hahnemann himself, who stands, and ever will stand high above all of us, our master, the man foremost, not only in his century, but in the history of a thousand years. All of what has been ridiculed, pitifully derided, proclaimed as folly, most of it childish prattle, shall not hinder me from doing honour to the man who is pitted against the world of superstition, and this flame shall forever be kept alive within me. May I be denounced should I have said one word too many! Gladly will I bear all the scorn that may be heaped upon me. It will be but an infinitesimal part of the mountains of mud that they have tried to pile upon his name. To be blessed and victorious in him will forever make life happy for me. My heart's desires, the intense longings in my soul, ever glowing with a warmer love, will find consummation in his service, in giving to the world what he intends. With all knowledge bestowed upon mankind there can be no other, none greater for me than he, until death. There can be nothing wider or higher than the heavens and what belongs therein. Often, have I not only felt and spoken this, but have put it in writing, as I do now, and will continue to do.

It was fitting that in darkest night, under the roof of heaven, this greeting was brought to me by one whose heart beats in joyous union with mine. The words were: "Hahnemann sends you his heartfelt greeting; gives you his blessing and wishes you Godspeed." Twice he told it to me; a third time and I would have embraced him, but the time had come to enter the stagecoach. It seemed to me as though the dark night had suddenly become illuminated by this message, received through my friend

Stapf. It was like a benediction upon my head, and my
feet seemed to touch consecrated ground. More greet-
ings in Weimar, and a parcel. Oken had sent a book on
botany, and to add to my pleasure there was a letter from
home.

We stopped over in Frankfort from six in the evening
of the fifteenth, until six in the evening of the seventeenth.
Much enjoyment was crowded into the forty-eight hours.
I took my passports to secretary von Carlowitz who received them with exclamations of delight when he saw
the signatures upon them of a dear friend, whose name
has escaped me. "Ah!" said he, "the signature of my
very dear N. N. I must introduce you to the ambassador." I made apology for my coat and shoes. "Not the
slightest bit of difference. You have come from my dear
N. N. Here his handwriting, the dear man! Come as
you are; you are on a journey. His handwriting! I will
show your passports to the ambassador and acquaint him
with your wishes. Your hand in welcome!"

I was kindly received by the Minister of foreign affairs,
who was politeness itself, without any show of formality.
His excellency, as also some of the servants in his house,
claimed knowledge of Frau Blum, my landlady in Dresden.
His Grace had the faculty of extracting information without the least discourtesy. We were invited to dinner. My
friend Weigel, occupied with affairs of botany, declined
the invitation. I went and enjoyed a perfect afternoon.
My host showed the liveliest interest in our undertaking
and was ready with advice, which, in most cases, came too
late. He thought we should have taken the Duke of
Weimar into our confidence, or at least since that was
too late, call on his son at Geldern who had shown great
interest in botany. But this we could not do. He mentioned the wife of a former governor in Surinam who
made her home in Frankfort, but who was temporarily
absent. After examining our passports he secured their
endorsement by the Dutch functionary, on the following
day, and our wishes were satisfied. Our departure had
to be made in some haste to avoid the chance of missing

our ship. I did, however, in all kindness, succeed in making arrangements for a stopover in Mayence where we arrived on the seventeenth and were given until the morning of the nineteenth, when we embarked in a fast sailing boat down the Rhine.

I realize, at the beginning of my departure, that among the many things in which I must learn to improve myself, is my handwriting. When I consider what little of extra care and restraint is needed to acquire a more legible hand, so gratifying to one's readers who so sweetly and patiently come to the task of poring over our correspondence, and what a torment it may become to those of our friends who must laboriously decipher what should inspire rather than weary them, I resolve at once to do better in the future. I well know the trouble I have had in reading my own writing, even when not of the worst.

Thinking and speaking have always come easily enough to me. Reading and listening more difficult. To the setter of type I must show leniency, for, should I undertake to sit too hard upon the setter, what more likely than that he might become completely upset. Hence I stand helplessly by, and misprints go before the public eye. Speaking of improvement in writing suggests improvement in style, which scarcely belongs here since I am not at present writing for publication. This, however, would not alter the contents of my letters in the least, excepting to give more attention to the systematizing of things under observation.

These thoughts did not come to me while sailing down the Rhine, in a dense fog which prevented one from seeing anything. I meditated then upon the realization of human desires and the anticipation of things to come. The people about us are talking of their travelling plans and are busy strapping their bundles.

I am reminded of plans my friend Dehmel and I had once made, after a long separation, to make a Rhine journey. I had had this desire, which grew to an intense longing, in the fall of 1824, when the days were cool and beautiful and the air filled with the singing of birds. It was in the early days when I had no money at all. only debts to be paid and no prospects. My booklet, *Poor Henry*, had now enriched me somewhat. and there were prospects of more to come from the sale of the *Water Sprite*. My heart was light as we set sail upon the green waters of the Rhine. Next fall, according to promise. we met again to make the journey together. and now once more, in the fall, sitting in the stagecoach, on my way to Frankfort, I was again to meet with my friend, who was to accompany me down the Rhine. This time in good standing and with better prospects for the future.

My mind is occupied with a long cherished resolve to write a treatise in which many wishes are to be realized. In this there is the charm of anticipation. I have in mind writing about the perfecting of certain attributes such as memory, and the like, which must be possible with leisure, and careful training. The way must lie clear before one, the victory certain or nothing will be gained. I have already dipped my pen into ink to write such a book. which, though not yet accomplished, is occupying my brain in leisure hours. Much of it still is in a fog like the one we are passing through. But more of this later.

As we neared Bingen, the fog lifted revealing the ancient castles. The Rhine flowed as always, and all was beautiful as before. We saw the vintners harvesting their grapes, the time for which had begun on the same day.

I thought of poets and their rapturous descriptions, sincere, not distorted, and of my own better hours in which I wrote verses. These, though not of great value, at least were true and not forced, if I may say so. I make mention of this because later, in my own way, I may be expected to describe some of the glories of the world. I cannot remember ever having been deeply moved. thrilled, or exalted by descriptions of the beautiful. For this reason I have never been able to either write or speak in glowing terms of things seen or experienced on a journey. I believe I might travel through Switzerland or Italy without writing a single intoxicating letter. I take delight in describing pictures of a room with its furniture, or of an

'individual to whom I have taken a liking. but these I
cannot associate with landscapes which for me retire into
a shade. I do not know why this is so. I have. however.
in a letter written recently, tried to make this clear to
myself. It is, as I understand it, the feeling of a definite.
distinct reality that I experience through the events that
occur in my life. Even events of great importance in one's
life, such as getting married, could not alter the case.
After all, things that happen, are but pictures come true
from what has passed in our minds in moments of silent
meditation.   Things that I have read, and others conceived in imagination, take shape and furnish material
for elaboration.   All vision is repetition *(Jedes sehen ein
wiedersehen)*. At present the actuality, the newness of
things, though they dominate me, do not disturb my composure.   There is no overpowering longing to see the new
world, such as some might feel in a burning desire to view
the tropics, long before they experience its scorching heat.
To me all outward experiences as well as my thoughts.
even when written with fervor, remain to be read peacefully on paper. I am calm, mostly smiling, seldom moved
to tears of joy or sorrow; and, in the latter case, only in
matters that touch the innermost recesses of the heart.

Our ship continued on its journey down the green royal
Rhine until, on the following day, we spied the blue Seven
Hill Mountains as they appeared in the background. I
felt sad as I said farewell to the blue hills so dear to me
from my childhood; dear as if they had been people. It
was the hills, more than aught else, that enriched my
youthful happy days; friends came later and singly. It
was only of late, and the time brief, that friends had
multiplied, and the hills were pushed into the background, but where they will forever stand, unforgotten.
It was the farewell to the hills that helped to make me
homesick as I took a long and lingering look behind. It
was among their rocks and valleys, forests and tree tops
I felt happy, and at home, before I was understood by
others. It was there I gathered my specimens, rested and
dreamed the dreams that were to brighten my future years.

Many things have happened since. are happening now, yet I feel that some day I will have a longing for these heights beyond all other things upon earth; from them to get other perspectives for my future. The next blue mountains to greet our eyes, in case we should not get to see the peak of Teneriffe, will be those in the interior of Guiana. At present I would not have the desire to look upon them; my heart must first grow lighter.

We arrived in Cologne by night. I could barely make out, by the dim light of the moon, the innumerable spires above the walls of houses that stretched along the banks. I said to myself, "This is Germany's Rome." There, in the distance, stood the dome like a gigantic ant hill, the magnificent structure which, in its entirety, I was never to behold. We wandered through the streets of the ancient city by moonlight; saw a large cemetery with many crosses. The general impression given was that of a city with many graves. There was just time to secure our passage in the stagecoach, and early next morning, which was foggy, we left the holy city, which, looking back from the lowlands, appeared blue in the distance.

I am reserving my impressions of my first day in Holland for another letter in which I will have more things to relate, for the benefit of certain persons.

We had travelled from Mayence to Coblentz, down the Rhine, on the nineteenth, arriving in Cologne on the twentieth, and left there early on the twenty-first, arriving at Utrecht at noon of the twenty-second, and at Amsterdam on the evening of the same day. Here good news awaited us. I have communicated some things about this great city, from later days, not intended for the many.

It turned out that we had travelled with unnecessary haste. On the morning on which I left Cologne, Weigel, who had remained behind, travelled alone to Brussels to obtain from the home-minister our passports and a letter to the secretary of the navy. My reason for leaving Weigel behind, was partly to save expenses, and partly to attend to affairs that might become necessary in the event of a hurried departure after his arrival. He soon followed, bringing with him a letter of importance to the Minister of Naval Affairs at the Hague. His funds. which had only held out to get to this place. necessitated another trip to the Hague. We are now prepared with the very best passports and letters of introduction to the Governor, all to our satisfaction. Likewise our business with the French Consul here has been most pleasant and satisfactory. We must say that we have been treated with even greater kindness than we could have anticipated . The first and more important point having been arranged to our satisfaction, we have to consider our second venture. our ship. The latter, as also its passengers who are to sail with us, appear favorable, and the passage costs reasonable. The company on board ship might not be all that could be desired, but we have our books which will help to make life supportable in our leisure moments.

While waiting here, in Amsterdam, we are getting acquainted with the city as far as bad weather and the necessity of keeping down expenses will permit. We have been kindly received in different quarters. We are mostly satisfied with the purchases we have made. The larger size of paper, thirty reams of blotting paper, besides other kinds, which we have found cheaper here than in Dresden. are packed to go on board tomorrow. Glassware is no dearer than in Dresden, of the same Bohemian quality. Our clothing for the voyage we obtained at a reasonable price from an honest dealer. Shoes were a different proposition, about which more later. With the tradesmen in general and their greed for money we had much contention.

Our lives take their course while waiting for favorable winds to come from the same direction as our money. A kind man brought us our first remittance; even left us the purse in which it came, since we had none. The morning after our arrival, as soon as the stores opened, which is late, we went shopping for the thousand and one smaller articles of greater or lesser importance, looking for the best and cheapest to be had.

We are fairly well at home now in the great city. We

eat at four in the afternoon, and if the company does not
provide entertainment for the evening, we return to our
room, to our books, papers and accounts. Much of our
time is occupied with reading, writing, drawing and the
like. Many of the rarer specimens of fishes from foreign
parts I would like to have gotten for my collection but I
had not the room for them, nor the price to pay for them.
All was new to me. I took particular interest in the dear
plants that grow in the sea, which I was allowed to see
and hold in my hands.

As soon as a favorable wind blows, many ships will
sail, some of them weekly until January; others later, at
the approach of spring, if wind and weather be favorable.
Our letters will be safely delivered. The first ship to return from the West, after we have arrived, will bring back
my second report to the place from which the first was
written.

I have been to the theatre. I was well entertained
though I could but understand a word here and there.
Most of the plays are translations, some from Kotzebue
and Ifland, who are still in vogue, others from the French.
I am eager to make acquaintance with some of the natives.
The language is very fine. It has a charm for an un-
spoiled ear, which makes impressive its serious side, above
all in what is child-like, as also its comic side which it
renders so charmingly. Its choice brevity in which it has
an advantage over the pure German, its softness and
fluency enable it to render smoothly sentences such, as
with us, savor of the strong arm and the rougher element.
It therefore better adapts itself to the more drastic come-
dies. One would think that comic opera would prosper
here. Both high and low Germans should become better
acquainted. By mutual acquaintance language would gain
considerably.

The actors here express themselves with intensity, their
work is keen and clever, yet always restrained. I have
not observed one of them to rant or yell. In general they
show thorough control in diction, but at times are inclined
to draw the picture too sharply, with a certain angularity

of gesture. One could wish to be a low German to write plays for them if but to hear one's words spoken so beautifully. In conversation, which is always extremely lively, and in their speeches they preserve the right inflections, not always the case with us, and they pass lightly and gracefully from one tone to another, which we are accustomed to hear only from masters. But one must listen to the actress to become thoroughly entranced with the beauty of the language.

In the much praised ballet there was little that was genuine. The male dancer, though nimble, was jerky and affected, with clownish manners. His gestures were awkward. Something might be said here about how far it might be possible to develop a language of bodily expression in gesture. But more of this another time.

The play was poor. If anything genuine has been written it has not endured. Nothing is left but sentimental trumpery stuff, the work of bunglers. To achieve something worthwhile in this line someone would have to be trained for the work by advice of musicians as well as dancing masters. It might be best to reserve the ballet for opera, where it rightfully belongs. Dancing, as practised here, is no less tedious than elsewhere. The art which the dancer has acquired by constant and laborious practice is wasted upon ugly, vicious and distasteful subjects. Let us hope that something better will take the place of the ludicrous children's dances in vogue; there nothing could be worse than a possible introduction of caricatures, such, for instance, as animal dancing. Even a trifling betterment would be welcome.

The Hollander has no ears, at least but very dull ones. Squawking of poultry in the streets, and noises of all kinds are constantly in evidence. Chimes of bells are most distressing. Without resonance one set interferes with another. Each spire, indicating the time of day, is out of tempo with the others. The jangle grates upon the ear and disturbs the dignity and holiness of the scene. Crying and shouting in the streets, seldom melodious, is always mournful. Music, of all kinds, is deplorable.

Among the abundance of folk songs one would expect some popular ones, especially those from the German and the French.

The written language of the Dutch is more characteristic than our own. Speaking the language is difficult for the Middle and South German; more so than the South German dialects, which sound affected from the mouths of foreigners, to us.

Paramaribo, Jan. 18, in the Evening.

Our ship has anchored in the Surinam River, at Fort Amsterdam, at the junction of two rivers, this 18th day of January, at 4 p. m. It was too late to get as far as Paramaribo on the same day. The captain had intended to send out notice of his arrival at that place. He took some of our travelling companions, whose home is here, together with some others, to the shore in his yawl. At last we will have an opportunity, the first in a long time, to have an evening to ourselves. I will, first of all, devote some time to writing and send what is finished with the first ship that sails. Another letter, supposedly a duplicate, is to follow with my next.

We have made a favorable and a speedy voyage. Most of the vessels that set sail before us have not yet arrived. Of the eight that left port with us only one caught up, on the last day. We met with adverse winds, on several occasions, to give us a taste of what might happen in a storm. Nearly always a stiff breeze arose to help us on our way. When other ships took in canvas our captain kept some of his sails up, thereby making headway. We were seldom becalmed, and luckily only for short periods. Absence of wind has retarded many a voyage at sea. The times when our ship lay idle, which was seldom, we profited by fishing for booty. It was not alone the enjoyment in beholding the sea, so quiet, mirroring the blue above, but it afforded rest and also opportunity to capture some sea nettles and fishes. It gave me great pleasure to examine and study these remarkable creatures. I made drawings, dissections, and learned new things about them not set down in the books.

As yet we have not found a way to preserve the medusae, which quickly perish out of water and dissolve. Their marvelous colors and construction vanish from sight even while under the process of dissection. Under more favorable conditions we will make further attempts to enlarge our collection of specimens and, by better preservative methods, get them ready for the market.

These occasional bright spots in the pursuit of natural science were the only rare ones in our voyage. In our next consignment the packages of written matter, somewhat meager, will furnish proof that a sea voyage, especially a first one, is not a favorable occasion for thinking or writing.

Weigel, who did not fare so well on account of being a botanist, is glad to know that the ship has touched bottom; doubly glad because, he himself, will again find ground under his feet on the morrow. Now that we have seen palm trees a new life opens before us. All looks serenely bright and hopeful and we feel as if immersed in a clear and luminous atmosphere.

Paramaribo, January 23d, 1827.

Although scarcely recovered from the fatigue of receiving social calls and making new acquaintances we are beginning to feel at home. Weigel and I are delighted with the new plants we have found and share, and on the first day we captured a bird-spider (*Aranea avicularia*) in our room. On the day before yesterday we purchased, at a reasonable price, a two-toed living sloth of unusual size.

The next ship is to sail in such haste that we are scarcely allowed sufficient time to write more than a short first communication. Soon as possible, which will be in about six or seven months, we will be looking for a budget of letters from home.

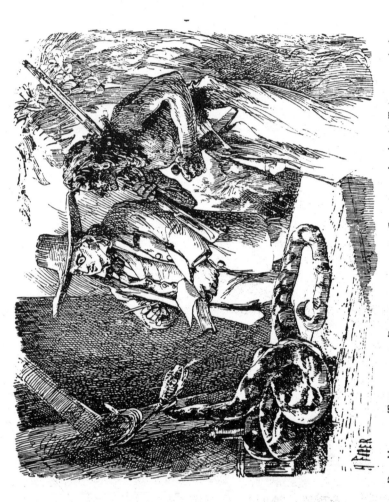

DR. HERING TAKING THE POISON FROM THE SERPENT. *Lachesis Trigonocephalus.*

Paramaribo, February 2, 1827.

My dear Dehmel:

I rejoice with you when I think what great pleasure this and the former letter will have brought to you and the folks at home. It may possibly arrive a day or so earlier than expected at your European shore where spring has come. It shall not bring new worries, at least such is not the intention. The worst is overcome: the most of our means expended. He (the father) is to forget the older worries. Former letters have given sufficient explanation. The next is to give an accurate account of weekly expenditures and of further excursions to be made. Until then only pleasant things.

The enormous wealth of plants, new varieties, easily pressed; the equally great abundance of rare insects are more difficult to obtain. Bird-spiders are to be caught by the hundred. Flying insects also. Lantern flies are scarce and only to be obtained in the interior.

I wished to prolong my stay here in the hope of having more leisure for scientific observation, for which, as it is now, I must steal the time. When it comes to the work of skinning, for which the time is limited, the work can be but tolerably well accomplished. Most of the bird skins, particularly those of the parrots, are exceedingly difficult to manage, because they easily come apart. The skin of a hummingbird offers no easy task to handle. To flay a tiger one requires the help of an assistant for a whole day, and for a tapir that of two quaymen the same length of time. May heaven soon send more of these monsters; I will be glad to take care of their hides. I hope there will be another consignment ready for shipment soon, even though it may not be of the choicest specimens. We, at first, make use of the most ordinary material and what is close to hand, as beginning and proof of our activity. Of insects there must be no less than ten thousand available for the first sending, otherwise it would not be worth the packing of them in boxes. The animal skins, in this climate, give us the most trouble, because they are so slow to dry, since this has to be done in ovens, and of these only bake ovens are available. This, with the arsenic, with which the skins are saturated, makes the process difficult, but ways and means must be found.

The biggest of enemies here to be met is the smallest. The small yellow ants, the length of a hyphen, are instantly on hand where they scent dead matter and they clean up with astonishing rapidity what they find. Poison they avoid, but eat around and beneath the spots that contains it. Insects find it hard to hide from these pests. Constant watchfulness and going the same round, from early morn till night, trying to restore what one had thought to be finished, is the only remedy other than quick transportation of the skins to Saxony and the cooler, fresher air of Europe. More soon.

Paramaribo, ... 1827.

My second report. Not a copy of the first, which was written under most unfavorable circumstances. I had, at that time, begun to sicken without becoming thoroughly aware of it until my condition became so weakened, in body, that I could scarcely walk, and had to lie down almost continually by day and night, the heat being very great at that time. I have completely recovered from the attack, which was of short duration. To my announcement of a safe arrival I may add that it is in no wise my wish to undertake soon another journey. Our affairs prosper.

We met with a very friendly reception from the governor, to whom we made our first visit, today. We are granted the privilege, which could not well be refused, to make expeditions through the colony and were promised letters to the officers at the forts situated in the innermost parts. To these places the governor's letters will admit us with the privilege of taking up our abode if we so desire. We are likewise provided with introductions and invitations to visit lumber, coffee, sugar, and cotton plantations in all localities, inland and on the coast.

There are very many Germans here who deem it an honour to support an undertaking, which, to my indignation, and to the shame of those in our country, be it said, was left to Hollanders to promote. As for the Dutch, they refrain from hindering, and try to look as if they too had some appreciation.

There is a young German physician here by the name of Husmann, who has a fine zoological museum to which we have access for observation. This man is for us a mine of wealth for advice. He shares the fruits of his own research with the utmost generosity. This intercourse, the only one of the kind that has come our way, will be a blessing.

W. has rented a house, which we share. I occupy the upper story, the part under the roof. We expect to move to another place shortly. My friend cannot get possession of his own under fifteen months. The houses here are very commodious, giving sufficient room to spread oneself.

Animal hunting is purely a matter of luck, depending upon the blacks and the Indians, and what they bring to our door. This means an outlay of cash although the things are dirt cheap at that. Trying to do the trapping ourselves is difficult and seldom succeeds. We have skinned a sloth *(Bradypus didactylus)* of unusual size. The large Iguana, its body measuring a yard and its tail two, we have caught alive. We also have a live marsupial mammal of a small variety, and a skeleton of a colibri.

We have added to our household a black servant, essential to our needs, and worth what he costs us. He carries our guns and containers on our expeditions into the bush, can shoot and manage wild beasts, helps with the skinning and has a good time in our service.

It is certain that the so-called bird-spider does not devour humming-birds, which is a fairy tale of the negroes. The colibri, of this region, does not suck honey from flowers, probably none does; it lives on small bugs which hide in the flowers.

Paramaribo, March 30, 1827.

I wrote you about our first reception here upon our arrival, and of our impressions and expectations, with a promise of writing again, after several weeks, a fuller account of our neighbors. In the meantime two months have passed.

I may assume that our present outlook is riper and gives more promise of continuance. Otherwise your answer, to this letter, could only arrive at a time when we would have to make preparations for leaving. I would much prefer a longer stay, as long as possible, not to miss too much in Germany.

Our reception here might well be called brilliant, its brightness being more of a subjective character than objective. There is on the whole a general desire to favor us. One cannot tell how long this may continue. At the present I have not the leisure to carry out my intention to describe all of the men and their families, or to give you a more complete picture of our social life. The time must come when there will be less work and then it will be possible to study the manners and customs of the country and its people. Social intercourse is expensive, but to live without it would cost more, with less of gain.

I will ask you to send a message to Carlowitz in Frankfort expressing our appreciation of all he has done for us. It was through his introduction to the colonies, in this foreign land, that we have everywhere met with so favorable a reception; at first from minister Clout in Holland, then by the governor here. Clout, who lives here, near the governor, introduced us to other people, influential residents of the town, one of them being Hayungen, counsellor of justice, formerly from Germany and an admirer of German literature. After we made his acquaintance he introduced us further, and himself favored us by sending us rare specimens he had collected. He accompanied us to Fort Amsterdam, nearby, which is in charge of Major Duersteler, who superintends the cordon of colonies, with their military posts, reaching to the

farthest boundaries. To accompany him on one of his
excursions to these distant places would give us an opportunity to study the natives, which is quite likely to
happen, for we have already received so many invitations
to plantations, some near, others distant, that we are
at a loss to choose.

In February we spent eight days on a newly laid out
plantation belonging to a Dr. Husmann, a young German
physician who came here to study natural history and to
secure an independent living. We were invited to call
and examine his interesting collection, and found his
conversation entertaining and enlightening. He has served
in both the German and Russian campaigns. Other collections were freely opened for us and we were glad to
take advantage of this privilege.

While getting ready, in March, to make a visit to a
more distant plantation there came a hurried invitation
from the major to accompany him on a journey to the
Saramacca, one of the wildest and least populated rivers.
The major, who had intended to devote eight days to this
excursion, stretched the time to almost fourteen, which
was agreeable to me, for I had a longing for such an
opportunity before leaving Germany. The major gunned
and helped to collect specimens while we advanced as far
as Fort Sarou and Fort Nathan, the former six days'
journey to the North, the latter on the coast. From both
places, although the time was short, we brought many
interesting objects. We profited by our experience on
this trip and will know better how to equip ourselves for
similar occasions in the future. This journey cost us
nothing. Other, similar excursions are to be made to other
rivers. While packing and putting things to rights there
came another, a still more important invitation.

The bush negroes, living in the more elevated regions,
are at peace with the colonies. They employ a runner
between them and the town and the Dutch have an official,
given the title of postmaster, to represent them. One of
the latter is stationed in the upper middle part of Surinam,
an eleven days' journey from here. This official is here

on a visit and appears quite anxious to have us visit his place. This we intend to do, God willing, early in May, for three months. There no longer are any Indians in that neighborhood. It might be one of our most important journeys and possibly the last we can make. I suppose taking with me a mulatto from here who is a good hunter, experienced in skinning. Things coming from there have a greater significance, so the gain of such an enterprise would outweigh what could be accomplished here in double the time.

We are doing well, as it is, and hope for continued success. I will not write again until after our return from the expedition. Before our departure we will send all the things, so far collected, at the next sailing of the N . . . There is not very much of zoological material at hand, but I will make a special report concerning the same. If this first export will but cover the cost of transportation I will be satisfied. I have several rare specimens but unfortunately not all of them are in the best state of preservation. The time for butterflies is not yet. Most of the birds are moulting, which hurts the skins. Many of the animals being good food, but hard to keep, are sent to the table to be eaten. However, not to mention other difficulties, the main impediment has to do with myself.

I have no other letter prepared, therefore kindly make it do for yourself and my folks. More next month, when, with the specimens, there will come a package of letters.

Paramaribo, Sept. 24, 1827.

I still owe you the promised report on the Moravians. You must long have desired to know about them. I have not forgotten how earnestly you admonished me to write soon and plenty about my "beloved missionaries." No less forgotten than one could forget your friendly and deeply impressive words from our conversations. I cheerfully set myself to the task of making my report. I would like to do so publicly, before all the world, only

I could not, in that case, do it so openly, or so cheerfully,
for I would then, to justify myself, have to do so apolo-
getically for fear of laying myself open to the charge of
being a sentimentalist, and thus lose influence with many.
I have met with intimations of the kind, here, as elsewhere in former times, when I was accused of mixing with
catholics, or at least of being inclined to mysticism. Sometimes I was rebuffed with the bald remark that young
persons should not act piously, which in older ones might
be excused; that the young were either hypocrites or senti-
mentalists, or at best weaklings who have sown their wild
oats, etc., etc. The majority here takes things for granted,
is indifferent, showing but little interest in things out of
the ordinary. It is an unhappy country in spite of its
many blessings and resources.

The aborigines, the Indians, as far as I may judge from
hearsay, and visits made to them, are far less impression-
able than what is told of Northern tribes. They are a
roving people, more disposed to follow the chase than
agriculture. They are far from being deceitful, and without taking much thought they look out for their immediate wants. The influence that the whites exert upon the
more friendly tribes might, perhaps, awaken their souls,
as happens in North America. As it is they see but little
good, and are lacking in experience. For their ready
wares they receive, in exchange, firewater, and when they
are drunk it is easy to coax from them the rest of their
belongings, for small pay. They frequently come back
for more whiskey but show little respect for the sellers
and cheaters. The few traditionary remnants left them of
God and higher beings, their feeble attempts at idol
worship, and their priests who are but slightly above the
rest of them, make it difficult for any more liberal education to find its way to them.

In politics they remain unnoticed, the people believing
them to be negligible, but they have, now and then, in
former times, been made use of against the bush negroes,
whom they dislike. The 'Moravians send missionaries
among the Indians, of whom some few who remain have

been baptized. What the rest, who remain unbaptized, think of these, I do not know, but probably they remain indifferent.

The negroes who were brought here, who constitute the majority of the population, are more recipient. They brought with them a larger measure of idol worship, but their language, originated here, is more picturesque, and with words continually added thereto, they are helped to communicate with the white people, which enriches their fund of ideas. A considerable number of them have been baptized although these are in the minority.

The bushmen, who were freed in earlier years, were at first inimical to the whites, but after receiving a greater show of kindness from these, they became more submissive; although on account of their native pride, more difficult to convert. They enjoy many privileges, carry on a trade in wood, but spend their money on frippery. An existing disposition to weaken them with luxuries and dissipation fails on account of their free forest lives, which bring them more of good than temptations abroad can do them harm. They are at discord with the whites and a burden to them. The latter live in fear of the bushmen, of which these are aware. The Moravians send their missionaries in the hope of making converts.

The slaves who are more numerous in the town, where they serve in various capacities, than on the plantations, particularly the outlying ones, and some of these who have been freed, are more approachable than the bushmen, with whom, however, they mix.

The so-called *Kleurlinge*, a mixture of black and white, mulattoes, are treated with more respect, and less work is required of them. These enjoy greater advantages, and a larger number from this class are given their freedom. Also most of them are baptized. Although more gifted by nature, mentally and physically, few of them are altogether free from objectionable traits. Nevertheless they are more ready to be taught. I regard them as being more capable and receptive. Through the influence of the Moravians they have become amenable to the law, and have the marriage ceremony performed according to custom.

The whites, with the exception of the higher officials who are legally married, live together in common law, a custom in Surinam sanctioned by usage. Foreigners who come here for commercial reasons, get rich and leave, employ housekeepers, negresses, mulattoes, even free born white girls. Only well-to-do white girls from the better classes, look for proposals and proper marriages. Many are the jests at the expense of the mulattoes for having the nuptial ceremony performed. I, myself, know of girls who would rather live out of wedlock with a man of wealth, than to be legally married to a poor one, and this by advice of their parents. As a rule, the numerous children from such alliances, are, in a measure, cared for and educated by their fathers, and are not allowed to suffer hardship, but in general, because the fathers have died, or gone away, or have changed wives the children are neglected, become poor, run wild and fall into evil ways. So it comes about that the white man is punished through his most sacred possessions, his children, to suffer for the crime of trading in human beings of which he is guilty.

The indolence of the coloured race makes it incumbent upon a householder to employ at least several servants, in small houses five or six, in large establishments as many as forty or fifty. All white children are raised by the blacks excepting in isolated cases where better educated white mothers assume the care of their children. Even the children cannot be kept from associating with the negroes whose language they learn to speak, a misfortune in itself, because upon the first language a human being is taught depends his higher development. As it is, the children not only remain dull and stupid but pick up many things, particularly bad habits, which stick to them and ruin their lives, not by halves, but wholly.

Such then is the soil in which heavenly seed should be sown. The sowers of the Word here are the Moravians, who, though much decreased from former times, are universally respected and loved. Plain honest folk, as you know them at home, living as one family, zealous without haste, simple in their ways, even more friendly than those I have met at home. The charge of hypocricy, with which the people at home are so ready, does not exist here. They are poor but contrive to make a respectable appearance in all ways, in a land where living is dear. They conduct a bakery from which we get our daily bread, also a tailor shop, by which they earn their daily needs and do good to the community besides.

More of these good people, in my next letter, and something too about others who are in the business of conversion. Also more about their activities, their sermons and teachings.

PART - III

LITERARY PRODUCTION

PART III

LITERARY PRODUCTION

The products of Dr. Hering's pen, principally in the form of essays, are scattered among numerous medical journals covering a period of over fifty years. The titles of these essays and the places where they may be found I have quoted, with the help of Mrs. Hering, after Dr. Hering's demise in 1880, so that all who wish to peruse what he has written, may do so by consulting the volumes in the Library of Hahnemann College. His later literary efforts were concentrated upon his larger medical works. An indexed review of these writings and larger works follows. They are complete in themselves so far as they have appeared, and are available to students and interested readers. They are links which, connected, form the chain of scientific research in which is summed up the experience of Hering's life. In earlier years, when cares were not so thick, nor duties so pressing, he wrote verse and light prose, fairy tales, satires and novelettes. A satirical vein runs through all of these writings, playful in the lighter products of his pen, but extremely biting and severe when in polemics, he felt called upon to defend the cause.

————

INDEX

Abbreviations

A. H. Z., Allgemeine Homoeopathische Zeitung.
Am. Hom., American Homoeopath.
Am. Hom. Rev., American Homoeopathic Review.
Brit. Jour. of Hom., British Journal of Homoeopathy.
Cor. Blatt, Correspondenz-Blatt.
H. M., Hahnemannian Monthly.
Hom. Clin., Journal of Homoeopathic Clinics (a part of American Journal of Hom. Mat. Med.).
Hom. News, Homoeopathic News.
Hom. Viertjschft., Homoeopathische Vierteljahres-schrift.
Int. Hom. Press, Internationale Homoeopathische Presse.
Med. Couns., Medical Counsellor.
N. A. J. of H., North American Journal of Homoe-opathy.
Quar. Hom. Jour., Quarterly Homoeopathic Journal:
St. Ar., Stapf's Archives.
Zeit. fur Hom. Kl., Zeitschrift fur Homeopatische Klinik.

─────────

A Collocation of Essentials to a good Drug Proving. 1854. *A. H. Z.,* v. 47.
A **Comforting Elegy at the Grave of Despair of all Medical Youths in our dear Country and other Nice Places.** Philadelphia, 1858.
A **Concise View of the Rise and Progress of Homoeo-pathic Medicine; historical treatise.** Philadel-phia, 1833.

A Criticism on the British Repertory. 1859. *Am. Hom. Rev.*, v. 1.

A Few Well-meant Words to Beginners, on our Materia Medica. 1864. *A. H. Z.*, v. 71.

A Golden Wedding in Philadelphia. 1865. *A. H. Z.*, v. 71.

A Historical Remark on *Euphrasia.* 1863. *A. H. Z.*, v. 67.

Allium Cepa. 1853. *N. A. J. of H.*, v. 3.

American Drug Provings. Leipzig, 1857.

American Drug Provings and Preparatory Work for Constituting Materia Medica a Natural Science. 1852. *Zeit. fur Hom. Kl.*, v. 1.

American Provings, advance notes. 1856. *Zeit. fur Hom. Kl.*, v. 5.

American Votes on the Question: German or Roman Type? Jena. 1871.

Anacardium as Anticriticum; No. 4 of New Hatchels. Leipzig, 1860.

Analytical Therapeutics. 1 vol. Philadelphia, 1875.

An American Protest Against Lutze's Publication of Hahnemann's Organon. 1865. *A. H. Z.*, v. 71.

An Answer to F. Freiligrath's Epistle to Audubon. Poem. Philadelphia, 1844.

Anecdotes from Life. 1863. *A. H. Z.*, v. 67.

Anecdote of a Patient in Search of Three Physicians to Agree Upon His Case. *Brit. Jour. of Hom.*, v. 4.

An Essay on Taste and Smell. 1865. *A. H. Z.*, v. 71.

An Example of Pathological Presumption. 1865. *A. H. Z.*, v. 71.

Annual Meeting of Homoeopathic Physicians. 1869. *A. H. Z.*, v. 79.

Annual Recurrences. 1852. *A. H. Z.*, v. 43. 1853. *N. A. J. of H.*, v. 3.

Antipsoric Remedies in Relation to Leprosy. 1831. *St. Ar.*, v. 10.

A Peal for the Jubilee, Schiller, Shakespeare, Humboldt. Philadelphia, 1859.

A Proposal for the Entire Annihilation of So-called

Homoeopathy by a Scientific Method; No. 3 of New Hatchels. Leipzig, 1860.

A Proposed Complete Materia Medica, a standard work. 1864. *A. H. Z.*, v. 69; and *Am. Hom. Rev.*, v. 5.

A Proposed Plan for Exchange of Homoeopathic Preparations. 1845. *A. H. Z.*, v. 29.

A Protest. 1872. *H. M.*, v. 7.

A Protest Against Falsifying History. 1853. *A. H. Z.*, v. 46.

A Reply to the "Open Letter" in vol. 44. 1853. *A. H. Z.*, v. 46.

Arnica, in Intermittent. 1868. *Hom. Clin.*, v. 2, p. 210.

Arsenicum Metallicum, Remarks on Provings. 1851. *N. A. J. of H.*, v. 1.

A Request for Information from Dr. Eidherr. 1864. *A. H. Z.*, v. 68.

A Review of Kleinert's "Sources of Physiological Drug Provings." 1863. *A. H. Z.*, v. 67.

Arum triphyllum in Scarlatina. 1868. v. 2, p. 273.

A survey of our Provings, arranged according to provers; an historical summary. 1845. *A. H. Z.*, v. 31.

A Survey of the entire Kingdom of Drugs. 1833. *St. Ar.*, v. 13.

A Warning Against the Parisian "Lachesis." 1863. *A. H. Z.*, v. 67.

A Way to Become Rulers of the Medical World. 1879. *Med. Couns.*, v 1.

Badiaga, Remarks on. 1866. *H. M.*, v. 2.

Baunscheidtismus; or, The Secret Discovered. 1858. *Zeit. fur Hom. Kl.*, v. 7.

Boundary, The Natural. Philadelphia, 1860.

British Repertory, A Criticism. 1859. *Am. Hom. Rev.*, v. 1.

Bromine. 1845. *St. Ar.*, v. 20.

Caladium Seguinum, A Proving. 1831. *St. Ar.*, v. 10.

Calcarea arsenicosa in Epilepsy, a note. 1849. *Brit.*

J. of H., v. 7.

Calcarea ostrearum., Case 168. 1868. *Hom. Clin.,* v. 2, p. 184.

Calcarea phosphorica, a resumé of provings and cures. 1871. *N. A. J. of H.,* v. 20. *History of Provings, H. M.,* v. 6.

Carbo vegetabilis, Note to Case 244, by Goullon. 1869. *Hom. Clin.,* v. 3, p. 10.

Caries of Teeth, Therapeutic Hints. 1868. *Hom. Clin.,* v. 2, p. 186.

Cepa and Euphrasia, a Comparison. 1869. *Hom. Clin.,* v. 3, p. 84.

Characteristics. 1867. *H. M.,* v. 3.

Characteristics, or Memory Cards. Philadelphia, 1866-67.

Characteristics and Therapeutic Hints. 1867. *Hom. Clin.,* v. 1. 1868. v. 2.

Chessmoves, A Reply to Roth's "Studies." 1863. *Hom. Viertjschft.,* v. 13.

Chlorine. 1845. *St. Ar.,* v. 20.

Cholera, So-called, on Board of English Ships. 1866. *A. H. Z.,* v. 73.

Cholera, Sulphur. 1871. *A. H. Z.,* v. 83.

Chronic Diseases, Preface to English Translation. 1845. *A. H. Z.,* v. 29.

Cistus Canadensis, Provings. 1866. *A. H. Z.,* v. 72.

Citation-Visitation, Incidental to. 1845. *A. H. Z.,* v. 29.

Coca, Practical Remarks. 1869. *Hom. Clin.,* v. 3, p. 142.

Collections of Symptoms, The Importance of complete. 1866. *A. H. Z.,* v. 72.

Complementary Relations. 1868. *Hom. Clin.,* v. 2, p. 210.

Complete Materia Medica. 1 vol. Philadelphia, 1873.

Conium, Case 62. 1867. *Hom. Clin.,* v. 1, p. 68.

Contagion and Miasm. 1833. *St. Ar.,* v. 13.

Correspondence. 1874. *H. M.,* v. 9.

Correspondence on Topics of the Time. 1879. *Med. Couns.,* v. 1.

Cough, Chronic, Case 265, Boenninghausen. 1868. *Hom. Clin.*, v. 2, p. 271; translation.

Critical Hodge-Podge. 1871. *A. H. Z.*, v. 82.

Critical Remarks on Dysentery. 1872. *H. M.*, v. 7.

Critical Remarks on the Scientific Communications on Snake Poison. 1861. *A. H. Z.*, v. 63.

Criticism on Case 9, *Porrigo Decalvans.* 1867. *Hom. Clin.*, v. 1, p. 14; on Cases 16 and 17, p. 19.

Cycles, Daily, in Diseases and Drug Effects. 1851. *N. A. J. of H.*, v. 1.

Desiderata of Our School. 1877. *N. A. J. of H.*, v. 26.

Desideratum, the Great. 1871. *H. M.*, v. 7.

Diagnostics and Remedies, the Study of. 1831. *St. Ar.*, v. 10.

Diarrhoea, Chronic, Case 121. 1867. *Hom. Clin.*, v. 1, p. 123.

Digitalis According to Baehr and Black's "Monography." 1862. *Am. Hom. Rev.*, v. 3.

Digitalis in *Menorrhagia.* 1869. *Hom. Clin.*, v. 3, p. 59.

Diptheria Cases. 1860. *Am. Hom. Rev.*, v. 2.

Disease Germs. 1872. *H. M.*, v. 8.

Domestic Physician. 1835. First German edition, Jena, Fr. Fromman. English editions, Philadelphia, Boericke & Tafel.

Doppelmops in Homoeopathy, No. 2, New Hatchels. Leipzig, 1860.

Dose, Repetition of. 1833. *St. Ar.*, v. 13.

Drugs, a Survey of the Entire Kingdom. 1833. *St. Ar.*, v. 13.

Drug Proving, a Collocation of Essentials thereto. 1854. *A. H. Z.*, v. 47.

Drugs, Several, their Action on the Well and Sick. 1834. *St. Ar.*, v. 14.

Drug Symptoms, Sifting the. 1865. *A. H. Z.*, v. 71; *Am. Hom. Rev.*, v. 6; *Brit. Jour. of Hom.*, v. 24.

Dysentery, Critical Remarks. 1872. *H. M.*, v. 7.

Eidherr, a Request for Information. 1864. *A. H. Z.*, v. 68.

Elegy. Satire. Philadelphia, 1858.

Epilepsy, *Calc. arsen.* as a Remedy. 1849. *Brit. Jour. of Hom.,* v. 7.

Essentials to a Good Drug Proving. 1854. *A. H. Z.,* v. 47.

Euphrasia and *Cepa,* Comparison. 1869. *Hom. Clin.,* v. 3, p. 84.

Experiment and Hypothesis. 1833. *St. Ar.,* v. 13.

Extracts from Letters from Surinam. 1828. *St. Ar.,* v. 7.

Falsifying History, a Protest. 1853. *A. H. Z.,* v. 46.

Flugblaetter (Flying Leaves), Novelettes. Sondershausen, 1864.

Fluoric Acid. 1845. *St. Ar.,* v. 20.

Fluoric Acid, Cases. 1845. *St. Ar.,* v. 3. New series.

Formica as a Remedy. 1871. *H. M.,* v. 6; *A. H. Z.,* v. 82.

Formica, the Ant. 1871. *N. A. J. of H.,* v. 20.

Fragmentary Contributions to Materia Medica and Therapeutics. 1851. *N. A. J. of H.,* v. 1.

Fragmentary Remarks on Study of Remedies and Diagnostics. 1831. *St. Ar.,* v. 10.

Fragmentary Reports of Symptoms. 1833. *St. Ar.,* v. 13.

Fungus Haematodes. 1830. *St. Ar.,* v. 9.

Future Investigations, a Guide. 1833. *St. Ar.,* v. 13.

Gelsemium nitidum. 1862. *A. H. Z.,* v. 64 and 65.

Germs, Disease. 1872. *H. M.,* v. 8.

Glonoine. 1849. *Quar. Hom. Jour.,* v. 1.

Gross's Comparative Materia Medica. Philadelphia, 1867.

Gross's Differential Diagnosis of Remedies. 1866. *A. H. Z.,* v. 72.

Gymnocladus Canadensis, Proving. 1851. *N. A. J. of H.,* v. 1.

Hahnemann's Analysis of Stapf's Case, Translation with Comment. 1868. *Hom. Clin.,* v. 2, p. 150.

Hahnemann and his "Absurdities," Seven Notes. *H. M.,* v. 7.

Hahnemann's Letter to Stapf on Fevers: translation.
 1868. *Hom. Clin.,* v. 2, p. 187.

Hahnemann in the Cradle. Philadelphia, 1855.

Hahnemann. The Requisites to a Correct Estimate of.
 1847. Hygeia, v. 22. 1851. *N. A. J. of H.,* v. 1.

Hahnemann, Saml. Life. Tract. Allentown, 1836.

Hahnemann's Three Rules Concerning the Rank of
 Symptoms. 1865. *H. M.,* v. 1. 1878. *Am. Hom.
 Rev.,* v. 2.

Hahnemann, Seven Characteristics of Method of Cure.
 Tract. Allentown, 1836.

Hausmann's Book, Lectures. 1868. *A. H. Z.,* v. 77.
 Announcement, 1867. *Hom. Clin.,* v. 1, p. 83.

Headache after Diarrhoea, Case 440. 1869. *Hom.
 Clin.,* v. 3, p. 114.

Heart Affections, *Spongia.* 1868. *A. H. Z.,* v. 76.
 1867. *Hom. Clin.,* v. 1, p. 133.

Heaven for Homoeopathy. A pamphlet. Philadelphia, 1869. *H. M.,* v. 5.

Hepar in Suppuration, Remark. 1869. *Hom. Clin.,*
 v. 3, p. 21.

Hepatic Enlargement, Case 307. 1869. *Hom. Clin.,*
 v. 3, p. 29.

High Dilutions, a Letter. 1847. *Brit. Jour. of Hom.,*
 v. 5.

High Potencies of Jenichen, Remarks. 1845. *A. H. Z.,*
 v. 29.

Hints by which to Form a Correct Estimate of Hahnemann's Organon. 1837. *St. Ar.,* vol. 16.

**Homoeopathic College and other Chairs, No. 1 of
 New Hatchels.** Leipzig, 1860.

Homoeopathic Hackels. Jena, 1846.

Homoeopathic News' Journal. Philadelphia, 1854,
 1855 and 1856.

Homoeopathy in Iceland. 1868. *A. H. Z.,* v. 78.

Homoeopathic Physicians, Annual Meeting. 1869. *A.
 H. Z.,* v. 79.

Homoeopathic Practitioner, What is Necessary to the
 Calling. 1832. *St. Ar.,* v. 11.

Lecture Introductory to Course on Therapeutics. 1864.
A. H. Z., v. 71.

Leprosy, Homoeopathic Treatment of. 1830. *St. Ar.*,
v. 9.

Leprosy, the Relation of Antipsorics. 1831. *St. Ar.*,
v. 10.

Lithium carbonicum, Provings. 1863. *Hom. Viertjschft.*, v. 14; *Am. Hom. Rev.*, v. 4.

Lobelia coerulea, Provings. 1871. *H. M.*, v. 6.

Marginal Notes to the Materia Medica. 1845. *St. Ar.*,
v. 3. New series.

Materia Medica, The Condensed. Philadelphia, 1877.
Second edition.

Materia Medica, Guiding Symptoms. 10 vols. Philadelphia, 1879.

Materia Medica, a Natural Science. Preparatory work.
1852. *Zeit. fur Hom. Kl.*, v. 1.

Materia Medica, Marginal Notes. 1845. *St. Ar.*, v. 3.
New Series.

Materia Medica, As a Natural Science. 1853. *N. A.
J. of H.*, v. 3.

Materia Medica, The New. 1865. *A. H. Z.*, v. 71.

Materia Medica, Our. 1865. *Am. Hom. Rev.*, v. 6.

Materia Medica and Pathology. 1853. *N. A. J. of H.*,
v. 3.

Materia Medica, Review. 1867. *Hom. Clin.*, v. 1, p.
11; Remarks, v. 1, p. 34.

Materia Medica, the Pathologizing of. 1854. *A. H. Z.*,
v. 47.

Materia Medica, a Proposed Complete. 1864. *A. H.
Z.*, v. 69. *Am. Hom. Rev.*, v. 5.

Materia Medica, Homoeopathic, The Study of. 1838.
St. Ar., v. 17.

Materia Medica, The Superficial and the Vital. 1864.
A. H. Z., v. 69.

Materia Medica, a Few Well-meant Words to Beginners. 1864. *A. H. Z.*, v. 71.

Materia Medica and Therapeutics, Fragmentary Contributions to. 1851. *N. A. J. of H.*, v. 1.

Mathematical Certainty. 1875. *N. A. J. of H.*, v. 24.

Menorrhagia, **Digitalis.** 1869. *Hom. Clin.*, v. 3, p. 59.

Miasm and Contagion. 1833. *St. Ar.*, v. 13.

Misrepresentations, Wilful. 1866. *A. H. Z.*, v. 73.

Moss and Mosquitoes. Philadelphia, 1863.

Myrtus Communis. 1851. *N. A. J. of H.*, v. 1.

Newer Provings. 1845. *St. Ar.*, v. 20.

New Hatchels. Leipzig, 1860.

Nosodes. Part I, 1877. *N. A. J. of H.*, v. 26: Part II, 1878, v. 27.

Observations on Solar and Lunar Influences and their Relation to our Materia Medica. 1874. *H. M.*, v. 9.

Obstetrics (Midwifery) in America. 1867. *A. H. Z.*, v. 75.

Offensive Odors from the Mouth, and their Treatment. 1873. *H. M.*, v. 9.

Organon, Preface to the First American Edition. Allentown, 1836.

Organon, Preface to the Third American Edition. Philadelphia, 1849.

Organon, Preface to the Fourth American Edition. Philadelphia, 1860.

Organon, Hints by which to Form a Correct Estimate. 1837. *St. Ar.*, v. 16.

Organon, a Protest Against Lutze's Publication. 1865. *A. H. Z.*, v. 71.

Organopathy; or, The Last Events of 1867. Philadelphia, 1868.

Origin of the Theory of Primary and Secondary Symptoms. 1879. *N. A. J. of H.*, v. 27.

Palladium. 1878. *N. A. J. of H.*, v. 27.

Pathogenesis and Patho-exodus. 1833. *St. Ar.*, v. 13.

Pathological Anatomy Viewed from its Useless Side. 1845. *A. H. Z.*, v. 29.

Pathology and the Materia Medica. 1853. *N. A. J. of H.*, v. 3.

Pathological Presumption, an Example. 1865. *A. H. Z.*, v. 71.

Pathologists and Therapeuticians, Remarks on their
    Dispute. 1831. *St. Ar.*, v. 10.

Plants, Relationship. 1845. *A. H. Z.*, v. 29.

Practical Remarks. 1867-69. *Hom. Clin.*, v. 1, 2, 3
    and 4.

Practitioner, Successful Homoeopathic; What is Neces-
    sary to the Calling. 1832. *St. Ar.*, v. 11.

Preparatory Attempt as Guide to Future Investiga-
    tion. 1833. *St. Ar.*, v. 13.

Prevailing Diseases, Treatment. 1873. *N. A. J. of H.*,
    v. 21.

Primary and Secondary Symptoms. 1876. *N. A. J. of
    H.*, v. 25. Origin of the Theory. 1879. *N. A. J.
    of H.*, v. 27.

Provings of Drugs, Suggestions for making them on the
    Healthy. Philadelphia, 1853.

Provings, Newer. 1845. *St. Ar.*, v. 20.

Provings, a Survey Arranged According to Provers.
    1845. *A. H. Z.*, v. 31.

Psorinum and its Chemical Rescue. 1852. *A. H. Z.*,
    v. 43; *N. A. J. of H.*, v. 2.

Psorinum, Remarks. 1833. *St. Ar.*, v. 13.

Relations of Drugs, Complementary. 1867. *Hom.
    Clin.*, v. 2, p. 210.

Remedies and Diagnostics, the Study of. 1831. *St.
    Ar.*, v. 10.

Repertory, a Plea for a More Complete One. 1831.
    St. Ar., v. 10.

Repetition, of the Dose. 1833. *St. Ar.*, v. 13.

Rhododendron and ***Rhus***, Diagnostic Remarks. 1868.
    Hom. Clin., v. 2, p. 247.

Rhus rad. and ***Ferrum*** in Cough. 1869. *Hom. Clin.*,
    v. 3, p. 84; *Hom. Viertjschft.*, v. 14.

Roth's Studies, a Reply. 1863. *Hom. Viertjschft.*, v.
    14.

Rule and Rules Again. 1865. *H. M.*, v. 1.

Sanguinaria. 1845. *St. Ar.*, v. 20.

Scarlatina, Comments on Case 227. 1868. *Hom. Clin.*,
    v. 2, p. 238; on Case 293. 1869. *Hom. Clin.*, v. 3,

p. 19.

Scarlatina. Arum triphyllum Cases. 1868. *Hom. Clin.*, v. 2, p. 273.

Scarlet Fever Epidemics, Reminiscences. 1845. *A. H. Z.*, v. 29.

Scirrhus of Tongue. Cases. 1868. *Hom. Clin.*, v. 2, p. 239.

Selenium, Fragmentary Proving. 1832. *St. Ar.*, v. 12.

Shibboleth, to What Purpose. 1862. *Hom. Viertjschft.*, v. 13.

Sides, The Rules of. 1865. *H. M.*, v. 1. 1878. *Am. Hom.*, v. 2.

Sifting the Drug Symptoms. 1865. *A. H. Z.*, v. 71. *Am. Hom. Rev.*, v. 6; *Brit. Jour. of Hom.*, v. 24.

Silicea after Vaccination. 1872. *H. M.*, v. 7.

Similar, What Do You Mean By It? 1834. *St. Ar.*, v. 14.

Similar, What is. 1845. Part I. *St. Ar.*, v. 20. Part II. 1845. *St. Ar.*, v. 3. New Series.

Skepticism. Tract. Allentown, 1836.

Skirmishes on our Eastern Coast. 1868. *A. H. Z.*, v. 77.

Smell and Taste. An essay. 1865. *A. H. Z.*, v. 71.

Snake Poison, Critical Remarks. 1861. *A. H. Z.*, v. 63.

Snake Poison, First Remarks. 1831. *St. Ar.*, v. 10.

Snake Poison as a Therapeutic Agent. 1834. *St. Ar.*, v. 14.

Snake Poison, The Effects of. Allentown, 1837.

Solar and Lunar Influences, Their Relation to our Materia Medica. 1874. *H. M.*, v. 9.

Song of the Bell. A parody. Jena, 1845.

Sore Throat, Case 120. 1867. *Hom. Clin.*, v. 1, p. 122.

Spongia in Heart Affections. 1868. *A. H. Z.*, v. 76. 1867. *Hom. Clin.*, v. 1, p. 133.

Staphisagria after the Operation of *Lithotomy.* Correspondence, 1880. *Med. Couns.*, v. 2.

Success, Our. 1866. *A. H. Z.*, v. 73.

Suggestions for Proving of Drugs on the Healthy.

Philadelphia, 1853.

Sulphur in Cholera. 1871. *A. H. Z.,* v. 83.

Sulphur in Gastritis. 1869. *Hom. Clin.,* v. 3, p. 115.

Sulphur in Headache after Diarrhoea. 1869. *Hom. Clin.,* v. 3. p. 114.

Symptoms, Fragmentary Reports of. 1833. *St. Ar.,* v. 13.

Symptoms, The Importance of Complete Collections. 1866. *A. H. Z.,* v. 72.

Symptoms, Where is the Proof to These? A Reply to Hoppe. 1851. *Hom. Viertjschft.,* v. 12.

Symptoms, Ranking of. Hahnemann's Three Rules. 1865. *H. M.,* v. 1.

Teeth, Caries of, Therapeutic Hints. 1868. *Hom. Clin.,* v. 2, p. 186.

Tellurium Against *Trichinae.* 1864. *A. H. Z.,* v. 49.

Tellurium, Provings. 1864. *Am. Hom. Rev.,* v. 5.

Terebinthinae oleum, Recommended for the Treatment of Malarial and Intermittent Fevers. 1877. *N. A. J. of H.,* v. 26.

Tetradymit, Proving. 1868. *A. H. Z.,* v. 77.

Therapeutic Hints. 1867-69.

The Voluntary System of Medical Education. Philadelphia, 1854.

Throat Affections, Therapeutic Hints. 1868. *Hom. Clin.,* v. 2, p. 175.

Trial of Dr. Pelleteer. Tract. Allentown, 1836.

Trichiasis, Suggestions. 1869. *Hom. Clin.,* v. 3, p. 132.

Trichinae, Tellurium. 1864. *A. H. Z.,* v. 69.

Vaccination, *Silica.* 1872. *H. M.,* v. 7.

Virchow's Verdict. 1872. *A. H. Z.,* v. 84.

Whitlow, Case 103. 1867. *Hom. Clin.,* v. 1, p. 102.

Wilful Misrepresentations. 1866. *A. H. Z.,* v. 73.

Zincum, Hepatic Enlargement, Case 307. 1869. *Hom. Clin.,* v. 3, p. 9.

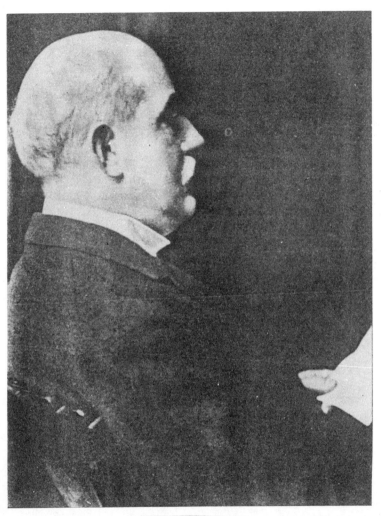

DR. CALVIN B. KNERR.

PART IV

DEATH OF CONSTANTINE HERING

Dr. Hering died at ten p. m. of July 23, 1880. The cause of his death was *angina pectoris*. The end came suddenly and unexpectedly. Dr. Hering had attended to office duties on the same day and had his family gathered about him at the supper table, under the elm tree in his garden. My home was then at Bryn Mawr, one of the suburbs of Philadelphia. I last saw my father-in-law seated at his office window where I placed into his hands a book on spiders lent me by Mrs. Furness, wife of the Shakespearian scholar, Dr. Horace Howard Furness, devoted patients of the doctor for many years.

When Dr. Hering had finished supper in the garden, after an hour's lively conversation, apparently in perfect health, he went to his study on the second floor to resume his writing. He was then working on the fourth volume of "The Guiding Symptoms." About twenty minutes before ten he was seized with an acute attack of the heart. There were only the wife and Mrs. Mertens, a friend of the family, present. His old friend and neighbor, Dr. Koch, Senior, was sent for in haste, but could give no help. When, shortly after, Dr. Bigler, Dr. Koch's son-in-law, arrived, Dr. Hering was already dying; his hands and wrists were cold, though he was perfectly conscious. He was restless and moved from side to side on his couch, suffering greatly from *dyspnoea*.

He very soon breathed his last, and before Dr. Raue, faithful friend and regular attendant, had arrived, who took one look at his dead friend and without a word passed out of the room in deepest grief. Just before the end Hering had said to Mrs. Mertens, a friend of the family, who was weeping by his side, "I am dying now," which were his last words.

At the autopsy, performed by Dr. A. R. Thomas, made on the following day, "Nothing abnormal was discovered in a healthy well-developed anatomy excepting a distinct calcification of the coronary arteries and some deposits of fat about the heart." The cause of death was pronounced to be *paralysis of the heart.*

Dr. Hering was laid away in Laurel Hill Cemetery in a private lot belonging to Curwen Stoddard, one of his oldest patients and faithful adherents, from which he was later removed to a lot in another part of the cemetery belonging to his son, Walter E. Hering. The funeral was held on the morning of July 28th. I quote the following account of this occasion from a Memorial published shortly after his demise:

"A large number of the relatives and friends, including many homoeopathic physicians from other cities and the greater part of the profession of Philadelphia, assembled at the house, where the services were conducted by the Rev. S. S. Seward, pastor of the Swedenborgian Church of New York City.

"The remains were placed in the rear parlor, and, according to the custom of the Swedenborgians, in which faith Dr. Hering was a believer, they were encased in a white cloth-covered casket and strewn with flowers. A number of floral tributes, placed around the room, testified to the affection of friends and relatives. Release from life and its cares is looked upon rather as an occasion for joy than sorrow, according to the articles of the Swedenborgian faith. The services were opened by the singing of Dr. Hering's favorite hymn, *Befiehl Du deine Wege* (Commit thy ways unto Him), by a quartette choir.

"At the conclusion of Mr. Seward's address the choir sang a hymn, composed by Karl Eduard Hering, brother of the deceased, entitled *Am Grabe* (At the Grave) and at its close the casket was carried by the selected pallbearers to the hearse in waiting and then conveyed to North Laurel Hill Cemetery. Here the cortege was received by the members of Concordia and Saengerbund singing societies, who united in singing hymns during the interment. which was very impressive, scarcely a dry eye being seen among the numerous persons surrounding the place of burial.

"As the dull thud of mother earth was heard, shutting away from mortal sight the remains of the departed, the relatives and friends slowly and sadly wended their way homeward, feeling bereft of as sincere a friend as ever lived.

"Doctors W. B. Trites, J. C. Guernsey and C. Mohr remained until the grave had been filled, and after paying a last tribute of respect and affection by placing on the new-made grave the floral devices stricken hearts had lovingly tendered, they too proceeded homeward, leaving all that was mortal of Constantine Hering to the watchful eye of his Creator."

MEMORIAL MEETINGS WITH EULOGIES.

A Memorial meeting of the homoeopathic physicians was held in Philadelphia on Sunday afternoon, October 10, 1880, which was duplicated in various places in the world where Homoeopathic physicians were to be found, not all meetings being held on the same day, that being found impractiable.

Mention is made of meetings for the special purpose of doing honour to Dr. Hering in the following places, by the societies mentioned:

Onondago County Homoeopathic Medical Society of Northern New York; Michigan College of Physicians and Surgeons; British Homoeopathic Congress; New York State Society; Homoeopathic Medical Society of Pennsylvania; New York County Homoeopathic Medical Society; St. Louis Memorial Services; Meeting in Kansas City, Missouri; University of Michigan; Cleveland, Ohio; Denver, Colorado; Minneapolis, Minnesota; Topeka, Kansas; Wilmington, Delaware; Washington, D. C.; Schleswig-Holstein, Germany; Paris, France; Canadian Homoeopathic Institute; Maryland State Society; West Jersey Society; American Institute Memorial Service; and a Tribute from Italy. Many notices appeared in foreign journals.

At a meeting of the homoeopathic physicians of Philadelphia, held at the old Hahnemann Medical College at 1105 Filbert Street, on Sunday afternoon, July 25, 1880, at five o'clock, Dr. John K. Lee was called to the chair, and on motion, Dr. H. N. Guernsey was appointed secretary.

The chairman, having called the meeting to order, requested Dr. Lippe to state the object of the meeting. Dr. Lippe then spoke as follows:

The sad event that has called us together on this occasion is the sudden and unexpected death of our old and venerable colleague, Constantine Hering. Before I offer for your kind consideration and approval, a series of resolutions drawn up for this occasion, permit me to express my sentiments, and no doubt the sentiments of all those who have known our departed colleague best.

Dr. Constantine Hering deservedly and undisputedly was considered the father of the homeopathic school of medicine in the United States. It is now almost half a century since he came here, attracted by the institutions of the Republic, and here he remained to enjoy for himself, and his chosen school of medicine the fruits of a republican form of government.

Even at that early day the name of Constantine Hering was well known, the world over. His contributions to homeopathic literature, beginning in the *Archives*, secured him an honourable place among the foremost standard bearers of the law of cure.

Fifty years have passed since this scientist made his first observations on the sick-making properties of the poison of *Lachesis trigonocephalus*, and this observation and the deductions drawn from them as to its health restoring properties, would alone have made him what he was—a shining light among medical men.

The beginning of a great work was then made, and soon we find him giving us the first works on Homoeopathy in the English language, while engaged in teaching the new healing art at Allentown in this State. Later we find him publishing his Domestic Physician as a textbook for those who could not avail themselves of the assistance of the then few homoeopathic practitioners, a work which was translated into almost all languages; we find him a large contributor to the homoeopathic journals, and especially defending the teachings of Hahnemann, protesting against multiplying departures from the methods of the Master. Notwithstanding his increasing professional duties, we find him continually adding to the Homoeopathic Materia Medica; his numerous monographs on old and new remedies being an heirloom to posterity, so that this worker shall never be forgotten.

We find him teaching the principles and practices of the new school in private and in public. The caller on him who earnestly desired to learn, found him ever ready to give the wished for information; we find his enthusiasm not diminished as he grew older; his fidelity to our principles was as firm as were the enthusiastic hopes he entertained for the perpetuation of our school of medicine. Always ready to advance the true interests of homoeopathy, he took especial pleasure in guiding the younger members of the profession, by explaining to them the great results obtainable for the cure of the sick by following, strictly, honestly and persistently the rules and directions to be found in the methods of Hahnemann.

As an individual who has known our departed colleague for more than forty years, who profited by his kind instructions and example, who with him. as one of the early pioneers. saw the almost miraculous growth of our school of medicine. I can only faintly express the grief felt when so noble and so self-sacrificing a member of our school is removed from among us.

His works will live after him; coming generations will profit by them, and like the present will honor his memory.

———————

Dr. John C. Morgan being called upon addressed the chair as follows:

It is honourable to mankind that we love to praise the dead. But it is no ordinary eulogy that we pass upon him of whom we speak today. A personal friend has been torn from us; our most venerable leader has departed. Nestor no longer lives. How shall we fitly recount his worth? And where begin?

The magnanimous generosity of Dr. Hering to his colleagues and pupils of this city ought not to be unrecorded. In one respect he was lavish—exceeding anything I ever saw. A man of such abundant literary productiveness, and of such great usefulness to the profession, and to the interests of Homoeopathy, could not have found much time for making money by practice. A large and select practice he always had; and he acquired a modest competency; only that. But I confidently venture the assertion, that no homoeopathic physician ever enjoyed intimacy with him, but he has not only been deeply instructed, but also more than once or twice surprised by his transfer to him of valuable cases, and of excellent families, who had applied to him. The practitioners of surgery and midwifery, especially, have reason to remember the unexampled friendship of Dr. Hering. Unflinching in devotion to law and principle; merciless, possibly, in denouncing license under the law of our art; upright and downright in his consistency; successful in his practice; classic in his teaching; to these traits he added the humanities which today bind to his memory that innumerable host, who, in all ways, are the better and the happier for his living; and above all that phalanx of true workers who oft times filled their exhausted pitchers from his neverfailing fountain of knowledge and encouragement.

I thought this morning of that unfinished work "The Guiding Symptoms". Who will take it up? Who will take up any of the work he has been doing? Upon whom shall his mantle fall? May we not pray that his mantle may fall upon all of us, and shall we not all take up the work upon which he has so nobly spent his life?

I must, for a moment, refer to another aspect of the subject—must allude to the lifelong hostility of some who are today reaping where he has sowed. For many years I myself was kept aloof from him, whilst practising homoeopathy, by the assertion of some who professed to know him, that he was dogmatic, like his master Hahnemann; that he was visionary, like his master Hahnemann; that he was unreliable and ultra, like his master Hahnemann. Great, then, was my surprise when I came to know him for myself.

I thank Providence that I have lived long enough to learn better of him, and of his master Hahnemann. I have ever found Dr. Hering most pliable to the force of sound reason, and thus ever open to conviction. I have never met a man so willing to take suggestions from juniors as was Dr. Hering. I have never met a man so humbly a learner from all sources; never met a man in the homoeopathic ranks who was so completely *en rapport* with all the departments of modern science.

Were there new discoveries made, who was so eager to grasp them as Dr. Hering? When the spectroscope was introduced, who knew it so soon, and so well, as Dr. Hering? When Hausmann, the professor in the University of Pesth, Hungary, published his great work, showing, from the homoeopathic standpoint, parallel lines of evolution of both organic beings and their organic pabulum —when, I say, that great book, hardly understood to this day, in Europe or America, appeared, who introduced it? Who, of all the homoeopathic profession, took up that book and interpreted it to the profession? Who, but Dr. Hering? In all these things Dr. Hering has been found in the very front rank of medical and collateral science; and I wish to give this testimony as one somewhat intimate with him. He was as far from being the dogmatic extremist—the visionary symptomist—he has been represented, as was possible; nay, who does not admit, now, that he was in the very front rank of the medical men of our day?

Dr. Hering's influence as a teacher in Homoeopathy is today felt everywhere. An incident will illustrate it. A very successful physician in Illinois, a graduate of the Philadelphia College, said to me that while a student he attended Dr. Hering's private lectures also and added—"I studied general medicine from a homoeopathic standpoint in the college; but I really learned *Homoeopathy* from Dr. Hering in that back-office of his."

Dr. Hering was not only, however, a teacher of men. He humbled himself in an unusual way. His love, I may say *reverence for children*, was characteristic and unique. The simplicity of his own heart found its counterpart in them. When the Homoeopathic Fair was organized in 1869, he insisted that a prominent place must be assigned to a "Children's Table," asserting that no good would come of the enterprise were the children left out. He poetically said that they, having lately arrived from heaven, have the angels still with them; and that they are ever nearer heaven than their elders.

He had convictions, strong convictions, why not? And he felt that he had a mission in life.

It has been said, "whosoever wishes to live in this world in comfort and in quiet, let him beware of a man with a mission." That is a true saying. Let a man who wishes to be at his ease keep at a respectful distance from a man with a mission. Dr. Hering was such a man. He was alive to the question mooted, and particularly to the recent departures from first principles from some in the homoeopathic ranks. He had the conviction that he should resist them to the utmost. He believed in his own mission. Only a few weeks ago he said to me, referring to recent departures from fundamental Homoeopathy, and his purpose to defend it, "The Lord has kept me alive for that."

A man with such a conviction of his mission and the divine origin of it, and with such a knowledge of his subject, might be expected to appear dogmatic. Coming in contact with generation after generation of dogmatic tyros, let us rather say, such a man could not be expected to pause in his great lifework, to come down, on command, and wipe away all the cobwebs woven by their experience, with a gentle hand.

Dr. Hering has been among us as a *teacher!* Let us then revere, for their great worth, his teachings, as we all do his memory.

Dr. Augustus Korndoerfer spoke as follows:

I scarcely know how to express myself on this occasion. In fact, I had thought that I should say nothing, as being truly unfitted to express the depth of my feelings, at the death of our old friend, Dr. Hering.

I have been intimately connected with him during a decade. From the first of my acquaintance I felt that he was my friend. He had a firm and abiding friendship, and even at times when it seemed as though he were not the friend that you thought him, it was that he might do you good.

I would like, in addition to what has been said, however, to speak more fully of his great friendship to the young practitioner. His knowledge, his labors, his wondrous store of information, we all of us know; but not all knew how uniformly kind he was to the beginner in medicine. Hours were all as minutes to him, if he might help the young men, and the labor was pleasure to him, if he could render assistance to them. I well remember, during the early days of my acquaintance with him, how utterly he abhorred the idea of keeping a secret from the profession; how earnestly he insisted on every member of the profession making known, in season and out of season, every fact which might tend to the healing of the sick or rendering assistance in the slightest degree to the suffering. It is this phase of his character which has attracted me more than any other, for he showed it so freely during the many years.

In regard to his work, it has been said by some, as intimated by Dr. Morgan, that his work was unreliable because dogmatic. I can only say that the man who says that, utters what he knows to be worse than a falsehood. It is infamous! Dr. Hering never put his pen to paper except where he had the fullest authority for the truthfulness of what he wrote. Every word and line he wrote bore not only the evidence of having been taken from some authority, but of being from his own authority, because he accepted the diction of no man.

It has been said by some that he made notes and memoranda of the most ridiculous experiences of physicians; but as the doctor remarked to me in reference to this: "Yes, I do take notes of everything; a great deal of which I only find fit for the waste-basket; but I take notes. There might be some truth in them which only the future will reveal." This exactness, this slow work, was simply the result of the overcarefulness that characterized him —his perfect desire to give everything, in its perfect shape, to the profession. This I learned from intimate acquaintance with him.

He lived in faith; faith in homoeopathy and the divine mission he was called to fulfill. And he left it almost fulfilled. He left it with the conviction that he could now leave it to be finished by other hands. He said to me only a short time ago that we had men left in the ranks who could go on and finish what he, for want of time, could not complete.

There is not one, here present, but feels his loss, and will continue to feel that a good, earnest, true man has been called from our midst.

At the request of the Chair, Dr. J. C. Guernsey read the following letter from Dr. A. R. Thomas:

Sunday, July 25th, 1880

Dear Doctor:

Having an urgent professional call to the country, one which will make it impossible for me to be present at the meeting called for this p.m., I desire to take this method of expressing my full sympathy with any action that may be taken with the view of doing honor to the memory of the illustrous and lamented deceased.

While all will admit the wide influence of the labors of Dr. Hering in the past, and the fact that this influence must extend far into the coming future, what more fitting memorial of our appreciation of his labors, on the part of the profession, than a united and vigorous movement for securing, what he has so long labored and prepared for, what this community and the country have reason to expect of Philadelphia—a permanently established and large general hospital.

During the life of Dr. Hering the ultimate purpose of every act or thought was the promotion of the one great aim of his life—the development and dissemination of the principles of Homoeopathy. No sacrifice of money, time, or rest was too great when required for this object, and now, that the largest and ripest fruit of this labor may be gathered, there remains a work for us to perform, and one that should command the united and hearty cooperation of every member of the profession.

Regretting that I am unable to join personally in the action of the meeting, I am,

Very truly yours,

A. R. THOMAS.

Dr. Pemberton Dudley said:

I feel that no words of ours can at all express what we feel at the loss, the profession and the world have sustained in the death of Dr. Hering. I think and know, that the homoeopathic profession should feel today very much as the passenger feels, away out from the coast, when the pilot takes leave of the ship; because whatever may have been the perfection with which the law under which we labor was developed by Hahnemann, it required something more than Hahnemann to establish the art and principles of medicine, under the law, throughout the world. Hahnemann was a man of research, as was Hering, but Hering was a man of different mould; the man to establish the new system in a new world.

The question is asked: Who will take Dr. Hering's place? Nobody will take it. The world does not need another Hering. Homoeopathy does not need to be established a second time in Amercia. We no more need another Hering than we need another Newton, another Kepler or another Washington. Homoeopathy is established now, and will go on doing universal good throughout the civilized world.

There were very few men, perhaps none, who could do the work that he has done. But there are other men, weaker perhaps, who can take up the work where he has left it. I believe that there is a Providence watching over homoeopathy; and I believe we should take the death of Dr. Hering as an evidence that God watches over our cause. It will occur to all that the death of Dr.

Hering fell upon an anniversary, fifty-two years from the day when homoeopathy was first introduced into the State: and his funeral occurs upon another, fifty-two years from the day when he first secured his *Lachesis*.

But we have other evidences that Homoeopathy is going right on with renewed vigor. There is a tendency in men to lean upon each other; but in order to strengthen a man he must be made to lean upon himself—to strengthen the spinal column put a weight upon his shoulders. I question whether we have not been leaning on him too much, and now that he is gone, whether we will not feel that there is more resting upon us; whether the rising generation will not feel that there is a burden resting on them that their predecessors did not feel; whether, when we feel that the death of Dr. Hering has severed a link between us and Hahnemann, cut us loose from the time when there was no Homoeopathy, it will not give us a new impetus that will carry us on to victories still more glorious than those we have already achieved?

Dr. Lee, chairman of the meeting, then said:

It is hardly necessary for me to say anything after the liberal expressions already made, of the high respect I have for the memory of Dr. Hering.

I felt, when the announcement was made of his death, that truly a great man had fallen. But perhaps, as Dr. Dudley has said, it may produce a distribution of labors which may lead to good. A supervising Providence never leaves a work that needs its protection; and I would merely express the exhortation: let us try and imitate the illustrious example set by Dr. Hering, who was willing to sacrifice fortune, and reckless of all personal interests to further the cause of Homoeopathy. If we all had his enthusiasm, victory would be far nearer than it seems.

Telegrams from a number of physicians in various parts of the United States expressing the great loss the medical profession had sustained in the death of Dr. Hering, were read.

A number of names of members of the profession, friends of Dr. Hering, constituting "The Old Guard" were named as pallbearers at the funeral.

These were: Chas. G. Raue, M. D., Philadelphia
     James Kitchen, M. D.,   "
     Ad. Lippe, M. D.,   "
     H. N. Guernsey, M. D., "

C. Neidhard, M. D.,   "
A. W. Koch, M. D.,   "
A. R. Thomas, M. D.,   "
J. H. Pulte, M. D., Cincinnati
Wm. Wesselhoeft, M. D., Boston
F. R. McManus, M. D., Baltimore
H. Detwiller, M. D., Easton
John Romig, M. D., Allentown
P. P. Wells, M. D., Brooklyn
Edw. Bayard, M. D., New York
John F. Gray, M. D.,   "   "
S. Lilienthal, M. D.,   "   "

Memorial meetings were held in many places through-out the world where Constantine Hering's name was revered.

At the meeting of the New York State Society, held in Brooklyn, September 7, 1880, Dr. P. P. Wells of Brooklyn, spoke as follows:

Mr. President: Before proceeding to read what I have written, it will be, perhaps, but just to myself to say that I was taken alto-gether by surprise last evening on receiving notice that I had been appointed to prepare resolutions commemorative of the death of our colleague, Dr. Hering. The time given in which to arrange my thoughts appropriately to so vast a subject and put them on paper, was so brief that it was exceedingly embarrassing. The interest that I have in the memory of that great man, and the many years of intimacy I have had with him, forbade my declining to attempt, as best I could, to present to you this morning the brief preamble and resolutions which I now read:

In Oschatz, in Saxony, on January 1, 1800, it pleased Almighty God to give a great blessing to the world of science, and to the world of suffering, in the birth of an infant, who afterwards be-came known as the man Constantine Hering. It pleased the same Almighty goodness to remove him from us, by death, on the twenty-third day of July, 1880. In view of the life and the labors which filled the space between these points of time there are to be mentioned:

1st. Gratitude to Him who gave so long life, and so great powers for good, to our friend, and brother, and that for so many years He gave it to us to receive inspiration from his great knowl-edge and generous spirit, becoming to us our leader and teacher, our father and friend, our light in the art of healing, and our example in his never failing devotion to the cause and interests of truth in all the time and circumstances through which he passed.

2nd. Gratitude to the memory of him by whose labors we have been so greatly enriched.

3rd. That in Hering, the philosopher, we remember his vast extent of knowledge, his vigorous pursuit and grasp of facts, his ready appropriation of these and his facile tracing of the relationship of new facts to old, and their sure reference to their proper place in the circle of facts known.

4th. That in him, as a teacher, we remember his clear perception of facts, and of just those his pupil needed first to know, and his skill in imparting them in the manner and sequence best adapted to meet these needs, and his heartfelt gladness in giving from his fulness to the wants of all who would learn. That he never was weary of adding to the knowledge of others from the vast treasures he had gathered in his long life of unexampled activity.

5th. As a physician, we remember his loyalty to his convictions of truth, and to the law of healing he had accepted from the great Master; his clear perception of the facts of disease and of the specification of the agencies he employed for its cure, and his never-failing or faltering endeavors to add to the number of these, and from these endeavors have come to us a knowledge of many of our most precious remedies.

6th. As an author, we remember the great number and excellence of the productions of his pen, each bearing in clear characters the impress of the individuality and genius of the writer, the whole making a series of unexampled extent, interest and value. We remember these as abounding in compact thought, with facts contributed to our knowledge, with suggestions of relationships of these to other facts and to each other; all so luminous with the effulgence of genius, and so astonishing by reason of the great labors they disclose. We remember that it is to these labors that the literature of Homoeopathy is indebted for more than half its wealth.

7th. As a man, we remember him as largely endowed by nature with the noblest qualities; frank, generous, affectionate, true, noble in his aspirations, loving the good and hating all that was mean, he has left to us a memory to which we can always recur with pleasure and profit. As the embodiment of great knowledge and learning, by his death he impresses us with a sense of our great loss, and we are constrained to feel, and to say, we shall never look upon his like again.

At the same meeting Dr. Samuel Lilienthal, of New
York, spoke as follows:

Will you allow me, in seconding these resolutions, to say a few
words about our departed friend. One thing which endeared him
to all those who were acquainted with him was the great encouragement he always held out to the young. There was no difference
manifested in him, no matter who it was that came. Anyone who
came to him poor went away rich. Another thing which I always
admired so much in Constantine Hering was that you never heard
him say, "Homoeopathy will go down". He knew, as one of the
founders of Homoeopathy, that the legacy was left in good hands,
and I am sure our young men will take pride in following such a
good example as that which Constantine Hering left to them. I
remember on one occasion he said, "I have no fears for homoeopathy; we shall mix with other schools, and I am pretty sure that
the others schools will come to us." Dr. Hering died in harness.
At six o'clock on the evening of his death he made his last prescription.

It was a beautiful trait in his character that he knew the great
resources of the Materia Medica and when others despaired he was
hopeful. His memory should be sacred to us.

MEETING OF THE HOMOEOPATHIC MEDICAL
SOCIETY OF PENNSYLVANIA

The President, John K. Lee, concluded his address
with the following words:

As an appendix to these desultory thoughts, I would ask your
permission to pay a brief tribute to our late colleague and collabor-
ator, the illustrous Dr. Hering. With natural ambition of a high
order, strengthened and developed by careful culture, he, in early
life, for the purpose of refutation, applied himself to the study of
Homoeopathy and as his logical mind advanced in this investigation
and he turned the clear light of reason upon its alleged principles,
and placed their proofs into the crucible of experience, the vigor of
his prejudice relaxed and gave way to convictions, and these convictions gradually hardened into firm belief; like Paul who went
out to persecute saints, he renounced his hostility and became the
champion of a new medical faith. Placing himself in communication with Hahnemann, he received a full revelation of this truth
and its corollaries, and imbued with the sentiments of his master,
and an ardent desire for their triumph, he sought an asylum in the

New World. where under the protecting aegis of our free institutions, he could accomplish his mission without embarrassment or interference.

Here, for nearly half a century, with untiring industry and zeal he prosecuted his researches. and from the perennial fountain of his pen flowed a continuous stream to fertilize the seed he had planted; and ere his great heart had ceased its pulsations. his eyes were ravished with a view of the waving harvest as a reward of his benevolent and useful labors.

Truly a great man has fallen—great intellectually, and great in simplicity and grandeur of character, greater still in the possession of those moral attributes which elevate man to that exalted plane where he can abnegate himself and make all personal considerations subordinate to the higher and holier interests of a common brotherhood.

His last moments were a fitting climax to his distinguished labors. since amid the undisturbed repose and endeared associations of his study, surrounded by his unpublished manuscripts and other evidences of his unremitting toil, he at once ceased to write and to live.

He requires no marble shaft to preserve the reward of his life or to tell the story of his achievements, for his history is the warp and woof of nearly every page of our literature; his memory will be cherished by thousands yet unborn, and his fame will only brighten by the lapse of time.

While we may not be able to receive the mantle that has fallen from his shoulders, we can imitate the brilliant example of his devotion to the cause he so ably espoused; and ere his lifeless form will have faded into dust and the wintry winds wail their plaintive requiem over his grave, let us renew our vows of fidelity to Homoeopathy, and endeavor to realize, as he eminently did that "He most lives who thinks most—feels the noblest—acts the best."

––––––––––––

At the conclusion of the address, a committee consisting of Doctors J. H. McClelland, Aug. Korndoerfer and H. Detwiller was appointed to draft suitable resolutions of respect, and in due time the chairman of the committee presented the following:

The Homoeopathic Medical Society of Pennsylvania, in an annual session assembled, with unanimous voice adopts the following minute:

The death of Dr. Constantine Hering. of Philadelphia. on the 23rd of July, 1880, is recognized as an event of signal import in the history of medicine. It marks the close of a life, remarkable for unflagging and long sustained industry in the cause of medical science and in promoting the good of his kind. With full recognition of his prodigious labors in the field of Materia Medica and Homoeopathic Therapeutics, the attainments of Dr. Hering, in general science and letters, entitle him to a high place among men of learning in this enlightened age.

This Society, therefore, records with willing hands its high appreciation of the distinguished dead, and with sentiments of high regard, offers heartfelt sympathy to the bereaved family.

THE NEW YORK COUNTY HOMOEOPATHIC MEDICAL SOCIETY

Dr. Edward Bayard, of New York, long an intimate friend, made the following address at a meeting of the New York County Homoeopathic Medical Society on October 7th, 1880:

If a great man is one to whom God has given large gifts, and who has cultivated them to the extent of his powers for the best interests of his fellow-beings, then Constantine Hering was a great man.

He was not a money-getter. His powers did not work in the direction of accumulating property. He did not care to amass this world's goods; but he wished to be rich in learning, especially in all that pertained to his profession.

He was logical, discriminating, a great lover of nature, and a close observer of her. He was a hard student, of unwearied industry. He sought Truth earnestly, and he found it. He made note of all his observations; hence he left behind him a large amount of valuable writing.

He was engaged at the time of his death in a great work, his "Guiding Symptoms" and would to God he had been permitted to finish that work; but it was otherwise ordered. I am told by those who knew his habits, that every sentence in that work was studied over, sometimes for hours, that its true meaning might be expressed. That he might lose no time, his writing desk and materials were placed close to the side of his couch, so that he could arise in the night, light the lamp and continue his work. As for recreation and amusement, he knew little of either outside of his profession.

While a subject of the Saxon Government he was commissioned to make collections as a naturalist in Surinam, South America. In the course of this study he found facts illustrating the truth of

Homoeopathy, and gave account of them to a homoeopthic journal in Germany. His government objected to this work as heterodox. Dr. Hering thought he ought not to be controlled, in any respect, in the service of scientific truth. Upon the instant he resigned his commission and sought a free land, where his thoughts, or the expression of them for the advancement of his race, would not be controlled. He found such freedom in this country.

This showed his noble independence of character, and his earnest search and love of Truth, which would not permit him to weigh against her a social position and a money consideration. He sought this New World to work, and to plow the field the providence of God assigned to him, with gifts to carry out fully and nobly his work, ere he was called away to be set in the heavens by the side of Hahnemann, Boenninghausen, Stapf and Jahr—a galaxy whose light will continue when the things of this earth and its monuments of brass and stone have crumbled.

Is it not wise and right that we should look into the sheaves of the rich harvest garnered by our late beloved colleague for our own instruction, and that we should examine into the principles that governed him in the profession and practice to which he devoted his life, and in which he stood out so eminently the acknowledged leader?

Dr. Hering made this the essential point of doctrine and practice to cure the sick easily and permanently, by medicines capable in themselves of producing in a healthy person morbid symptoms similar to those of the sick. He sought no other cure, nor recognized it as one, unless it was under the law proclaimed by Hahnemann. He sought no palliation, except under this law, believing that it hindered and endangered a perfect cure. He believed that the morbid condition of tissues are the result of the dynamic disturbance, and not the cause of disease. He was therefore a Vitalist—believing the disease to be the disturbance of the vital force, and its equalization the state of health. He believed that the totality of symptoms, subjective and objective, are the only indications for the choice of a remedy. He did not believe that prescribing on the pathological states, nor diagnosis where the vital powers were tending to those states, were sufficient to effect a cure. The symptoms in their totality alone were the only guide for a cure to him.

He believed that the only proper way to ascertain the disturbing properties of medicine upon the vital force is to prove them on the healthy; that thereby only the true expression of that disturbance can be observed. And he believed that in order to obtain and secure the highest curative results, medicines must be administered singly, and in a dose just sufficient to cure, because he knew that all action is followed by reaction (there is no exception to this law); that all action on the vital powers is, by an inherent law, followed sooner or later by reaction, which terminates in cure and health. Hence an overdose must, by its intensity of action, delay or prevent reaction and cure.

I remember on a certain occasion, early in my practice, I told Dr. Hering of my suffering. He asked me the remedy I had taken, and seemed to think it well chosen. He then asked the dilution. I told him the third. "Ah", said he, "you have stopped it; perhaps not made a cure." He shook his head and seemed disappointed. He said no more: but he caused me to reflect that it might well be so—that I had thrown an obstacle before the diverted vital force—that I had stayed its forward movement by a shock which had injured its reactive powers—as a boulder thrown in front of a carriage wheel in motion not only stops it, but also cripples the wheel.

Dr. Hering believed that when he produced the impression at the right point, and in the right direction, the force must be permitted to be exhausted: therefore he waited. Shorter or longer the time he waited, his eyes wide open, and his observation on a stretch, looking for that action which is to end in equalization.

Dr. Constantine Hering was a true Homoeopathist. He believed in Homoeopathy and lived up to it. He believed that the highest results in his art were obtained by close individualization alone: not by generalization.

I loved him for his simplicity and directness of character; for his large brilliant inquiry after truth, and for his resting on principles derived from a patient examination of facts.

He enriched our Materia Medica by his severe labors. I will not name the many remedies he has proven, arranged and published. You know them all. The diligent student of our Materia Medica must have observed how full, exact and characteristic. He took his great master, Hahnemann, as his model, and we only hope that those who have the direction of arranging and publishing his writings will give them to us just as he set them down. Then we shall feel that the seal of reliability is placed upon them.

When some patient astronomer, who night after night has been watching the stars, brings to light some unknown planet, to do him honor the newborn world is called after his name, and the discoverer is never to be forgotten. If the astronomer is worthy of distinction, what shall we say of the man who brings to light a new remedial agent to relieve suffering humanity, ward off death and bring back health? He, methinks, has done a greater work. And so the great discovered of *Lachesis* will be gratefully remembered by those who know how to apply this remedy in all its varied forms, for which in the provings he suffered; and his only suffering was from the seal set by *Lachesis* from which he never fully recovered. That suffering was a crown of glory for him.

Constantine Hering showed in his death his medical principles, and showed that if the homoeopathic law, the law proclaimed by Hahnemann, was followed, a man would live longer and die easier than under any other practice; for he that is filled with disturbing drugs must die as the hunted fox, torn and rent by the bloody mouths of a pack of hounds. But he that follows the practice of our beloved colleague, will have sleep rather than death. The forces equalized, he has rest. He ceases to exist, by the withdrawal of his life by the Giver of life, like some locomotive running smoothly upon the track, after exhausting her fuel, slows down and stops— not thrown from the rails by broken machinery and rushing to ruin with terrible violence.

At six o'clock in the evening he made his last prescription to a patient, observing to his wife with great animation and interest, that this patient had been prescribed for by many physicians, and he believed he should help him. Then he went, as he was accustomed, to take his evening meal with his family, which he greatly enjoyed in that social circle under an arbor in his garden. At eight o'clock, the meal being over, Dr. Hering said he would retire to his study and his couch. His devoted wife went with him to aid him in preparing for bed. He said to her: "I believe I shall sleep." She left him to his repose. At nine-thirty he touched his bell, which summoned her at once to his side. He remarked that his breathing was embarrassed; accompanied by constant yawning. He asked her to get a book in his office that he might examine this symptom. She did as directed; but, being alarmed, sent for a physician. He tried to select a remedy, but too late; a short time after his last words, "I am dying now," were spoken, he passed into that sleep which knows no waking. The great physician demonstrated the benign, gentle, but controlling influence of the action of the great law to which he devoted his life. Thus died Constantine Hering, dear to Homoeopathy, and to be forever honoured by its true practitioners.

———

Dr. Samuel Lilienthal said:

For the little that I am, the little I ever accomplished, the little reputation I have gained, I have to thank two men, who have gone home to do more precious work in higher spheres—I mean Carroll Dunham and Constantine Hering.

The day I made the personal acquaintance of Father Hering will never be forgotten, as long as I live. In the beginning of the year

1870. I had received an invitation from the faculty of the Hahnemann College, in Philadelphia, to deliver a lecture during the
preliminary course. Our mutual friend, Dr. Raue, introduced me
to the Father of Homoeopathy in America. With that even, cheerful smile on his face, he looked at me attentively, and then, with a
sonorous laugh, he addressed Raue: "I thought I would see a young
man before me, and now that hardworking Lilienthal is as grey
as I am." I soon found myself at home, in the full sense of the
word, in his company, and when after that lecture we met at Raue's
house to spend a few hours in convivial conversation, Constantine
Hering was the life of the whole company.

It is just ten years ago, perhaps eleven, when the firm of Boericke
& Tafel bought out Mr. Radde, in New York, and seriously intended
to give up the *North American Journal of Homoeopathy*. Hering
would not listen to it. "There is your editor," he said pointing to
me; "and we must support him." Relying on this great support,
not in words but in deeds, I accepted the trust and Hering never
disappointed the readers of the Quarterly. In fact, this was one
of the great traits of this great and good man, that his word was as
good as his bond, and as number after number appeared for the
last ten years, he kept on cheering to the last; and now that he has
departed, I consider it my duty to collect from the old German
literature the writings of our Father, and give them to you in that
old Quarterly of mine.

During the Centennial World's Convention in Philadelphia,
friend Raue was again my host, and one day, visiting Papa Hering,
he requested me to invite some congenial spirits and meet that
night, quietly, at Raue's. Though it was the night of the big ball
and it rained in torrents, the old man came to 121 North Tenth
Street according to promise, and I can never forget the happy hours
passed there. Hering and Dunham were sitting on the sofa together, Dunham asking and Hering answering, and we, a dozen or
so, listening to that interesting conversation. The rain had stopped;
it was a clear night, and when we broke up Hering was so happy
he would not ride home, and invited us as his body-guard, to accompany him the short distance. The next morning Dunham and
myself compared notes at the Continental Hotel, and, Dunham
said: "We felt better for having spent such an evening, with such
a master, and we envied the physicians who could (night after
night) enjoy such a privilege."

It was my habit to make, year after year, my pilgrimage to this
holy shrine, and I always left it highly satisfied with my gain. I
learned my lessons in liberality and charity from Dunham; I
learned from Hering to value the opinions of others, and to despise
those who preach one thing and practice another. Any falsity

was an abomination to his straight-forward manner, and the language he then could use, was more forcible than elegant.

He always felt happy in the midst of the young and rising generation, and none ever left him without an encouraging word. Envy was unknown to him, for he knew that he had done his duty to humanity, and no one was more pleased than Father Hering with the increase of our Homoeopathic literature. The one great fault which this master had, was that he tried too much, began too much, as if life would last forever. His restless mind knew only work, work, work, and if tired of one thing there were many wakeful ganglia in that large brain, suggesting more work to be performed, and to be accomplished. For this reason we find in that glorious room, up stairs, and in those safes treasures garnered, which he intended to give to us, piece by piece; but three score years and ten, perhaps four more, the allotted time, is not enough, and though a gracious Providence spared him for so long to us, the clock has run down.

Let us honor the memory of Constantine Hering by continuing those masterly works which he mapped out for us during his lifetime.

Thus, though departed, he still lives in us and with us.

Remarks of Dr. Timothy F. Allen:

Some of our colleagues can speak of the departed hero, whom we commemorate this evening, as a fellow-laborer, as one with whom they toiled in their earlier as well as during their more mature years.

To me, he seems like a pioneer, one whose labors were to be built upon, one who prepared the way, hewed straight paths through the thickets and let light into dark places.

This feeling toward him had birth when one winter's evening, twenty years ago, my revered preceptor, Dr. P. P. Wells, took me to a meeting at the house of Dr. Joslin, the elder, on the corner of University Place and Thirteenth Street. How vividly I remember that evening, the calm, philosophical Joslin, the earnest Bayard, the positive Wells, the dogmatic Reisig, the keen-eyed Fincke and the enthusiastic life and centre of all—Hering. I was the only young man present, fresh from the University, full of the teachings of the scholastics, full of the old-time prejudices of my father.

That group of men, that enthusiasm of Hering, the whole tone of thought was so different from that of the schools, that I was forced to believe in a vitalizing truth in Homoeopathy. I ventured one little remark to Dr. Wells during the evening. Dr. Reisig was

explaining some preparation of *Castile soap*, which he considered
a specific for burns. He was in the habit of applying it locally
and of giving a potency internally, and Dr. Hering was combatting
the local application. I asked Dr. Wells, almost in a whisper,
"But does it cure?" "Cure", thundered Reisig, "of course it does."
Hering looked at me, smiled, and said, "That was a good question."
My heart warmed toward him, and from that time we were friends,
though he did not always approve of my way of doing things.

Hering was always searching for truth; he despised no contribution to his large knowledge, however humble its source; he
proved all things and held fast to that which is good. One cannot
but be impressed by the avidity with which he sought for the truth,
while reading his earlier contributions to homoeopathic literature.
His first article is in the *Archiv fuer Homoeopatische Heilkunst*,
for 1828, a letter to the editor, Dr. Stapf, from Surinam, dated
September 28th, 1827. Prefacing the letter the editor remarks:
"These communications from Dr. Hering, of Dresden, who is well-
known to several readers of this *Archiv* and highly esteemed as a
zealous naturalist and warm friend of Homoeopathy, now, for more
than a year journeying to South America studying the natural
sciences and medicine, deserve a place in this journal on account
of interesting notes concerning the diseases of those countries and
their homoeopathic treatment; they will also be peculiarly welcome
to those more nearly related to him, giving, as they do, information concerning his life and doings."

First he gives us a careful analysis of seasickness and his experience with *Cocculus*, 12th, followed by *Staphisagria* 30th. In
succeeding communications he relates his experience with Leprosy,
the symptoms of which he studied most carefully. The enthusiasm
with which he took up the study of *Psorinum*—the provings of
which Hahnemann reluctantly, and after patient investigations
allowed to be published—was characteristic of the man; now was
his restless mind content. He seemed to see boundless possibilities
in the "Nosodes," and took up the fascinating, but fatal doctrine
of Isopathy, and enlarged, embellished and generalized from it, till
he found the bottom of soft, slimy ooze, which he then struggled
out of and hastened to wash clean off his skirts. In his latter years
he saw clearly that it was fatal to Homoeopathy, and, like a true
savant he retracted all he had said in its favor.

I can testify, with thousands, to his large heartedness, to his
never failing generosity. In the special work on Materia Medica
which I have undertaken, he has always been ready, even anxious,
to help me; from the time when I translated his provings of
Aloes, Apis, etc., for the *American Homoeopathic Review*, to my
latest task, I am proud to acknowledge with gratitude the en-

couragement and assistance of Dr. Hering. We differed in some things and he has bereated me soundly for differing, but his help continued.

His faith in the homoeopathic law of cure was boundless; his faith in his friends almost equally boundless; by nature, trusting as trustworthy, he gathered from everybody. and his shelves, groaning beneath the weight of the harvest, testify to his unwearied industry.

We shall do higher honor to Constantine Hering by imitating his example. Could he have desired more than that? There has never been a time in the history of Homoeopathy when it was more necessary to hold fast to the first principles of our faith; never a time when more were inquiring the way to save the sick than now, and shall we relax our firm grasp upon what we know to be right, for the sake of gaining popularity? Hering knew, as we know, that the chief principles of Hahnemann are laws of nature. Let us then imitate him. Let us be enthusiastic. Let us be scientific. Let us be industrious. Let us seek the good that is in everyone and help one another. So shall we honor Hering.

Dr. Joseph Finch said:

Mr. President: I wish this evening to add my humble testimony to the worth of the great and good man who has gone from us.

In regard to the death of our friend Dr. Constantine Hering, there can be but one sentiment, one feeling, viz., that of loss, irreparable loss, the extent of which we do not realize tonight, but shall more and more in the days to come.

The immediate circle in which he lived and moved has parted with its brightest light and its sincerest friend; and those who have only known him through the medium of his zealous labors with his pen, missing the profoundness of his research and the unusual clearness of his statements, will gather up and cherish what he has given, with a double care.

Homoeopathy has lost her eldest son, her clearest-sighted pioneer, her bravest defender. He was her Nestor in America. and when she writes his epitaph many words will be required, each a picture in itself, to describe the hero she has lost, the friend she has buried.

His unparallelled devotion to Homoeopathy was not the outgrowth of fidelity to a school, nor could it be justly attributed to the impulses of an ambitious nature. It was founded in the deepest conviction of an earnest heart, and stimulated by a manly love of truth.

He was not partisan in feeling. He was not a hobbyist, but a scientist that commanded the admiration of his friends and the respect of his foes. But he has gone, and our grieving shall be tempered by submission to the will and wisdom of that Divine Providence which gave him to us at the first, which sustained him so long and well in his professional career, and hath in the full harvest-time gathered him so peacefully to the garner of refined and ripened life—his home in the skies.

Dr. C. Th. Liebold said:

Mr. President: I am not a convert to Homoeopathy; I have been brought up in the faith. In fact, among my earliest recollections is the magic relief of a very severe pain by two or three diminutive sugar pellets, administered after careful selection, in "Hering's *Homoeopathicher Hausarzt*", (Domestic Physician) by my parents. I have never wavered in my faith; neither the ridicule nor the scientific contempt of greater or lesser medical and non-medical lights has ever, for a moment, been able to extinguish the memory of the fact that it did help. Not that I have ever remained faithful to the smallest possible pellets or to any other "dictum" about the "dose", but nothing has struck me more forcibly or made me a more confirmed homoeopath than the attendance on lectures on Allopathic Materia Medica. On one side the advice never to give more than just enough to cure; on the other from Arsenic down to Zingiber, how much a patient could possibly bear without doing him serious harm, and so-and-so much will kill a large dog, while so-much will finish a puppy.

Reminded to present also my mite at this memorial meeting, I rummaged among my old papers and found a copy of a letter addressed to Dr. Hering, nearly fifteen years ago, soon after I had settled in this city. The occasion was a letter written to a mutual acquaintance but indirectly to me, inquiring about information on some questions concerning the eyes. The first was the dilatation of the pupil by atropia to facilitate ophthalmoscopic examinations, and whether it would not cause permanent mydriasis in some cases? The second: what was really the cause of the sparkling of the eyes (Augenglaenzen)? The third: what are the crossed rhombic lines in the field of vision? It does not matter about the answers, I only hope to be able to follow. Some years later I remember he asked my opinion about that mischievous but plausible humbug of dry-cupping of the eyeball.

The last years have brought some antagonistic views to light, about the enucleation of a diseased eyeball in certain cases, to prevent the loss by sympathetic ophthalmia of the other sound eye; in regard to which I will only say that every oculist will be glad to learn that medicine will be able to prevent permanently such a disastrous result. All such controversies not only do no harm in the end, but are absolutely necessary to elicit the truth, and if they are conducted in the sole interest of the truth, they will benefit both sides. I do not believe that his hottest, but honest opponent, will ever say that Constantine Hering ever had any other aim in view in his whole life. Blessed be his memory among us, always.

Dr. J. W. Dowling said:

If anything could be added to the perfect happiness that exists in Heaven, I should say that our dear old patriarch, brother and friend, as he looks down upon us from his celestial and eternal home, is rendered supremely happy at listening to the kind words which, with stirring eloquence, have been spoken, and which have come from the hearts of warm friends and admirers to whom his memory is still fresh and dear.

It seems as if nothing was left for me to say. Those who are my seniors—who have known him perhaps longer than I—have justly sounded his praises, have pictured his virtues, his honesty, his earnestness and zeal in advocating a cause dear to him, not for advantages he himself derived, but because of the benefits it conferred upon suffering humanity.

This is not an occasion for mourning, but rather of rejoicing. It is true he has left us; his earthly remains have been laid in the ground, but why should we be sad? Was he not with us half a score of years beyond the allotted time of man? Should we not rejoice that this long, this spotless life had been one of usefulness and of unremitting labor in the cause he loved so well—to the very last? Should we not rejoice that the results of those labors of his later years are living, and will live to aid us and our children in the work to which our lives are being devoted? Should not we, who respect and love him, rejoice that through his long and active life, not a truthful word had ever been uttered that could reflect upon his character as a man—as a christian—and that at the last his death was peaceful, calm and free from protracted suffering? Should we not rejoice that his sorrows—for he had sorrows—sorrows hard to bear, too, are at an end, and that there is before him an eternity of happiness? For I believe of such as he is the kingdom of heaven.

The following note was sent by Dr. B. F. Joslin:

I am being prevented by a cold from being present at the meeting this evening, but I desire to contribute one word of praise to the memory of the illustrous Hering.

I wish to say, that if in his long and useful life he had but given us the proving of *Lachesis*, he would have been entitled to the everlasting gratitude of mankind.

Dr. Egbert Guernsey said:

It is my misfortune never to have had a personal acquaintance with Dr. Hering, but the magnetism of his mind was so diffused through all his works, that a personal acquaintance was hardly necessary to know the man. Were I asked to write his epitaph, I should say, as was said of Sir Christopher Wren, beneath the stately dome of St. Paul, reared by his genius: "Look around you!" Dr. Hering can have no nobler epitaph than his pure, almost blameless life, and the broad catholic spirit and the earnest scientific research found in all of his public works, which have placed him in the first rank of profound, practical thinkers in the medical world. Aside from the scientific value of his life's work, we are forcibly struck with that spirit of christian kindness and charity, which we shall do well to imitate. He was, in every sense of the word, a christian gentleman, and illustrated in his life and writings how a man can be truly great and noble when divested of bitterness and selfishness. By none will he be more deeply mourned, and his memory held in greater reverence, than by the younger workers in the field, who looked to him as father and friend.

Dr. George S. Norton said:

Having known Dr. Hering for several years, both in a professional and social way, it gives me pleasure to record my appreciation of him as a physician and as a man. In his home life there was much to admire. Wife and children were devoted to him, and he to them. His hospitality was well known and it always gave him great satisfaction to see his friends gathered at his table; all were made welcome, and all could not help but to enjoy those delightful, instructive talks with the gifted Father Hering.

One of his chief pleasures and relaxations from work was on a Sunday afternoon, when a circle of old friends assembled in his reception room, and over their cigars and coffee compared experiences and discussed various subjects. Neither hot, cold, nor stormy weather interfered with those social gatherings.

Of his investigations and teachings of our Homoeopathic Materia Medica. I need not speak, as his extensive knowledge, diligent researches, and practical additions to this important department of medicine are known to you all—yes, not only to us, but to all in every land and clime who have studied the law of similia.

It therefore seems to me as if the most comprehensive and fitting eulogy to his worth is expressed in the words: Constantine Hering, a Father to Homoeopathy.

Dr. Alfred K. Hills:

It is with no small degree of effort and embarrassment that I attempt to find words in which to express my respect for one so great as he is whose memory we meet tonight.

As we younger members of the profession glance reflectively over such a life as that of our late colleague, it inspires us to greater energy in the living of our own. His was filled not only with the most industrious effort, but he gave freely of what he had and without the asking, to all those who chose to avail themselves of the results from his researches.

With him nothing professional was secret, could not possibly be kept as such, and he had the greatest abhorrence for any who attempted this practice. His precept always was, make everything known that may, by any possibility, be of service to another.

We could scarcely find his equal in the world of science, as a student, and few have originated more than he.

What greater epitaph could be placed over his resting-place than the words *"Lachesis"*, *"Glonoine"* and "Guiding Symptoms of our Materia Medica". Certainly no one individual could hope for more than this would express.

Our appreciation of his devotion to that cause which we all hold so dear, justly emphasized by many, cannot be repeated too often by those who love and cherish his memory.

Let us, therefore, emulate his example in our faithfulness, and then we may hope for that reward which is vouchsafed only to such.

Remarks of Dr. L. Hallock:

Dr. Constantine Hering may, I think, be regarded as next to Hahnemann in the value and amount of his labors for the interests of Homoeopathy.

Every reader of the periodic literature of our school must have been surprised at the number and variety of his contributions.

Nothing but talents of the highest order, united with earnest zeal and tireless industry, could have furnished so many and so valuable practical essays as he has given to the profession. Besides his large and systematic works, the numerous additions to our Materia Medica furnished by his incessant labors, have placed our school under everlasting obligation to respect and to honor his memory.

Among these additions *Lachesis* has long been prominent as one of the most valuable remedies at our command. More recently his elaborate and minute articles on the history, effects and therapeutic value of *Lyssin* evidence an amount of patient research and self-denying devotion truly surprising in one so occupied in active professional duties. The thoroughness of his work is well illustrated in the extended pathogenesis of this potent remedy by experiments upon himself as well as upon others, until, as he expressed it, "terrible forebodings warned him of the danger of further trials." Such bold and self-sacrificing labors for science and humanity certainly deserve our admiration and gratitude. The writings of Dr. Hering seem designed to be clear, forcible and practical, and when from their frequent novelty and boldness they were sometimes received with adverse, or doubting criticism, were defended with the energy and ability of conscious integrity.

Remarks of Dr. E. Carleton, Jr.:

Mr. President: In response to your request to speak, I will offer my humble tribute to the character of our departed friend, by saying that I felt love and reverence for him.

I remember, as if it were but yesterday, the first time we met. It was in his office as physician and patient. He stood and looked at me calmly, while I related my symptoms. Then, silently turning to his desk, he prepared three powders and handed them to me with directions: I left him in wonder, for my case had troubled the physician who had sent me, and I had expected a long search. The remedy produced a violent aggravation, and I recollect that wonder temporarily gave place to a state of mind akin to resentment.

Recovery followed, and so did my promised report to the doctor. The recital of the success of his prescription caused his face to smile all over, which ended with a hearty, genial laugh and he said, "That was *Aloes*; it was low; it was the five hundredth." Then seating himself and motioning me to a chair, he went on to relate how he had suffered similarly when proving the drug, and made me promise to write out and give to him a history of the case, which I afterwards did, and informed me that the medicine had been potentized for him by Doctor Fincke, from a choice bit of crude material furnished by himself. He then enlisted me in the search for a pure drug that he had not been able to procure, for a proving. When we parted I had learned to place a high estimate upon him. He was a noble man.

Soon after that we met again in the college lecture room, as professor and student of medicine. His subject was *Natrum muriaticum* and as the golden words fell from his lips, I made every endeavor to preserve and profit by them. It was my good fortune to hear his lectures upon various drugs, which in the hands of many prescribers have verified the provings, and demonstrated his sagacity in arranging them. I have often thought of him when difficulties would beset me in the sick-room; and I knew that his contributions to our literature have enabled me to save lives. For this his memory is sacred to me.

But, Sir, I must not detain you with my extended remarks. You do not care to hear more of my personal experiences. It is enough to say that I loved and revered Constantine Hering; and when he died, I felt that I had lost one of my best friends.

PHILADELPHIA MEMORIAL MEETING

A large memorial meeting was held on Sunday evening, October 10th, 1880, at the Hahnemann Medical College, in Philadelphia. The following report was submitted on behalf of the County Society:

We recognize in the decease of Dr. Hering the loss of one pre-eminently adapted by nature and education to be a leader in the early struggles and sacrifices of a new medical dispensation. Cultured in literature and in general science, learned in all the medical wisdom of the allopathic fathers, careful in the formation of his opinions, zealous for the advancement of his chosen profession and ambitious to excel in the practice of his art, we yet find him fearlessly investigating the principles of a new system, accepting without reserve and without hesitation the overwhelming testimony to the truth of homoeopathy, flinging aside the temptations of professional honor and political preferment, fearlessly asserting his "liberty of medical opinion and action" in the presence of an arrogant and intolerant profession and in the face of his king, and deliberately casting his lot with the derided and persecuted pioneers of a new and hated system, devoting all his talents and energies to the perfection and dissemination of the newly-discovered art of

healing, laboring with heart and hand and brain for its establishment over a whole continent; unswerving in his adherence to its
teachings, unflinching in its defence and untiring in all labors for
its advancement. he seemed ever to realize that he had been raised
up for this, his heaven-appointed work. We rejoice that he was
permitted to witness the vast results toward which his own Hercu-
lean labors had so largely contributed. the shaken foundations of
the old medical superstructure. the triumphant vindication of the
once despised system of Hahnemann, the establishment of its hospitals, its colleges and its journals, the organization of its societies
over the whole civilized world, and the spread of its beneficent influence by thousands of educated physicians into millions of homes.

We, his fellow members of this Society, among whom he walked
and taught and labored for so many years, who enjoyed his intimate personal acquaintance and counsel, are proud to express our
appreciation of his personal character, and his abounding services
in the cause of progressive medicine, the cause of suffering humanity. We shall ever hold his name, his work and his worth in warmest remembrance, and our posterity will rise up to do him honor.

As expressive of the feelings of the Faculty of the
Hahnemann Medical College, the following was communicated by Dr. O. B. Gause, Registrar:

We have contemplated the death of our venerable friend and
co-laborer, Constantine Hering, M.D., Emeritus Professor of Homoeopathic Institutes and Materia Medica, with unfeigned sorrow, believing that the Hahnemann College has lost its brightest light,
and the Homoeopathic school its most profound and learned ex-
ponent.

Dr. C. Pearson, of Washington, spoke as follows:

It was not my good fortune to be as intimately acquainted with
the deceased as many who may be present this evening, but my
acquaintance was sufficient to induce me to travel over a hundred
miles to meet with you. his more immediate neighbors, on this
memorial occasion, and deplore with you the worth we have lost.

That Dr. Hering should not live longer in the body was not at all
strange; for eighty years he has seen the seasons come and go;
over half a century he had devoted to the relief of suffering
humanity. he had heard the call for help come up from a thousand
tongues, and in response to this. he had endured the summer's
heat and the storms of winter.

With the key of energy and application, and the lamp of knowledge, he penetrated the *arcana* of nature, and searched through her storehouse for the hidden remedy, which, when discovered, became the property of the entire world; his humanity was co-extensive with the race, which he left wiser and better for having lived and thought:

> A life thus long for others' comfort spent,
> Is human nature's grandest monument.

The end is not yet. Hering still lives, like the dynamic property of his *Lachesis;* and a hundred years hence the child will be born that will bless his name for the relief this medicine affords.

But he has gone to that great institution of learning, where we, his pupils, will, ere long, like irregular school-boys, be dropping in one by one.

And who then shall say so much of us? No one; and yet I hope it may be justly said of each and all, that we contributed our mite of influence to that reform of medicine which portends to the afflicted a brighter and happier day.

But while we aspire to this, let us not forget that change is not always improvement, that belief is only temporal, while truths are eternal, that these are the golden particles that glitter in the sands of time; and the friction of years but adds to their lustre. If we cannot furnish another to that cluster of diamonds Hahnemann discovered, and Hering cut and set in his starry crown, let us not wilfully or ignorantly tarnish their brightness. If we attempt to travel the road they trod, let us be careful which end we take, for they certainly tend to opposite results, and it is better to be right with a minority, than with the majority wrong.

Fourscore years is a ripe age to attain, and yet it is far too short to reform a world; truth is of slow growth, and requires care and painstaking, and if it rise again when "crushed to earth," more than one generation may be required for it to do so.

Those truths then left us by Hahnemann, and so ably promulgated by Hering, Boenninghausen and other pioneers gone before, should be guarded by us with jealous care, and as we too will soon pass to "that bourne from which no traveller returns," may the young men who succeed us realize that "truth is ever the same, that time alters it not, nor is it the better or worse for being of ancient or modern tradition."

It may be possible that no improvement could be suggested on the order of nature, but in some respects it seems unfortunate that the knowledge and experience accumulated during a long life of patient industry, could not be bequeathed to others to be used and added to during their natural lives, and then to pass like a landed estate to the next of kin; but this seems not to be a part of the programme, or panorama of human life, but whoever would excel in knowledge and usefulness must do so by his own individual efforts. And however economical of time, his life, however protracted, will be too short to attain perfection.

We are only prospectors in the field of science. One finds a treasure here, another there, these become the support of the indolent, the wealth of the wise, and the sport of the ignorant; the patient toiler in the mine of knowledge is rarely appreciated. Few take him by the hand and wish him Godspeed; he is called visionary, foolishly demented. Sir Joshua Reynolds says: "present and future time may be regarded as rivals, and he who solicits the one, must expect to be discountenanced by the other," and as men are the creatures of the age in which they live, not its creators, it is not difficult to see why they should desire, and court the commendation of their own times more than that of succeeding ages; for with such tenacity does mind cling to the dead traditions of the past, that the iconoclast is rarely popular during his lifetime; but it is the bold adventurer on unknown seas that tells us of other continents; and future ages build his monument.

"So runs the world away."
"We are such stuff as dreams are made of,
and our little life is rounded with
a sleep."

It is unfortunate that among the unnumbered millions

"That strut and fret their hour upon the stage
And then are heard no more,"

so many should be "poor players," hence, when "after life's fitful fever" a good man sleeps well, it becomes so difficult to fill his place.

But though a standard-bearer in our cause has fallen, our flag must not be lowered, and when we too shall have followed him, others, I doubt not, will close up the ranks, and still keep it floating in the sunlight of eternal truth.

Hering's earthlife is ended, his conveyance was ready before ours, and he is still in our advance; we shall miss him, but:

"He hates him
Who upon the rock of this rough world
Would stretch him out longer."

"The night dew that falls though in silence it weeps,
Will brighten with verdure the grave where he sleeps;
And the tear that we shed though in silence it rolls,
Will long keep his memory green in our souls."

Dr. Ad. Lippe then spoke as follows:

Like children who have lost their father, we meet here this evening to express our grief over the loss we suffered by the death of Dr. Constantine Hering.

As mourning children we vividly remember what the departed was to all of us; we remember how he instructed us, how he taught us by precept and example, the way to obtain a perfect knowledge of the healing art, how he advised us to study the writings of Samuel Hahnemann; and we remember with gratitude his ceaseless labors in the field of Materia Medica.

Dr. Hering was chosen among many able medical students at Leipzig to write a pamphlet, and in it to expose the follies and absurdities of a new system of therapeutics by Samuel Hahnemann, and with the honesty of purpose which always guided him through life he undertook that task; his first step was to study Hahnemann's *Organon of the Healing Art,* and then he tried the correctness, or the falsity, of the teachings by the experiment.

The only true test, the experiment, convinced him that the follies and absurdities of the prevailing allopathic school of medicine were exposed by Hahnemann, that a rational system of the healing art was revealed to the world by him. Homoeopathy had slowly gained ground in those days. The medical student who, in 1824, dared to declare his conviction of the truth of Homoeopathy, over all known systems of medicine, had to be a brave and fearless man.

Persecution followed Dr. Hering at once; his friend and benefactor who had expected him to ridicule and to demolish Homoeopathy, summarily dismissed him; distressing privations followed, but his faith was firm and not to be shaken by early personal adversities, no more than the progressive development of homoeopathy could be retarded by innumerable adversities and persecutions which all early adherents of it had to suffer. Finally Dr. Hering overcame these obstacles and he found a true friend in Professor Schoenlein, the father of a well classified pathology, and protected by him, the young student graduated at Wuerzburg. After teaching natural sciences and mathematics at Blochmann's Institute at Dresden he obtained an appointment from the Saxon government as naturalist. We find him at Surinam, in South America, making collections for the Museum of the Academy of Natural Sciences, at Dresden. As an eminent naturalist the Saxon government provided for him, but he was, almost against his will, compelled to practice the healing art in Surinam. The Saxon government demanded that all of his time be devoted to his appointment as naturalist, and were displeased with his practice and the papers published by him in the homoeopathic journals; he had himself dismissed from the government service and was again thrown upon his own resources.

It was there and then, that Dr. Hering obtained the few drops of the poison of the Trigonocephalus Lachesis, and there and then that he published the first provings made on the healthy (on himself) and earned the everlasting gratitude of the profession, who thereby were enabled to cure sicknesses formerly considered incurable.

Again we find him devoted to the teaching of the healing art at the Allentown Academy, (near Philadelphia) the first public institution of the kind chartered by a liberal government. The unselfish, self-sacrificing apostle, regardless of his own individual interests, resolved to fulfil his self-chosen mission to its full extent, and accepted a much smaller compensation for his laborious work to which he devoted all of his time and energies, than was accorded forty years later to the Secretary of the American Institute of Homoeopathy.

The teaching of students of medicine, the publishing of Hahnemann's *Organon*, and a *Materia Medica*, with a *Repertory*, in the English language, the proving of drugs and the publication of the medicinal virtues of Trigonocephalus Lachesis occupied his time. He finally had the gratification to see the diplomas conferred by the Allentown Academy upon its graduates, the first homoeopathic diplomas ever conferred, accepted at home and abroad. Dr. Wahle presented his diploma to the Papal government when he came to seek permission to practice Homoeopathy in the Papal States.

Later, Dr. Hering returned to Philadelphia, after Dr. William Wesselhoeft had been appointed President of the Academy.

With a large clientele which he found in Philadelphia, this indefatigable man added much to the further development of our healing art by the proving of new remedies and by perfecting and rearranging many proven ones. Not less active was he in guarding our school against innovations and perversions. Many posological papers were published by him in the Homoeopathic Journals, his witty sarcasm silencing those who tried to modernize Hahnemann's plain teachings. He never rejected, *a priori*, apparently advanced ideas till he had patiently investigated the proffered claims of their superiority over established principles and rules accepted by the early followers of Hahnemann, but when no convincing proof of the correctness of such innovations could be established, either by argument or by the test of experiment, his powerful pen was brought into requisition and he very soon silenced these bold writers. One of his last acts was the signing of a paper declaring his unswerving faith in the essential principles of homoeopathy, and finally saying: "If our school ever gives up

the strict inductive method of Hahnemann. we are lost and deserve
to be mentioned only as a caricature in the history of medicine."
(North American Journal of Homoeopathy, August, 1880.)

As children who have here assembled to mourn the loss of a
father, we can do no greater honor to his memory than to always
remember this parting instruction and warning; and on this solemn
occasion, let us resolve never to depart from the strict inductive
method of Hahnemann, a method our departed friend followed
most faithfully for more than half a century.

Dr. Henry N. Guernsey then addressed the meeting as
follows:

In rising to offer this tribute of respect to the memory of our
departed colleague, allow me to dwell for a little while upon the
early reminiscences of my acquaintance with him, which dates back
to the days of my medical pupilage.

In the autumn of 1842, I matriculated in the Pennsylvania
Medical College, which then occupied the very building in which
we are now assembled, and I soon made the acquaintance of Mr.
Husmann, a fellow student, who was then a private pupil of Dr.
Hering, and later became his brother-in-law. My friend soon introduced me to the distinguished subject of this memorial, whose
office at that time, nearly forty years ago, was located at the North-
west corner of Eleventh and Spruce Streets.

During the session Dr. Hering frequently came to our dissecting
room to examine the viscera of the cadavera that he might the better establish the truth of some of his theories.

In my mind's eye I now see as I saw him then—his erect and
commanding figure, his eager and piercing eye, his massive brow,
his well-shaped head, with long, black hair, and his whole appearance so clothed with dignity as to render him apparently unap-
proachable.

At our first interview, however, I discovered my mistake; for he
proved so genial, so friendly, and so communicative, that we
fraternized at once. Thus, I am proud to say, our fraternal relations continued to our last conference, which was only a few hours
before his demise. During all these years it has been my good
fortune to have free access to him, even to his private study, at
almost any hour.

His active and inquiring mind led him to continually search for,
and gather up, all facts, particularly if new and of recent occurrence. As an illustration, I will mention the following circumstance.
A short time after I had located in Frankford, I was quite astonished to find Dr. Hering at my door, early one morning, inquiring

for the residence of a person who had been stung by a bee, whose sufferings had been published in the daily papers. I at once took him, in my carriage, to the house of the sufferer, where he carefully noted down every face and sympton developed by the bee sting. This case proved of great value in making up the pathogenesis of *Apis mellifica*, but it cost Dr. Hering the fatigue of a sixteen mile drive, besides the loss of time to his professional duties of nearly the whole day. We all know the value of time to a physician in full practice. But for him, when in quest of knowledge, everything else had to give way; time, money, strength, sleep, and all else were sacrificed for the sake of science and homoeopathy. "Anything and everything for our cause," he was often heard to say.

Dr. Hering, as consulting physician, has many times driven to Frankford to advise me on a bad case of sickness. How mightily he would apply himself to find the proper remedy! He never resorted to any makeshift; but firmly relying upon the unfailing law of the Similars, he would persevere until the true *Simillimum* was found, and the cure effected. As an invariable rule, the more dangerous the case, the more mightily would he apply himself to the letter and spirit of the law bequeathed to us by Samuel Hahnemann.

After my removal into the city proper, in 1856, the frequency of my visits to him increased, while my confidence in, and reliance upon my dear old friend's judgment, were vastly heightened. His abiding faith in the true law of cure was exemplified in the treatment of his own person and that of his family, when ill, as well as in the treatment of all of his patients. Everybody was treated according to the same principles, and everybody shared equally with him one of the greatest blessings a merciful Heaven has vouched to mankind.

I will briefly refer to one or two of the many instances, which might be cited, to illustrate this point. Some years ago he suffered from a very painful attack of hemorrhoids, which confined him to his bed. Dr. Lippe had prescribed *Causticum*, one dose, and admonished him to await the action of the drug for three days. The improvement appearing but slight, as the prescribed time drew near its close, he began to doubt that the true *Simillimum* had been found; so he took up his books and brought his own great mind to bear upon the search for a remedy. Finding no better one, he concluded to await the full expiration of the time, as agreed upon. Soon afterwards he fell into a sweet sleep, lasting several hours, from which he awoke, well. He enjoyed telling of this triumph of the single dose, and the high potency, as an encouragement of all true healers to go and to do likewise.

Again, when one of his daughters was very ill with diphtheria, by my advice he had given a single dose of *Lachesis*, but which was followed by so little improvement in twenty-four hours, that he was sorely tempted to either repeat the dose or to change the remedy. But as the little patient was no worse, he concluded to wait twelve hours longer; at the experiation of which time he had the satisfaction of seeing her greatly improved.

He was ever faithful to the true cause he loved so well, because he believed it to be true. As with all true men, believing, with him, was synonymous with doing.

About seventeen years ago Dr. Ad. Lippe was greatly prostrated by an attack of typhoid fever. So fearfully did the disease rage that I feared he would not recover. As was my custom in all such bad cases, I repaired to Dr. Hering, who had not yet seen the case, and told him my fears. Dr. Hering suddenly dropped his pen, and giving me one of his searching looks, apparently to see if I was in earnest, said with great emphasis, "Dr. Lippe must not die yet; I will go with you."

For over an hour, with book in hand, he applied his great mind to the case and finally declared *Silicea* to be the remedy. Dr. P. P. Wells, and the late Carroll Dunham, who had been summoned, came in later and confirmed the wisdom of their teacher's choice—for they too, had taken their first lesson in homoeopathy from Dr. Constantine Hering. *Silicea* stayed the ravages of the fever; its subject made a rapid recovery, and Dr. Lippe stands among us tonight, a living monument of one of Dr. Hering's good works.

And so it ever was with our lamented Father of homoeopathy. in this country. I never knew him to deviate from the true line of action in his efforts to heal the sick, or to relieve the dying. For he knew this to be the best, and indeed the only safe means that could be employed.

Dr. Hering, above all men in our ranks, best understood the art of acquiring wealth, that real wealth which far transcends the value of such material dross as gold or silver.

Look at his *Lachesis!* Is not this alone a work worth living a lifetime to accomplish? Surely it would be a sufficient consolation at the close of anyone's life to be able to say, "I have done thus much for the good of humanity."

Dr. Hering's notebook was always at hand, and ever and anon. wherever he might be, or with whomsoever conversing, he jotted down observations, precious "nuggets" as it were, to be deposited in his big strong-box so soon as he had retired to his private study. As yet, only a few peeps into that box have been granted to his heirs, for, are not we his heirs, and are we not to receive our respective shares of his valuable legacy *pro bono publico?* And we trust that all this will be dealt out to us, in good time, by the publication of his invaluable work, *The Guiding Symptoms.*

Never did the slightest feeling of jealousy cross his mind. If any of his patients became restive and called upon other physicians, his first inquiry, on missing them, was, "Where have they gone? If to another homoeopathic physician, then I am satisfied; there is no loss, but rather a gain to our cause." He was large-hearted and liberal, seeming to take in the whole profession as one man and considered himself as one of the least.

As an observer, none equalled him. On entering the sickroom, for instance his all-seeing eyes took in at once the condition of things and his mind had often decided upon the proper course to pursue before a question had been asked; his interrogations, later, were often more to confirm and to place on record than to elicit facts for decision. Intuition was a powerful element in his mind, and this was cultivated to a high degree by his truthfulness of character, and his good thoughts and feelings toward everyone he knew. He never plotted evil and never sought revenge, but was as innocent-minded as a child. He reached out in all directions for truth, and wherever his investigations extended, all Nature seemed to yield up her treasures to him, for she found no corrupt or opposing influences in his mind to operate against her. Truth ever responds to the true-minded truth-seeker; and never was she better treated, never less perverted, than by Constantine Hering.

But, his race is run, and he has left us. He was almost the last one of Hahnemann's pupils to remain upon this earth. Hahnemann and his faithful contemporaries are now reunited in a nearly completed phalanx, to stand enshrined in our memories as the noblest representatives of the cause they lived for in this world. It was a needful and an orderly step that our good doctor should go to the end, that he might be more fully conjoined to, and continue to labor with those faithful and powerful allies on the other side. And he departed, was almost translated, in the Lord's own good time, and now we may reasonably expect a fuller, a more powerful and a more general display of the real Hahnemannian principles than ever before.

Let us profit by his example and cherish in our memories the truths which came worded from his tongue.

Dr. Robert J. McClatchey spoke as follows:

If I have a proper understanding of the object and scope of this meeting, it is to afford an opportunity to those who loved, and who revere the memory of Dr. Constantine Hering to testify their respect for his memory, and, at the same time, to give evidence in some way of their appreciation of his character as a man and as a physician; so that by the contributions thus made, the world may be able to know what was thought of our departed friend, by those who knew him best, and are most capable of estimating him at a proper value.

Upwards of thirty years ago Dr. Hering wrote as follows, in an article entitled *Requisites for a Correct Estimation of Hahnemann,* published in the *Hygeia,* vol. 22, p. 296.

"If we would form an estimate of a man who belongs to history, an estimate which shall itself lay claim to a place in history, and rise above the fleeting interest of ephemeral productions, we must found it upon a full consideration of the whole life and labors of him to whom it relates.

"Thus should the historian accompany his hero to the time when a friendly beckoning hand withdraws him from things without, his senses close to page and speech, unfold to sources of joy and hope, and departs, at peace with himself, with God and the mantled world.

"Then let the estimate follow—not in the work—not penned by the laborious biographer, but formed in the inmost soul of him who shall have read and weighed the whole."

It has seemed to me that there was no more marked trait in Dr. Hering's remarkably pronounced character than his steadfastness of purpose, in his endeavor to carry out to the utmost every task laid before him; and there is, in my opinion, a unity of purpose distinguishable through all of his work, and characterizing it, in a marked degree, as well as exhibiting this steadfastness.

Those of us who had the privilege and pleasure of personal intercourse with Dr. Hering, well know what an instructive, and even fascinating conversationalist he was. And we now know that, while pursueing a subject in this way, his vast learning would often lead him away from the path that led directly to the subject under consideration, into what, at a superficial glance, seemed mere nothoroughfares of thought, that led no-whither. It would soon prove that these were, instead, pleasant and beautiful by-paths, which led directly into the main pathway, and which had served simply as an agreeable and momentary diversion, but not in any way distracting attention from the end in view. Even in such matters as those, of every day occurrence, and coming up in the way of chance, and every day conversation, he exhibited the utmost steadfastness of purpose. How much more marked, then, might we expect to find this steadfastness in his life's work.

I can liken Dr. Hering's life to nothing more appropriate, I think, than by comparing it to a magnificent and grand piece of music by a Bach, a Handel, a Mendelssohn or a Haydn, in which, whatever variations are introduced, the original theme is recognizable throughout and at all times, and which gives to variations their tone, their key, their character and their power.

The theme of Dr. Hering's life music consisted in his desire and striving for the elevation of his beloved homoeopathy to a position among the sciences; to place it upon a scientific basis and to make its workings those of an exact science. Refer to this man's life and labors. Consult his writings, as I have done, from his earliest to his latest, and you will see, as I have seen, that he had this constantly in view, and was steadfast in his wish for its accomplishment, and no matter into what no-thoroughfares or byways he may have strayed, he never lost sight of his great goal.

There was nothing meritricious about Dr. Hering. Whatever work he did was for homoeopathy and the truth, and without reference to pay or reward. He was always accessible and always willing to teach all who wished to learn what he considered to be the better way, but he never indulged in that very agreeable, but by no means useful pastime of "damning those he had no mind to." He afforded the fullest respect to the opinions of others, and largely for that reason, he and his opinions always commanded respect.

The amount of work he did was simply enormous. He was an earnest and a patient toiler, who, as we are informed, died almost with his working-harness on. In his work, whether in verbal communications, through books, or through journals, he supplied enough of wisdom, of learning and of other requisites to make first class reputations for a score or more of doctors.

His works were grandly conceived and as grandly executed, and of course there was surplusage. To him and to his works are applicable the words of Schiller:

"How many starvelings a rich man can nourish!
When monarchs build—the rubblish carriers flourish."

So then our greatest has departed. That melody of life, with its cunning tones, which took captive ear and heart, has gone silent; the heavenly force that dwelt here victorious over so much, is here no longer; thus far, not farther, by speech and by act, shall the wise man utter himself forth. The end! What solemn meaning lies in that sound, as it peals mournfully through the soul when a living friend has passed away. All now is closed, irrevocable; the changeful life-picture, growing daily into new coherence, under new touches and hues, has suddenly become completed and unchangeable. There as it lay, it is dipped, from this moment in the aether of the heavens, and shines transfigured, to endure even so—forever. The weekday man, who was one of us, has put on the garments of Eternity and become radiant and triumphant.

The man whom we loved lies in his grave; but glorious, worthy; and his spirit yet lives in us with an authetic life. Could each one here vow to do his little task, even as the departed did his great one, in the manner of a true man, not for a Day, but for Eternity! To live as he counselled and commanded, not commodiously in the Reputable, the Plausible, the Half, but resolutely in the Whole, the Good, the True:

"Im Ganzen, Guten, Wahren resolut zu leben!"

Dr. Bushrod W. James made the following remarks:

We, the intimates, associates and friends of Constantine Hering, and residents of the city of his adoption, assemble together tonight, as do his friends in other cities, all over the land, and the Homoeopathic world, to say a few words of meed in honor and to the memory of a great and good man.

We are not here to erect a monument, for that his life has done for us, in his works, his writings and in his teachings.

His labors are known; his virtues need no further description, his good qualities of heart are impressed upon all whom he conversed with, his professional skill was undoubted, his steadfast purpose of benefitting mankind was a guiding star in his life; he was always at his post of duty, and he filled the post, allotted to him by the Great Architect of the Universe, with faithfulness and cheerfulness of disposition.

His mission was, first, that of a standard-bearer of the new system of medicine and later he was acknowledged a superior officer in the warfare between the medical opponents. He lived an eventful and useful life, and died with honors and glories surrounding him.

Every age has its progressive spirits; men that are born to leave a name inscribed upon the roll of time, deeply cut in letters of gold, and whose acts stand out in plain relief and beauty among good deeds of others. Our fallen companion was truly one of those so honored.

He was liberal in his prescribing, not bound to any excrescent ideas; he read Hahnemann's works as he did his Bible, and he tested all that was there advanced, and held firmly to all that was valuable in the Organon of Homoeopathy as written by Samuel Hahnemann, and like him was not afraid to stand up boldly for its truths, at all times.

He was not one to fetter the dose or to limit the size or repetition of the same: he allowed every physician his own judgment in such matters, but unswervingly exercised his own. While thus liberal he adhered strictly to the law of *Similia* and to the selection of the remedy according to the totality of the symptoms. He was most careful in the proper and thorough examination of all of the symptoms of his patients regardless of the time and trouble involved in the questioning, knowing that success depended upon obtaining a true picture of the disease. He believed in a general knowledge of all branches of medicine of both schools, for he says: "No one can be a successful disciple of Hahnemann who is not well versed, as Hahnemann himself was, in the learning of the medical schools, and it would be just as impossible for him to act judiciously without having a knowledge of anatomy, physiology, pathology, surgery and materia medica, together with chemistry and botany, as for a man ignorant of navigation and seamanship to carry a vessel safely into port."

He was free in giving advice to learners, and would sit by the hour and converse with any member of the profession who desired to have the benefit of his wide experience with our homoeopathic remedies, and his mature judgment in the proper selection of the remedy, in complicated and obscure cases, was often thus sought. Even I, when a student, with a number of others, paid frequent visits to his house, at his request, to hear from his lips (without desire of recompense) the unfolding of *materia medica* and clinical experiences of this large-hearted, generous disciple of Hahnemann.

No toil was too arduous, no time thus spent was considered lost, no research on his part was thought burdensome, no careful study was left undone that would enable him to present to students of homoeopathy, in or out of the profession, clearly the doctrines of the homoeopathic practice.

He was a constant student and arduous laborer in the cause. He fought for a higher medical education all his medical life; he directed many a battle; he passed through the lifework campaign; he was on the upper outlook of the mountain peak of knowledge himself, and he saw the desire of his heart realized, the victory won, the world acknowledging the truths of homoeopathy and its educating influence upon the profession and the people; and today we place the laurels upon the brow of one of Hahnemann's most trusty and worthy generals.

Dr. John C. Morgan pronounced the following eulogy:

Ripe, full of days, and rich in worthy doing, so departed our friend, our teacher, our patriarch, Dr. Constantine Hering; and so we would speak of the loved and lost. Deep in the human soul, today, as ever, survives that earliest idea of worship—the homage of the Past—overlaid and encrusted, indeed, with the glory of the ᵥPresent, but warm and vital, ever awaiting the artistic touch, the seer's interpretation, or the tension of public or private grief, or triumph; for occasion to glow, bright and beautiful, in the sunlight of the human affections.

Are the Fathers in honor? Then do the children rejoice, with front erect, bold, forceful. Are they in contempt? Then do the children cringe, falter and fail.

Time was when ancestor's names were household gods; time was, when citizens, blameless, devoted, venerable, invincible departed life for the land of shades, only to be deified—we know better now, do we not? But in the grand old days, the heroes lived evermore, caring for the commonwealth, guiding counsel, directing war, upbuilding the state; as demigods adored, with sacrificial honors. Insult offered, even to the statues of heroes, was insult inflicted upon the state; nay more—whoso refused homage, was the enemy of the state, and of his people. In the Christian ages, the church has ever done likewise by her saints; revered, even when unadored.

Hero-worship! Is it commendable? Ancestral glory? Is it nothing worth? Antiquity! Is it venerable? Let the potent conservation of "the medical profession" answer. Let the large and respectable clientele of that old guild, reply; that army of devotees who bend the ear to hear, and the knee in devotion, as medical antiquity is exalted and its heroes named; justly exalted—truly named. The heroes and their deeds—their thoughts, their words— these are indeed immortal! 'Twere but a bootless venture, were we, their legatees, to turn the ungrateful back upon those mighty dead.

But the long, long past stretches forward unto this day. Homoeopathy writes beneath that noble galaxy the names of a new constellation—a group of heroes as glorious as they; few in number, but of imperishable fame. Antiquity overtakes us. Hahnemann, Gram, Jahr, Boenninghausen, Buchner, Hausmann, Grauvogl, Henderson, Quin, Jeanes, Beebe, Temple, Williamson, Dunham, Gardiner, Payne, Hempel, Hering; these have gone over to the reunion of the great. One by one has the heroic Past inscribed them upon her scroll. We, too, are acquiring a history—short, it may be in time; but long in all that makes time venerable; ages old, in the truth spoken, and in deeds performed.

Ye Homoeopaths, behold these your heroes! Measure the territory; glory in the fame they have won for you; emulate their exalted worth. Mark well, too, the noble souls who yet remain with us, to pile still loftier mountains of grand doing upon the heights attained by them. Behold our fast rising Olympus, our moving Pelion, our trembling Ossa, upheaved by their giant shoulders, and say, if we live not in the heroic age ourselves—the age of the pioneers—the age of laborious sowing—the age of iron, of the power of law, in the history of medicine, as of universal progress! Let us know what is our birthright—recognize the heavenly afflatus inspiring our own heroes—erect our own Palladium—build our own Pantheon—perceive the vision of our Olympian court—cherish worshipfully our own hastening antiquity—and condemn the threatening oncoming of an untimely age of brass; of an early and slovenly reaping; of glib and lively egotism, and, it may be, of reaction.

What care we for that—or for them? That is the meteyard of our own domain. They fought and labored to win it; their posterity enter in and possess it. Homely and trite is the proverb—and true as trite. "'Tis but an unclean bird who befouleth his own nest." He is but an unworthy homoeopath who would asperse his own professional ancestry. And for what? To conciliate the medically ungodly? To win opponents, never generous, never just? (I except individuals). Rather let us learn their politic wisdom. *Fas est ab hoste doceri.* The compulsion of history alone can win them; each full-mailed warrior, like the ancient Spartan, must fix the boundary of his estate, only with the point of his spear! Each must be a hero, each hero panoplied in the armor of truth, sent down from heaven at the prayer of Samuel Hahnemann; claiming the whole continent, moving forward—forward—upward, evermore!

Constantine Hering thus fought the good fight, and has conquered. The hero has taken his Olympian seat! The glory of the ancients is his. His deeds and his memory remain to us. Thus he fought, and thus he won. By that sign may all we prevail!

And as we look backward upon the more than half a century of his struggle, may the lesson of his life be to each of us, at once an inspiration and a new point of departure; may each emulate the courage, the patience, the industry, the truth, the faith, of these grand fifty years of his doctorate; remembering ever, that for us, as for all, the path of true honor lies oftenest through valleys of obloquy, to hills of difficulty, mountain-high; our only sustenance, ofttimes, the soul-power within; ofttimes unresting, ofttimes alone.

"The heights by great men won, and kept,
    Were not attained by sudden flight;
But they, while their companions slept,
    Were toiling upward in the night.

We have not wings, we cannot soar,
But we have feet to scale and climb
By slow degrees, by more and more,
The sunlit summits of our time."

The life of our departed friend was the realization of this song
of our national poet; for

Thus did our Hering toil and climb—
Thus proved his life-work true, sublime—
Thus wrought, thus fought, thus won; then died,
Nay lived anew, and Death defied.

Sage! Teacher! Hero unexcelled!
Thy name shall be in homage held—
Thy work endure, while time shall be;
Thy praise befits Eternity.

Dr. Martin Deschere, of New York, was the next speaker, who said:

I too was permitted to press his hand once in my life. My longing for that moment to come was more than compensated by the
happy hours which I spent in his sacred study. Those few hours
were blessed. They truly belong to the happiest ones of my life.

Many of you, who knew Dr. Hering intimately, are better able
to speak of his personal traits than I am.

To my mind the object of this personal meeting should be the
collection of those thoughts which characterized the man for whom
we mourn tonight. For within us he planted the seed of his wisdom; unto us he left the great work of his life as a sacred inheritance—the search after truth. Therefore we can honor him no
more than by following in his footsteps, by marching onward from
where he stopped, by fighting with his weapons for our beloved art.
And here we must ask the important question: What was the mission of Constantine Hering? It was to make homoeopathy universal; to proclaim its truth to all mankind.

The history of his life tells us how far he has succeeded. He
has spread homoeopathy over nearly one-half of the globe.

But is homoeopathy universal? It is not. And here begins the
work which he left for us to do, as far as our power permits, with
all energy and force, just as he did himself. This is the inheritance which he has left us and which we must hold sacred.

If we look, today, at the number of homoeopathic physicians
in the United States, with its flourishing colleges, its numerous
societies, its well-conducted hospitals and dispensaries, we might

be inclined to think that nothing remains to be done, that all is good, and working for itself. We might be inclined to think that homoeopathy is really becoming universal.

But look at Europe. Look, in particular, to Germany, where stood Hahnemann's cradle, where homoeopathy itself was born, where Constantine Hering was consecrated to the cause.

I hold in my hand a letter addressed to Dr. Hering, by a man, who, from pure devotion to homoeopathy, begs a few articles to be written in defense of homoeopathy, for a German periodical. In this letter the position of homoeopathy in Germany is painted in the most pitiful colors, and Dr. Hering is requested to write a treatise on the success of our cause in America, that it may open the eyes of the public across the Atlantic.

The one who wrote the letter is not a physician. He is a man who has witnessed the great blessings of homoeopathy among his friends, and who cries for help in behalf of his fellowmen throughout his country.

The letter never reached him, to whom it was addressed. It arrived in Philadelphia a few days too late and was sent to me, with a request that I should fulfil the demands expressed in it, for it carries a plea of great significance.

Just at the moment when our great counsellor departed from us, this voice calls from abroad for help—help in our good cause.

Homoeopathy is not yet universal. The iron chains of prejudice, of scientific idolatry, of despotism hold it in their tight grip.

From this country of freedom, alone, liberty must come to homoeopathy throughout the world. In the name of Constantine Hering let me beg of those gentlemen who will visit the World's Convention, to be held abroad next summer, to remember this meeting, to keep sacred Hering's inheritance, and to fight, for homoeopathy in Europe.

I trust to their wise counsel that by some means they may plant a nucleus containing sufficient life from which to develop a giant in aid of homoeopathy abroad. The World's Convention held here, which Dr. Hering instituted, was a great step toward the universality of homoeopathy. And in working thus with the true spirit of progress we shall honor our immortal Hering.

It is a sacred debt we owe, and we must pay it.

Dr. Constantine Lippe, of New York, followed with these remarks:

Allow me to offer my tribute of respect to the memory of my namefather. As an individual loss, his departure leaves a great void.

It was my custom, on my visits to Philadelphia, to call on our friend and spend some very profitable hours with him. His uncompromising adherence to the strict principles of homoeopathy, as taught by Hahnemann, helped me, in a great measure to be certain that these principles were true, for in his long and successful practice, he, by adhering to those principles, could, and did, cure cases of disease, entirely unmanageable by any other course of treatment.

Dr. Hering was one of the best friends I ever had, genial, cordial; and never was a visit paid him, by me, but he was ready and willing to share his great knowledge on any subject inquired upon. He took great pleasure in imparting his information, gained by his close studies and long experience.

He completed his life, full, long and useful, and dropped to sleep to wake without the wornout frame which had become enfeebled.

"That bodies should be lent to us while they can afford us pleasure, to assist us in acquiring knowledge, or in doing good to our fellow-beings, is a kind and benevolent act of God. When they become unfit for their purposes, and afford us pain instead of pleasure, instead of an aid becoming an incumbrance, and answer to none of the intentions for which they were given, it is equally kind and benevolent that a way is provided by which we can get rid of them. This way is death." So wrote Benjamin Franklin in 1756.

Our friend has departed from the earth-sphere, but his memory will be held in dear remembrance.

Dr. Charles B. Gilbert, of Washington, D. C., expressed himself in this wise:

Having been a member of Dr. Hering's household for some months, and having had some opportunities for observing the inner life of that great and good man, there is one quality to which I wish to refer.

As I was hurrying across the country from the West to attend the funeral, to relieve somewhat the madness of my thoughts, I took up a little book that had been put into my hand by a friend just before I started; it was the little story by Edward Everett Hale of the *Poor Men of Lyons*, as they were called—how they had given up wealth and position to spread the gospel; their appeal to each other was—"For the Love of Christ," and the answer was—"In his name."

"Verily." I said. "Dr. Hering was a Poor Man of Lyons indeed. and a prophet among them.

On the day of the funeral, as I stood by the door receiving the hundreds who came to view the face of their benefactor, and saw among them scores who could, in their poverty, only have called on him "For the Love of Christ," I could not help thinking: These are of "The Poor Men of Lyons." The tears that rolled down their cheeks told louder than words that the answer to their appeal had been—"In his name."

I cannot find words to express my individual sorrow and my indebtedness to him on whose monument no fitter motto could be engraved than this—"He loved his neighbor as himself."

Reminisiscences by Dr. C. W. Boyce, of Auburn, N. Y.:

We speak today in memory of the late Dr. Constantine Hering. of, I cannot say, Philadelphia, because he belonged to the world.

You have selected me to say something in regard to him, not because I am more competent to do it than the rest of you, but from the accident that I had been thrown more into his society.

In order to explain how my acquaintance with him began, and why it continued, I must commence several years before I first saw him.

The name of Dr. Hering is so closely associated with Lachesis—. in my mind, that when one is mentioned the other is almost sure to come up with it, and to a great extent, with me, homoeopathy depends upon Lachesis—for its glory.

It was by homoeopathy that I became acquainted with Lachesis. and it was by Lachesis that I came to know Dr. Hering. In 1846 I first became practically acquainted with homoeopathy, and began to practice it in preference to the ordinary method. It was not until several years after that the wonderful healing powers of homoeopathy were fully revealed to me. I had a case of typhoid fever which had continued unchecked for twenty-one days. At this time there seemed no chance for the patient to recover. Hope had been abandoned. when, during the night follownig the twenty-first day. Lachesis was given every two hours. Next morning there was a complete change for the better. The tongue was moist, the delirium greatly lessened. From this time on convalescense progressed until health was restored. This case was never forgotten. but in my daily rounds it was a long time before I saw another such result. It came, however, in a case of gangrene. A woman discovered a small spot on the calf of her leg. which gave her a great deal of uneasiness. and it rapidly increased in size. When I saw her, she was in bed, and the spot measured three inches in diameter; it was rapidly increasing in size, and she grew sicker and sicker. Lachesis was given and in a few hours the progress of the disease was checked. In a few days the entire piece of flesh which was affected fell out, leaving a hole reaching to the sheath of the muscles; but this healed kindly in a short time.

These cases were treasured up in my memory. Soon after this, a case of aneurism of the aorta, where the patient was obliged to sit by an open window day and night to get all the air possible, was wonderfully relieved by the Lachesis.

Again followed a time of professional drudgery, without striking results, when again I was startled. A woman, who was nursing a child, was aroused at midnight by the cry of fire. She had only time to grasp her child and rush out of the house in her night-clothes. It was winter-time, and she went into snow to her knees. She stood about in this undress until the house was consumed before seeking shelter. The result was that she did not get out of bed until the following summer, and then only by the help of Lachesis, which, in nine days, not only took her out of bed, but set her to doing her housework.

Now, to me, homoeopathy was fast coming to mean Lachesis, but I was soon to be aroused from any security I felt in the practice of even homoeopathy. A great grief came upon me. My only son sickened, and died within a few days. During his sickness I could not see that anything given medicinally had produced any effect. The disease went on unchecked until he died. On the day of his funeral the twin sister was taken with the same disease, and only after a severe struggle was saved. Disheartened I asked: Is there any remedial virtue in medicine? My experience with Lachesis answered this question affirmatively. Then came another question: Has my practice of medicine been a success? On comparing results with other physicians whose death-roll I knew, I found that my success or failure, whichever it might be, was perhaps that of a fair average. This did not satisfy me. I asked myself another question: If occasionally I could obtain such results as I did from Lachesis, why could I not get them from other remedies? Where should I seek for the answer?

I had been practising homoeopathy for several years, and preferred it to allopathy from which I had turned. During these years of practising I had not seen, in either practise, any such results as came from the administration of Lachesis.

Two steps had been taken; I had found homoeopathy, and I had found Lachesis.

I knew, or believed that Dr. Hering had been the one who introduced the remedy. So the next step, in my progress, was to seek ·Dr. Hering. I wrote to Dr. Hering, asking him whether I might call upon him and hope to find him unoccupied long enough for me to get some information that would help me in the practise of homoeopathy. I was impressed with the idea that by seeing and talking with Dr. Hering I would be able to go and acquire what I wanted. I did not wait for an answer to my letter, but went, at once, to Philadelphia, and called at his house on the same evening of my arrival.

I found Dr. Hering entertaining a number of physicians in his garden, which, for the occasion was lighted by tapers placed in the trees. The garden was full of little tables, which held refreshments, and which were served after the German style.

On announcing myself at the door, as being a physician, I was ushered into the garden, along with the rest. After being there a short time I learned which was Dr. Hering. I saw a large man with long gray hair which fell down to his shoulders, and with a beard, likewise gray which reached to his breast. As I watched him, first speaking to one, then to another of his guests, I almost wondered why I had ventured there. He was always the centre of a group of interested doctors. Presently he turned to one of the tables, fortunately near where I stood, and took some bread and cheese. Now, was my opportunity; I stepped before him and announced my name. I wondered how I would be received. All at once he laid down his bread and cheese and taking both my hands he said: "Oh! Dr. Boyce, I am glad to see you," and calling his daughter, cried, "Here, Odelia, is Dr. Boyce; keep him until all these go away; I want to talk to him." Odelia fulfilled her father's desire, and gave me my first introduction to Limburger cheese.

I have always thought that she, and Mrs. Conrad Wesselhoeft, who was her companion for that evening, must have enjoyed the scene when I first essayed the eating of some of this cheese. It was made up of the most inviting little balls, ornamented with greens. Dr. Hering again took up his bread and cheese and began to eat, and following his example I took one of those beautiful little balls and a piece of bread. The balls looked so nice, and withal so small, that I put the whole of one into my mouth and began to chew. Imagine me standing before Dr. Hering with this in my mouth trying to hold it and at the same time wishing to keep him from turning to someone else, and you can have some faint idea of my first acquaintance with Limburger cheese! I was finally obliged to turn away from him, behind the neighboring bushes, and spit it out. On turning back again I caught a glimpse of two pairs of eyes set in countenances convulsed with laughter.

This was my first introduction to Dr. Hering, and to Limburger cheese. I was with the doctor until late into the night and nearly all of the next day, and the next, and so on, until I was ashamed to take up any more of his time, and excused myself on the plea that I must go home.

In about another month another great calamity seemed to be impending. My eldest daughter was taken with diptheria. It went on to the corupy stage. This was at a time when I had never seen a case recover in which the larynx had become involved. The disease had first shown itself on November 1st. You all know how this disease progresses, and how anxious we all are when we have such cases to treat. This one progressed until the eleventh day, slowly but surely getting worse, when I wrote to Dr. Hering, giving minutely the symptoms and condition, saying that on the thirteenth day, when I knew he would have the letter, I would telegraph the symptoms, if the patient were still alive. This I did, and soon had the reply: "Give Lachesis." The case began to mend from this time, and finally recovered entirely.

In December, 1863, another claim came to me in my immediate family. To give a correct account of this case I must copy it as reported at the time. "A child of twenty-one months, with light hair, blue eyes and light complexion, took cold on Christmas day. During the night of the 26th there was fever and rapid respiration. At 11 a. m., on the 27th, the child had a spasm lasting fifteen minutes. From this time, until January 8th there was continued fever, greatly increased at night, with a pulse of 150. The respirations per minute were seventy on actual count, and at no time less. Generally there was a red spot on one cheek, which frequently changed sides. When one cheek was red the other generally was pale. All of this time the left lung was impervious to air. Auscultation revealed slight bronchial respiration but no vesicular murmur. The right lung was not implicated; there was constant cough, yet much increased at night. The case had gradually, but surely, become worse, up to the 8th of January, when the right lung began to be affected. On this day the child became uneasy and restless, throwing itself about in all directions and positions in its efforts to get breath. The face grew dark, there was constant spasmodic cough with labored breathing; the little thing in its agony striking at the mother for control. When it fell asleep for a few seconds at a time the throat became so dry that a condition resembling croup came on, and all the sufferings were increased."

This fearful condition was rapidly hurrying the little sufferer to its grave. All of the remedies prominent in similar conditions had been given; including Lachesis 200th, without result. At this juncture Lachesis 12th, (three pellets) was given, dry, on the tongue;

immediately (the pellets had not entirely dissolved on the tongue) the cough stopped and the breathing was relieved, for four hours. At the end of this time the cough gradually returned with all of the sufferings (in a diminished degree) when another dose of Lachesis 12th produced the same decided relief, this time, lasting for sixteen hours. Four doses in twelve hours so changed the condition that the child slept nearly all of the night, and air passed freely again to all parts of the previously obstructed lung. During the autumn of 1863 and up to January 1864, there seemed to be severe sickness nearly all of the time, in my family, and twice during that time, Lachesis had helped me out.

In the summer of 1864 I again visited Dr. Hering. I was received with the same cordiality, and made at home in his house. At this time the old faculty of the Homoeopathic Medical College of Pennsylvania had become tired of bearing its burden. The trustees of the college offered this charge to Dr. Hering, or at least so that he, associated with his friends might have control and direction of it. They accepted the offer and associated themselves together and formed a new faculty, which gave its first course of lectures during the winter of 1864-65. Doctors Hering, Lippe, Guernsey and Raue were Professors in the College and Dr. Hering invited me to attend its course of lectures in that winter. This I accepted. When, in October, I presented myself at his door, ready to follow his instructions, he said to me: "Now, here you are at home; come every day at three o'clock in the afternoon and take coffee with me; at this hour I have my noonday rest and I allow no one to disturb me."

Every day at three o'clock found me at his house where I spent this hour with him. All this time he did the talking, spoke of homoeopathy and almost everything else. It finally came about, that almost every evening, found me at Dr. Hering's house where I met some one or more of the above named professors, and often all of them. There I spent the winter, virtually in association with Doctors Hering, Lippe, Raue and Guernsey. These four were like schoolboys learning their lessons. Every night they met at Dr. Hering's house and related the experiences of the day, and when any new result was reached they all noted it, and Dr. Hering recorded it in his manuscripts.

A close friendship with these men was begun in consequence of the publication, in May and June, in the *American Homoeopathic Review*, a periodical which all of these were interested in maintaining, by giving a minute account of all the results I had obtained by the administration of Lachesis as a curative agent. Those of you who remember the controversy, at that time going on as to whether there was any remedial virtue in Lachesis, can appreciate the pleasure with which this publication was received by these men, all of whom were positive, both from helping to prove it and of making use of it in practice, that it was a great curative agent. Hempel had fulminated his anathemas against it, declaring it inert. Others had condemned it.

This report detailed cases in actual experience, where such wonderful results were obtained that no one could make answer to them excepting that he said, "I don't believe him." I stood ready to prove every case and bring witnesses before any court, and take their sworn statements to the truth of what I had written. Dr. Hering felt, and always said that this was the turning point with Lachesis, and at once called me the man who had saved it.

Often as I came into his house, he would cry out, "Here comes the man who saved Lachesis." He loved to tell me about the capture of the snake, and how he took the poison, and how he had proved it. We were to go to the Academy of Natural Sciences and see the original snake, preserved in alcohol.

What great results often follow small affairs. In this case the publication, of what seemed to me, only an ordinary report of cases cured, was followed by the lifelong friendship, and even gratitude, of one of the greatest benefactors of the human race; for so I consider the discoverer of a remedy which will produce such wonderful curative results as does Lachesis.

During the winter which I spent in Philadelphia, and so much of the time at Dr. Hering's house, just at Christmas, I received a message from home, that Mrs. Boyce was severely ill, and that I must go home at once. On my arrival, I found a case of typhoid-pneumonia of a serious nature. After studying the case carefully I gave Phosphorus, but, feeling anxious, I telegraphed to Dr. Hering the condition, and again received help from him. He was ever ready to do anything in his power for anyone who suffered. In about ten days I was able to return and finish the winter course.

Another circumstance shows the constancy of Dr. Hering's friendship. Some time before the College Commencement I wished to go home, but this was against the wishes of Dr. Hering. He said: "You have been here thus far, now stay for the Commencement." On the important day Dr. Hering invited me to accompany the Faculty and take a seat with them on the platform. When the ceremony of conferring degrees was concluded by the president of the college, and each recipient of a diploma had been given a bouquet of flowers, I noticed that Mrs. Hering had another which made me wonder why it had not been given to some one. I also noticed that the Dean of the faculty held another sheepskin, but I had no idea that this had any significance for me. But soon the Dean stepped out upon the platform and began to speak. I heard

my name called, and in the confusion which followed, I managed
to stand up and hear whatever of his speech I could. The purport
of it was that the Faculty of the Homoeopathic Medical College of
Pennsylvania had unanimously voted me the special degree of the
college, and that the association with me through the winter had
been such as to give them great pleasure, at this time, in conferring the degree upon me. Then Mrs. Hering gave me the bouquet which I had noticed in her hand, and then came the con-
gratulations from different members of the faculty, and I was
glad to get out of the Hall.

Altogether this was the happiest, as well as the most instructive
winter I ever passed. So many memories cluster about these men,
and those whom I had met at Dr. Hering's, that I must stop and
think of them. There was our noble Dunham, our Damascene P. P.
Wells, our loving Jeanes, our lion-hearted Lippe, our beloved Raue,
and our accurate Guernsey. Doctors Dunham, Gardner, Jeanes,
and now Father Hering are gone. Those who are left of the Old
Guard are well worthy of our love and respect, and as we drop
a tear upon the graves of those who are gone, let us not fail to
cherish a warm love for those who are left to bear aloft the standard of pure homoeopathy.

Many times since 1865 I have visited Dr. Hering, and was always received with the same warm welcome. These interviews
were full of instruction and friendship. I wish I could describe all
of the many reminiscences I retain of him, but this I cannot do.
With your patience and indulgence I will give you a few of the
incidents as they occurred during these visits subsequent to 1865.

For several years, after 1865, I visited Dr. Hering every summer
and was always welcomed as warmly as before. In his home (a
double house, Nos. 112 and 114 North Twelfth St.), on the first
floor, were four rooms, besides kitchen and laundry, and one small
room off the dining room. The two front rooms were his reception
rooms. The north room was the ladies' room and the south, his
ordinary business room. This last was evenly divided across between the two windows by a couple of desks, behind one of which
the doctor stood, with pen in hand, ready to write down symptoms,
or, when seated, to look up the remedy from his books; at the other
desk sat his assistant. Many a time I have seen the space in front
of these desks full of patients, even extending out into the hall, in
fact all over the lower part of the house, awaiting their turn for an
audience. Behind his desk Dr. Hering stood passing upon one,
then upon another until all were served, after which he would go
out in his carriage to visit patients.

The other two rooms on the first floor were, respectively, a dining
room and a reception room for visitors and in which to see his

women patients. This room was about twenty by thirty feet: on one side, the south, were shelves full of clinical notes behind a red curtain; on the north side, closets for microscopes and books; on the west end, giving into the garden, were two large windows. In front of one stood a good-sized aquarium; at the east end were folding doors of solid mahogany separating it from the ladies reception room, in which were oil paintings, a marble statuette of Hahnemann on the mantel, and a marble bust of his friend, Karl Formes, famous opera basso, on a pedestal. Over the folding doors was a portrait of the original serpent, the *Lachesis trigonocephalus* from which was taken the poison for his provings.

As I remember it, half erect, with the rest of its body coiled, and the mouth open, it seemed a formidable reptile. I have wished that I had a photograph of it. In my office there is a representation of the South American lance-headed viper which a water-color artist made for me from a description in Jahr's *Pharmacopoeia*, but it does not resemble the portrait Dr. Hering had made for him, of the genuine *Surukuku snake*, the *Lachesis trigonocephalus* from Surinam. People often come into my office, and after looking at my picture, with a shudder, exclaim: "How can you bear to have that ugly thing here?" Ah! that to them ugly thing, to me is a thing of beauty! I never tire of looking at it. As I look at it I am reminded of the remedy *Lachesis* and I seem to see one of my children, if not two, who were saved by it, and as I continue to look I see here one, and there another, who only for this beneficent virus in potentized form would have passed over to the majority. I rejoice that Dr. Hering lived to introduce this remedy into practice.

Once when I visited Dr. Hering there was a stranger who answered the bell when I called, who ushered me into the reception room. There were several patients there when I entered. Dr. Hering took no notice of me whatever, but went on with his examinations and prescriptions until he got through. During all this time I sat there watching him, but he did not show that he had ever known me. When the last patient had passed out and my turn came he said: "Come into our room; I can't see you here." He wanted to hear something more about *Lachesis*. During the time I sat in his reception room he would not allow himself to be diverted from his purpose, even so far as to recognize me, but kept steadily on until he had made his prescription for the last one, when he immediately dismissed all from his mind, and gave himself up to friendship. I really thought that he had forgotten me, and said so. "No," he said, "I never let one thing interfere with another."

At one time, when I had called early in the morning, I found him in his study, on the second floor, where his manuscripts are kept. This room on the second floor, was over his business room.

It was here that he shut himself up and generally admitted no visitors excepting intimate ones on rare occasions. Here Raue, his intimate friend, came unfailingly for a short talk every morning. This room was lined with shelves, filled with books and manuscripts, which he needed in his work of book making, principally material for his Materia Medica. At one end of the room, the north side, there was a large iron safe for special manuscripts, and this was full. Dr. Carroll Dunham, prized friend and frequent visitor to this room, once said that his highest ambition would be gratified if he could but edit Dr. Hering's manuscripts. I am not sure if I heard Dunham say this, but, if not, it came direct from him through his next friend, Dr. Henry M. Smith. It was in this room that on a couch placed beside his writing desk, he slept and where he began work long before others in the house were awake. Here he would sit, half dressed, and wait until Mrs. Hering came to help him into his clothes to come down stairs to meet his patients, which was about ten o'clock. For his breakfast he had much earlier, a couple pieces of zwieback, with a cup of coffee, or hot chocolate prepared by himself over an alcohol lamp. He never seemed to know when it was time to get ready for the day's business.

On the particular morning when I was in this room Mrs. Hering came with a bowl of water and some towels for the doctor's toilet. When he came to change his night dress for his day-shirt I thought it time for me to retire, and was about to pass out of the room. "Oh, don't go," he said, "I am not a woman!" I remained until his toilet was completed and then he went down to his office.

Dr. Hering's mind was constantly occupied, and he was either talking, writing, or listening. He was a good listener if one had anything to say of value. I well remember the time when first I saw him to have any conversation with him. I happened to speak of an effect produced by *Euphrasia* on the nasal mucous membrane, and some use of this remedy in measles. At once out came his pencil and paper and down it went, subsequently if approved to appear in his portfolio. He always carried with him tablets of paper, about three by four inches in size, on which he wrote all he observed, or heard. On these he also noted his cases. I don't think I ever saw him too weary to tell something which would help others in homoeopathy. I don't remember a time that he was the first to say good night.

The great desire in Hering's heart, through all the time I knew him, was to publish a complete Materia Medica. During the winter I spent with him he tried to consummate this wish and issued a prospectus for publishing the work, both in German and English, in the same book. He offered it at the exact cost of printing and paper for five thousand copies. Some money was raised for this

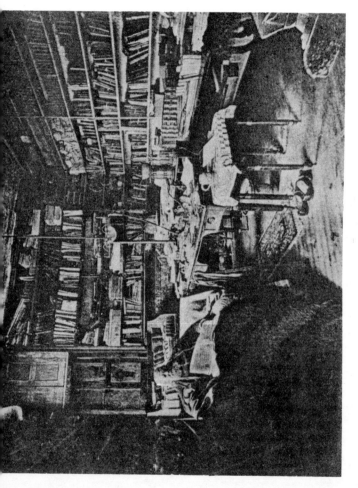

Dr. Hering in His Study.
The Second Floor of 112-114 North 12th Street,

purpose. how much I do not know. Although this project fell to the ground, I know that he was happy in making the effort. Those who sent the first instalment of five dollars had their choice, either to take the money back or receiving a copy of Gross' *Comparative Materia Medica*, a work which he had translated; I presume they all took the book. Later he made another attempt to get out his Materia Medica in a periodical, and through this he issued several pathogeneses in the *American Journal of Homoeopathic Materia Medica*. This came to an end all too soon.

At last the desire of his heart was to be gratified, and his *Guiding Symptoms* began to make its appearance under such auspices that a certainty had been reached. And now, instead of the enterprise falling through, and thus disappointing him, he passed away. Like Moses on the Mount, viewing the promised land which he was not to enter, Dr. Hering at last had a view of the consummation of that which he had been looking for so many years. This work is in loving hands, and it will be completed, before long, I hope. His expression to me about this work, full of enthusiasm, was: "When this comes out, what a grand thing it will be. Nothing ever published can compare with it."

What a life his was! A life of desire to benefit others. Laboring on, even to the last hour of his life. If I were to be asked what was the chief trait in his character, I should say that it was a desire to aid his fellows, with perfect confidence in those whom he trusted.

It will be presumptuous in me to attempt to give an estimate of how much Dr. Hering knew, since this will be told so much better than I can do, by his many associates. I only knew, that there seemed to be no subject which he did not appear to understand. and frequently, when with him, he would start out to talk upon his favorite theme, homoeopathy, and from this pass on to some other, perhaps music, where he seemed to be equally at home. Once, I met at his home a favorite opera-singer, Karl Formes, I think, and as I listened to their conversation, I could see that Dr. Hering was as conversant with operas and opera music, as was this professional singer. I well remember this meeting, for I was surprised to hear Dr. Hering talk and to have Formes listen to him. Afterwards. when listening to the singing, in opera, of this artist. I found myself wondering whether Dr. Hering, too, might not have been successful as an opera singer, if his pathway had led him to it. That same evening, when we were alone together, he gave me. as I now see it. about all the information I possess in regard to opera. He knew the history of all the artists who were successes in their line.

At times he would talk of the future life and what he expected in it. It was, to him. only another step in progress. We are to take up our lives and go on in the future just where we lay it down here.

Our pursuits are to be the same, only the incumbrances are to be removed. I don't think I ever heard him hesitate in this regard.

He seemed to have reflected upon this subject, and to have settled it in his mind just as definitely as any other subject he undertook to study. He believed that we carry with us our preferences and our distastes, and that we will exercise them there as here. I have no doubt he expected to gather students about him in the other world and go on increasing in knowledge forever.

In 1876, at the time of the World's Convention of Homoeopathic Physicians there was a large number of physicians present from all the States and from abroad. Dr. Hering's time was very much taken up by calls from a great many of these strangers, all of whom wished to see Dr. Hering. I began to fear that I should not enjoy a visit to him on this occasion, when, one day, the day of Dr. Lippe's dinner at the Union League Club House, Dr. Hering said to me, "Come here this afternoon and go with me to the dinner; I shall not go unless you go with me." I was told that he seldom went out alone now, and as he desired me to go with him, and for fear that he might not see me at any other time, I did not fail to go. We took the cars on Twelfth Street at his door and rode to Walnut Street, where we took another car and rode to Broad Street, near the Club House. It rained hard all the time, but this did not disturb him. He talked all the way about that first winter when the new faculty lectured, and of the class, all of whom he seemed to look upon as his children. Some of these he met at the dinner table. He seemed very happy all of the evening, but was glad to get home again. When I left him he said: "Now, when you come to Philadelphia again we will call on Dr. Lippe together, and I shall not go until you go with me." At this time, I saw him but once more, and then only for a few minutes. He said: "There are so many here now to see me that I have no time for you, but I am hungry to see you just the same."

There was always a chair at his table for me, where I learned to like cheese, but I did not wish it in two ounce doses, without bread. I can vouch for the flavor of Limburger cheese, when taken in small quantities, and as a flavor to bread or crackers.

In 1877 I was again at his house, when he invited several of his friends to supper with me, in his garden. He seemed more fond than ever of calling around him younger members of the profession, and this afternoon, I think, there were at least ten or twelve of them. He was particularly pleased that so many came to see him. When he invited me to this supper he said: "I want them to see the man who saved *Lachesis*." After they had gone he talked about the first time we met, in the same garden, and how unexpected the meeting was. He had received my letter asking to be allowed to call on him for instruction in homoeopathy, only a day or two before the meeting. He said, then, that it had been the chief pleasure in his life, viz., to impart to others what he knew.

We expected then to make our call upon Dr. Lippe, but were prevented. This called up the time when Lippe was very sick with typhoid fever, the time of his visit to him, and Hering taking down the Materia Medica, looked it through and found the remedy in *Silica*, which saved Dr. Lippe to homoeopathy.

When I left, Dr. Hering said: "Come again next year." I said: "Yes;" and fully expected to have done so, but did not, and never saw him again.

In writing these reminiscences I have given them as they recurred to me. On reading them over I wonder if his friendship for me was any closer than for others. Sometimes I feel that I was more than ordinarily a favorite, but when I recall the memory of those whom I have met at his house, I can not pride myself on this. I will not undertake to name these others, but as I remember what Dr. Hering said of them, I can but think that had I not wanted instruction in homoeopathy I should never have found the way to his heart, and so must give the honor to homoeopathy, instead of to myself.

This morning a postman brought me a letter, postmarked Philadelphia. On opening it I read, "Enclosed I send you a lock of father's hair." How glad I was to get it, I will not undertake to tell, but I will say that I will cherish it, as a memento of that dear old man, who for so many years honored me with his warm friendship.

The President, Dr. John K. Lee, spoke as follows, after relinquishing the chair to Dr. Henry N. Guernsey:

We have listened with intense interest to the narration of the personal reminiscences of Dr. Hering and have been touched by the glowing eulogies upon his life, and it may seem superfluous and redundant to pay a further tribute to his revered memory.

But whilst he has been extolled for the greatness of his intellect, his profound erudition, his untiring research, and his devotion to his profession, still the portraiture is incomplete, because it does not include a delineation of his moral qualities. And these, according to their development, either add grace and dignity to intellectual endowments, and link man to his Creator, or else dim the splendor of his achievements, tarnish the lustre of his fame and spread a pall of darkness over his grave.

In this respect. I am happy to affirm, it is not necessary to prevaricate or to enfold Dr. Hering in a mantle of charity, since his moral nature expanded in beautiful harmony with his mind and blending, each reflected the glory of the other and formed a well-rounded symmetrical character, always grand, because underlaid by simplicity and fidelity to truth.

A single instance in his history, related to me by one who was admitted to his confidence and privacy, will illustrate the elevation of his moral sentiments, his magnanimity and abhorrence of the least departure from the path of rectitude, and honor. Some years ago, the relator, during a conversation with Dr. Hering he remarked, "J - - - - is stopping with me. He is a man of wonderful ability, but I have lost all regard for him. At supper, last evening, in a burst of feeling, he said: 'How badly it makes one feel to be convinced of error!' I felt indignant at such a sentiment, and replied: 'No, not if he be moved by proper motives. The only feeling of an honest man should be—How glad I am to learn the truth; and from that moment I lost all regard for the man!'"

The thought here expressed is so lofty, grand and pure, that I will not impair its force by verbal comments, but leave it to penetrate your minds to influence your lives.

Dr. Joseph C. Guernsey addressed the chair as follows:

Mr. President: I do not rise to eulogize Dr. Hering, or to recount his many good works in the advancement of our cause. There are many here, tonight, who can do, and have already done, more justice to that than I can do.

I merely wish to present an interesting memento relative to his medical graduation. It is a translation from the Latin of the subjects of his Thesis, which he defended, as was the custom, in public disputation before graduating at the University of Wuerzburg, in the year 1826.

The following preamble is printed, in Latin, on the cover of the Dissertation:

"Johann Lucas Schoenlein, Dean *pro tempore* of the gracious order of physicians, Doctor of Philosophy, Medicine and Surgery, and public professor in ordinary, etc., etc., with all due courtesy, invites the noble vice-rector of the Academy, the senate fathers, the professors of all grades, the academic citizens, finally men of letters and the patrons of letters, to a public disputation, to be held March 22nd, at 9 a. m., by the very noble, illustrious and learned man, Herr Constantine Hering, Saxon, under the presidency of Cajitanus

Textor, Doctor of Philosophy, Medicine and Surgery, Aulic Councillor to the August King of Bavaria, and Public Professor in Ordinary, etc., etc., for the purpose of duly obtaining the highest honors in Medicine, Surgery and Obstetrics.

INAUGURAL DISSERTATION

On

Psychic Remedies

Theses

I

Springs are living fossils.

II

I hold that there are nerves in the placenta.

III

The "ganglion petrosum" is to the ear what the "ganglion ophthalmicum" is to the eye.

IV

The olfactory, optic and acoustic nerves are apophyses of the cerebrum and cerebellum, not nerves.

V

The old man is the perfect man.

VI

Materia Medica is to Hahnemann what Pathology was to Hippocrates.

VII

Such as life is, is disease.

VIII

The rational system is not merely the better, but the only one in pathology.

IX

I deny psychical diseases.

X

Any disease may be removed at any stage.

XI

No one has yet appeared to refute Hahnemann.

XII

Homoeopathy is heterostheny, and its fundamental law: *Contraria contrariis.*

XIII

In the struggle of vital forces as a foundation rests every vital effect.

XIV
There is only one normal position for the foetus.

XV
The resurrection of the dead is the highest ideal of
medical art.

XVI
Not to deliver individual men from particular diseases, but to
deliver the whole human race from the cause of disease,
is the ultimate goal of medical science.

INAUGURAL SUBJECTS
I. *President's Question:*
The checking of traumatic hemorrhages.
II. *Candidate's Subject:*
The Medicine of the Future.

Dr. Charles Mohr then rose and made the following
remarks:

I approach the subject of anything relating to the life and work
of Dr. Hering with a great deal of diffidence.

But, on this occasion, I cannot, consistently with any sense of
duty, neglect saying a word or two in regard to the manner in which
Dr. Hering treated the stranger student and the younger practitioner of homoeopathy.

I remember the first time I ever saw Dr. Hering. It was on an
evening after I had attended a lecture in this room, and I was
somewhat perplexed about a case I was treating and thought I
would like to hear what he had to say in relation to what had best
be done.

I later went to his house, rang his door bell, was shown into his
office, and when I told him my purpose of seeing him, he at once
extended his hand and gave mine a hearty shake and said: "Sit
down." After he had waited upon two or three patients he was
ready to hear my story, which I related. I think it was more than
an hour before I was ready to leave him. He gave me his opinion
as to the nature of the case, and what I might expect, and what,
in hi- judgment, was the proper remedy, and I wondered that the
man, without the least idea of receiving any remuneration, should
take so much time and trouble to give to me, an utter stranger, the
knowledge I desired; and when I rose to say good-bye and express
my thanks, he again extended his hand, and shaking mine with a
hearty grip, he said in that same tone, which, after that became
very familiar to me, "Well, come again!" And I did go, again and

again. and never saw Dr. Hering in my life that I did not learn
something to profit me and those who came within the influence
of my professional life.

ST. LOUIS MEMORIAL MEETING

At a St. Louis Memorial Service held October 10th,
1880, Dr. Charles Gundelach read a biographical sketch
from which the following extracts are a part:

Dr. Hering's life-work was Materia Medica. He made provings
of the most of our remedies in present use, introduced many new
and valuable drugs, and published his remedies and experiences in
different works, here and abroad, and was, during all his years of
practice, a very diligent contributor to the periodical medical literature in America, as well as in Germany. Of his publications should
be mentioned his *Domestic Physician*, first published in 1835. The
work passed through seven editions in America, two in England,
thirteen in Germany, and has been translated into the French,
Spanish, Italian, Danish, Hungarian, Russian and Swedish
languages.

The Effects of Snake Poison, 1837.
Suggestions for the Proving of Drugs, 1853.
American Drug Provings, 1853 - 1857.
Translation of *Gross' Comparative Materia Medica*, 1866.
Analytical Therapeutics, Vol. I, 1875.
Condensed Materia Medica, two editions, 1877 - 1879.
Guiding Symptoms, a ten volume work, the third of which he
    began just prior to his death, was completed by his Literary
    Executors, Doctors Raue, Knerr and Mohr, now out of print.

In person, Dr. Hering had an imposing and dignified appearance. He was tall, and wore spectacles; beard full and hair long
and curling. Dr. Hering was married three times. First in South
America, where the mother of his first child, a son, now living in
Paramaribo, died after giving birth.

After returning to Philadelphia, from Allentown, he married a
girl of German parentage with whom he had three children, only
one surviving; a daughter, married and living in Boston. After
his second wife had died, during a visit to Germany, in 1845, he
married Therese, the daughter of Dr. Buchheim, a celebrated allopathic physician, by whom he had eight children, six of whom, and
their mother, survive him.

Dr. Hering enjoyed good health until about ten years ago, when,
at the ripe age of seventy, he occasionally suffered from attacks

of asthma. Even to the last day of his life, he was in comparative good health, having attended to his patients during the day, the last one just before retiring. Later in the evening, in his study, while engaged in literary work, (on his *Guiding Symptoms*) he was suddenly attacked with paralysis of the heart and died within twenty minutes, with none of his family present but his devoted wife and Mrs. Mertens, a friend of the family; this was on Friday evening, July 23rd, 1880, he being in the eighty-first year of his age.

Dr. W. A. Edmonds followed with these remarks:

In surveying a great and noble life, like that of Dr. Hering, we very naturally incline to be inquisitive as to the peculiar point, or quality of character which may have resulted in so much usefulness and prominence.

Undoubtedly the great beaconlight of his lifework and the charm of his character, was his enthusiasm; the enthusiasm of conviction, and especially his conviction as to the theoretical and practical truth of homoeopathy.

By enthusiasm, we understand that particular emotional glow and warmth of delight experienced upon the attainment of new knowledge, or a new idea. All of us have greater or less experience of such emotion; but so soon do we turn aside into the avenues of sordidness and selfishness, to see what of gain or position may be made out of the newly-gotten idea, that the sensation, like the sparkle and aroma of the newly uncorked vintage, wastes with the touch of early use.

A pure and unalloyed enthusiasm is not found in companionship with avarice, ambition and untruthfulness. The purely selfish intriguer may be impelled by his desires to heroic efforts and deeds of daring, but is ever a stranger to that holy poetic fire which warmed and illumined the pathway in the life of our distinguished comrade. To say, then, that he was enthusiastic, is to say that he was truthful and loyal to his convictions.

Peculiarities of organization and modes of life, as before intimated, render enthusiasm with most of us an ephemeral affair. With our dear departed friend, this activity was in ceaseless motion, ever present. He loved the truth for itself, and for its usefulness to humanity; he loved it as the young mother loves her newly firstborn; and as the love grew older, it grew stronger and warmer, until, in the very last days of a long and eventful life, it shone with a phosphorescent glow and undimmed splendor. His unselfish love of the truth, and devotion to conviction, was "a thing of beauty, a joy forever." With all my soul I bow with reverence and adoration in the presence of a life so resplendent with loyalty to truth, or at least that which he believed to be true. Hundreds of practitioners, the country over, evince much of his brainpower and industry, but for want of his mental warmth have never approached his eminence. There seemed to be a charm and magnetism about this element of his character, which sent him, at a bound, away ahead of all competition. When new knowledge, or a new truth, had set his head and heart fairly aglow, he never halted to inquire what might be the consequence of its adoption; whether it would bring gain and position, or loss and disparagement.

In the earlier years of his life, he was requested, by his preceptor, to furnish a paper in refutation of homoeopathy. Most young men, under such circumstances would have set to work in quest of material to furnish the desired refutation and thereby receive the approbation of his superior. But he, with a true nobility of soul, went straight to the side of homoeopathy to ascertain what might be said in its favor, with the result of his immediate conviction and conversion, instead of the contemplated refutation.

At a later period of his life, he, with another, was sent abroad by his government for scientific purposes. Very soon he was detected by one of his medical associates in the promulgation and practice of homoeopathy. At once his conduct was reported to his superiors. He was ordered to confine his attention to special objects of his appointment.

Promptly he closed his portfolio, set his papers and accounts in order, tendered his resignation, entered upon his lifework in the teaching and practice of his profession; and so continued to teach and to practice, through good or evil report, praise or disparagement; living long enough to see the hated heresy a power in the civilized world, and a boon to humanity in the ills to which flesh is heir.

In tracing his life and character, we find a striking parallel to that of the dramatic life of the illustrious Apostle Paul, who had but to know the truth of his convictions in any given premise, and he was ready to brave all the perils and hardships of fire, famine, stripes, imprisonment, shipwreck and martyrdom in its vindication. The trials of our friend were less literal and corporeal, but the social and official ostracism of his early days, were scarcely less trying to a sensitive and noble nature.

Who shall estimate the results of such a life as its benign influence radiates and ramifies down the chambers and corridors of time, through ceaseless future ages, until our efforts at comprehension are paled and wearied as in an attempt to grasp infinity.

"If a man die, shall he live again?" Let us, our friends, in this, our hour of bereavement, accept such a life and character as a great and mighty revelation in behalf of the soul's immortality. The good Father never made such a life to go down in one eternal night of annihilation. In the matter of what we call his death, we recognize the breaking up of the casket in order that the jewel may have a new setting, to fit it for the glories and splendor of the great beyond, where it is destined to glow and sparkle with an ever increasing brilliancy, through the countless cycles of an eternity of which we may talk and write, but of which our present finite powers can have but a poverty of expression or appreciation.

Our friend in the flesh has gone; we shall see his face here no more forever. For eighty long winters and summers did he continue the voyage of life, and when his mortality went down in the Jordan of death, he went down as some gallant ship, with sails unfurled and banners flying, with the inscription high over all: "Homoeopathy as a truth once, always and forever."

Dr. S. B. Parsons prefaced the reading of the following poem by saying:

The theme of this poem was suggested by an incident in the life of Dr. Hering, which was, that in the early part of his professional career, in Philadelphia, he was called to attend a little girl, an only child, who had been given up to die by the physicians that had seen her.

Dr. Hering was summoned to the case, not because the parents had any faith in the homoeopathic mode of practice, but they had heard of him as a gentleman of culture, a man of scientific attainments, and hoped something might be found in his treatment that would restore their loved one to health.

Dr. Hering's treatment was successful, and when his little patient was out of danger, and able to talk and laugh with her mother, the parents overwhelmed him with expressions of gratitude, complimenting him in the warmest terms on his skill and ability, and drew a bright picture of his future life and the high eminence he would someday attain in his profession. When they had ceased, he thanked them kindly, and replied: "I am nothing, God is great!"

C ould we draw the veil aside
    From the night of infant state,
  Mortal eyes would see the guide—
    "I am nothing, God is great!"

H appy childwood—morn of life—
    Chasing shadows drawn by fate,
  Knows but faintly in the strife—
    "I am nothing, God is great!"

E ver smiling, sunny youth,
   Weaving webs to captivate,
  Then unfolds the spirit's truth—
    "I am nothing, God is great!"

R esting on the fair mid-land
   'Tween the in and outer gate,
  Budding manhood's thoughts expand—
    "I am nothing, God is great!"

I n the bloom of life's bright day,
   Lurid storms may devastate;
  Through the darkness beams a ray—
    "I am nothing, God is great!"

N earer draws futurity,
   Nor asks the pentinent to wait,
  Clearer sees maturity—
    "I am nothing, God is great!"

G ently comes life's winter day,
   When the heart seems desolate;
  In true faith will be its lay—
    "I am nothing, God is great!"

The following tribute was paid by Dr. J. Martin Kershaw:

As the majestic river passes to the far off sea beyond, so has the life of him we have come to honor, gone to the unknown country. Like the grand old oak, ever erect and noble, he bore all the storms of adversity and beclouded sunshine, throughout the scores of years that were his to work in and to be faithful.

Towering above his fellows, working and waiting for what he knew was truth, he was rightfully and indeed a king among men in his God-like work for humanity.

The truth, the pure snow white spotless truth was that for which he labored and toiled, from the early springtime of life until the frosty winter of old age had come upon him, when, full of years and full of honors, he crossed over to that land the Deity has given to those who work faithfully and well.

His priceless treasures he has bequeathed to us and to the multitude of God's sick and suffering creatures, in every clime and country, and the world is richer and better today, because Constantine Hering lived and worked in it.

In the quiet city of the dead, where countless weary toilers sleep, the sad song of the autumn winds is heard above the resting-place of him for whom we mourn tonight; but the earnest lifework, and the more than human deeds of the departed, still live for us and the coming worlds of people.

Dr. C. W. Spalding next addressed the meeting as follows:

There are epochs in human history that are occasioned by the discovery and introduction of new principles, or laws, which, in their operation have a direct relation to human happiness and the welfare of society. Not that there is anything absolutely new; for all things exist potentially in the Creator from eternity; and are called new, when they come into actual existence in the material universe.

The discovery and announcement of the law of *"Similia Similibus curantur"* constitutes such an epoch. Upon this great basic verity, has now been founded a school of medicine differing from all previous schools, in the adoption and application to practice, of this therapeutic law. The fundamental principles of medical science are the same in all schools of medicine; the differences being chiefly in their systems of therapeutics.

In order that the beneficent of a new therapeutic system should be made available for the alleviation of human suffering by the removal of diseases, it became necessary to develop and establish, by study and experiment, a system of medication in agreement therewith. Homoeopathic Materia Medica has arisen from this necessity. The proper presentation, and the ultimate establishment of new ideas in the minds of men, or of new methods in their habits of life, call into activity the labors of a class of minds peculiarly fitted for the performance of their definite tasks. As the knowledge of the discovery of this new therapeutic law was disseminated, it arrested the attention of such medical minds as were endowed with sufficient independence of thought to allow them to be open to conviction; and prominently among these was the man, whose life, and not whose death, we are now assembled to commemorate. His first study of the new system was occasioned, we are told, by his being assigned to refuting it. This is not the first time that the individual, chosen by his fellows, as the one most capable among them of disproving the new ideas, has become an able instrument in establishing them upon surer foundations and of spreading among mankind a better knowledge of their transcendent merits.

In relating the new law to practice, the great problem to be worked out was the ascertainment, by trial, of the specific action of drugs upon the human system, and subsequently the orderly arrangement of the great mass of experimental knowledge thus obtained into such form as to render it readily available in the practice of medicine. For the successful accomplishment of this important task, it was requisite that individuals peculiarly qualified by nature and education for this particular work should devote their lives to its development and perfection. In this arduous labor Dr. Hering has spent the best years of his life. To him, in very large degree, the homoeopathic physician is indebted for the completeness of our system of medication. Patience, industry and untiring perserverence have been brought to the work, and if any man, more than any other, is entitled to be called the apostle of Homoeopathic Materia Media, that man is Constantine Hering.

Dr. J. P. Frohne then spoke as follows:

The gentlemen who spoke before me have eloquently dwelt upon the merits of the departed as propagator of homoeopathy in this country.

Therefore, allow me to remember and make mention of his love for his native country, of which, especially during the Franco-German war he bore brilliant testimony; celebrating the victory of the German arms most solemnly at his own house. He thus manifested that he was proud of being a native of Germany, of that country which sent many a great man over the ocean to sow the seeds of German thought and German art among distant nations.

The departed has shown his love for his native country, and his interest in science by a multitude of articles printed in homoeopathic journals, here and abroad. His essays are as genial as they are instructive, and his memory is, in due appreciation of his merits, this day celebrated in the cities of all Germany.

And wherever, upon the face of the world homoeopathy has gained permanent ground, the name of Constantine Hering will be known, and be ever memorable, since he has, by his works, secured for himself an immortal name.

To but very few of us mortals is granted to do as much for suffering humanity as he has done; for Providence had laid in him the talents of a true therapeutist, as well as those of an author, of which during his long life, he has made the most salutary use, saving the lives of thousands, who, in the sense of gratitude lament his loss.

The life and works of our Hering ought to be a shining model for us younger physicians; and may his memory be everlasting!

The following remarks were then made by Dr. Charles L. Carriere:

Grand is the celebration of today! The fact that all homoeopathists of the world join in a Memorial Service of one so universally known, esteemed and beloved as Dr. Constantine Hering makes this celebration one of the grandest of the kind. It is proper, therefore, that on this occasion everything should be thought of which may add to the honor of our departed friend.

I have chosen to occupy the few minutes allotted to me, to draw your attention to the fact that Dr. Hering was not only a man of great culture and a most successful practitioner of the Healing Art, but, in addition to his excellent qualities and his superiority, he was also on the progressive path of a christian; not a christian by name only, but one who did believe in Jesus Christ, our Saviour. Still, his faith differed from the generally acknowledged doctrines of the church of the past. As he had left the old school of medicine and adopted the doctrine of "similia" and became one of the founders of homoeopathy, so he also left the old church and became a receiver of the doctrine of the New Jerusalem. Thus he was one of the beginners and promoters of the New Era, both in Medicine and Religion.

A German paper, referring to his departure from this world, says: "Dr. Hering was made acquainted with the doctrines of the New Church soon after his arrival in the United States; he received them with warmth and zeal; he was of the opinion that the action of the homoeopathic remedies would, at some time, be established by the doctrine of Correspondence." It may be proper here to state that the doctrine of correspondence is a doctrine of the New Church (as taught by Swedenborg). The paper referred to also states: "He occasionally mentioned that in his house the first German Christmas-tree, in the whole large city of Philadelphia, spread its brilliancy."

The words "German Christmas-tree" were probably used because it is claimed that the Germans introduced that custom into this country.

In looking at Dr. Hering as a medical man and as a religious man, we see that he was not led by blind faith, he was not bound to the doctrine of his predecessors because they were believed by them, or for reasons that they were the old and acknowledged doctrines of the world; he would investigate for himself, and be a rational believer of that which he accepted as truth. His religious belief differed as much, and even more, from the generally accepted doctrine of the church, as his homoeopathic theory and practice differed from the old school of medicine.

The difficulty of three persons in the Godhead, and how to make one of the three, did not trouble his mind, for he knew and fully understood that the Trinity was embodied in the Divine Humanity of Christ, and that there is but one God in but one person. Nor was it difficult for him to solve the apparent contradiction of the literal sense of the sacred Scripture, neither the apparent contradictions of scriptural statements with the developed facts of this age; for he well knew that the word of God is infinitely higher than human thought or language, and that in the inner life of these literal forms we find an inexhaustable fountain of the Divine Wisdom from which we may drink and never thirst.

From his knowledge of the spiritual world, and the relation between this life and the life to come, he knew that man, as a spiritual being, continues to live, that death is only the departure from one world to another; that it is but the material body that dies, and returns to the earth from which it was taken, there to remain and to rise no more; but that man himself will never die.

When, he, therefore, at the last moments of his earthly life, spoke the words "I am dying," he knew that it was but the material form that had fulfilled its mission and would cease to exist, but that he, who had for many years, in and through that body, accomplished great good to this world, would not go from this land of the living to the silent repose of the dead, but from the land of first development and preparation to that of eternal perfection.

Dr. C. W. Taylor expressed himself next in these words:

"The air is filled with farewells to the dying and mournings for the dead." Hourly, in some graveyard, the yawning earth is closing around the inanimate forms of loved ones. We are summoned but once to join the innumerable caravan moving on into the "silent land."

When the summons came to Constantine Hering, it found him ripe in years and intellect—fourscore years replete with benefits to his brother man. Quietly, as a child, he sank into that last dreamless sleep and was borne to "the garden of the slumberers."

He whose soul panted for communion with the great and good, and reached forward with eager struggle to the guerdon in the distance, has passed away.

A flower is plucked from one sunny bower, a breach made in one happy circle, a jewel stolen from one treasury of love. A harvester

has disappeared from the summer-field of life, and his funeral
winds, like a wintry shadow along the street. A sentinel has fallen
from his post, and is thrown from the ramparts of time into the
surging waters of eternity.

His heart was hopeful and generous, his life a perpetual litany—
a Maytime crowned with flowers that never fade.

> Deck not his couch with sombre shrouds,
>   It is not death, but only sleep.
> That kisses down his eyelids now;
>   Then why should we in sadness weep?
> He has but gained the needed rest
>   From weary toil, from care and strife.
> His fittest meed of praise will be
>   The grandeur of an earnest life.
>
> Take each the lesson to his heart,
>   And in his earnest struggles know
> That he strives best, who strives for truth,
>   Though faint and weary he may grow.
> You may not reach your highest aim,
>   Nor tread the heights that Hering trod,
> But do your duty—in that lies
>   The path that leads you nearer God.

Dr. C. H. Goodman related the following incidents:

My relations to Dr. Hering were only those of pupil to teacher,
for it was my privilege to sit under his instruction during the medical season of 1868-69 in the Hahnemann College of Philadelphia.

I can see him now as he hurried into the lecture room, his long
hair flowing over his shoulders, and his eye aflame with zeal and
enthusiasm. What scrupulous attention to detail; how minutely
and analytically he dwelt upon the symptomatology of each drug,
carefully weighing and balancing every expression and utterance!
His mind was so full, so teeming with facts and information, the
hour was too short to impart them to his hearers.

During my calls at his residence, I was particularly impressed
with his having recourse to his Materia Medica at every prescription. My examination hour with him was one of the pleasantest I
ever passed. The subject of my thesis being of some interest to
him, he discussed it fully and took occasion to enlarge upon his
own peculiar views of what constitutes Health and Disease, and of
the analogy between the latter and drug-provings. He narrated to
me at the same time his experience in curing with *Antimonium*

crudum a large corn on the foot of a sea captain. "Why," he re-marked with a merry look, "In a short time I was consulted by all of the captains in the navy, and they all had corns on the soles of their feet, and I nearly lost my reputation because I could not cure all of them!"

My last sight of him was on graduation-day, as he sat on the stage of the Academy of Music, beside Dr. Raue, to whom he was especially devoted, completely wrapped up in the music of the orchestra, which was rendering an air from the opera of *Der Freischuetz*. He was nodding and bending his head in unison with the music, apparently oblivious to all his surroundings, smiles of pleasure brightening up his venerable face as the harmonious strains fell upon his ear.

So was he completely attuned to, and in harmony with the world, and profession to which he devoted his life and best energies, and he fell, like the ripe fruit from the tree and was gathered into the garner of the faithful.

Dr. Philo G. Valentine next recited some verses, cleverly expressing in rhyme, Dr. Hering's life-story from the cradle to the grave.

Dr. G. S. Walker then delivered the following oration:

Constantine Hering is dead. The great Healer has passed from the realm of wounds and diseases. The Antagonist of Death, and his Conqueror on a thousand hard-fought fields, has yielded at last, when the issue of the struggle was but his own life. Invincible in his conflicts for others, he was mortal only when he struck in his own behalf. And death has gained a splendid prize. If the old chivalric theory be true, that all the honors of the defeated belong of right to the victor, Immortal Death has seldom, in all ages, from the issue of a single fight, won so large a spoil.

The mighty Physician, whose visits to the couch of suffering were as the Angel of Heaven's mercy, and whose prescription was Healing's potent spell; the calm, all-furnished schoolman—then the Champion of the Old School—who laid his boyish lance in rest against the Black Knight of Medical Heresy, and, doomed to dis-memberment by his Client, was saved by his Adversary, and thence consecrated all the energies of his redeemed strength to the new banner of "Similia"—bearing it in triumph, through both Hemis-pheres and in every clime, under the Southern Cross and Northern Pleiad, and planting it, with his dying hand, on the very citadel of the Enemy; the great Teacher, whose graduation thesis was "*De Medicina Futura*," and who founded the first College of our Order in the world; whose name lies at the foundation of our Medical Literature, side by side, with that of the immortal Hahnemann; the Poet, whose creative genius found and grasped, and whose sense of harmony set in eternal order and beauty, the great original truths of our system; the Seer, whose prophetic vision pierced the sullen shadows of the Infinite, and brought within the apprehension of common men a revelation of the Divine; the Laborer, whose untiring energies knew no pause or recreation, save in added and deeper toil; the Hercules, who cleansed the fouler than Augean Stables of Medical Science, and encountered and slew the Nemean Lion of Medical Orthodoxy; the gentle, generous, brave, great-hearted, wholesouled Man, whose qualities were no more simply great than his attributes were sublimely splendid; all these have gone down in that last desperate struggle, in closed lists, where his only second was a woman, whose loving hand and tender strength were all unable to hold back from the heart the icy grasp of Death.

Constantine Hering is dead, and all the orphaned Children of Affliction weep, and all the generous and noble of earth have sympathy in their sorrow and are partakers of their grief.

In the effulgence of his larger and brighter fame, we are sometimes inclined to forget that Hering was preeminently the Physician. Let us tenderly and gratefully, in sympathy with the wide circle of his bereaved patients, remember this fact tonight. Nature and education combined to render him the great Healer. His temper was generous, ardent, tender, affectionate and high. The pathematic was amongst the strongest forces of his grand nature; and it was always a wisely regulated and perfectly governed force.

High over all that wealth of sympathy, delicate, and susceptible as ideal women's, sat the intelligent and regal Will, rendering it subservient to the great end of his presence in the sick-room. And what a presence there! His stately form—his flowing locks and beard—the pure white light of cultured intellect shining on his lofty forehead and flashing in his earnest eye, mellowed and softened by the roseate hue of deep and hearty kindness—his mere appearance was the Harbinger of Hope to the Couch of Despair. And then his manner! Quiet, not soft; gentle, not weak; firm, not hard; confident, not rash; serious, not solemn; the gravity of simple earnestness, combined with the assurance of abundant resourses and an armed disciplined Intelligence; it was the finished perfection of the bearing of the Typical Physician, and had, in itself, a healing power.

His Method of Diagnosis was the analysis of exclusion. He ascertained, with the utmost care, and minuted with the greatest

exactness every characteristic symptom. This group of hostile
appearances he attacked with all the energies of his powerful mind.
One after another, he cast out and trampled under foot every false
and specious probability, until he stood, at the last, face to face
with his great enemy—the actual, the imminent and the dangerous
Dynamic Force; and against this, when found, his Arsenal of
Provings rendered him almost invincible. He was never hasty or
empirical in practice. He cared nothing for the man—whether
rich or poor, or high or low,—but everything for the patient. It
was a hand-to-hand fight with Disease; in which, once engaged,
he thought only of his Antagonist, and would neither surrender or
be beaten. Of course, his success was great, if not unexampled.
By his own person and individual prescriptions, he snatched from
the hand of Disease and Death unnumbered and innumerable
thousands; and indirectly, by the influence of his discoveries, suggestions and teachings, he was undoubtedly the most valuable factor
of his age in the grand multiple of Health and Life. His patients
venerated, trusted, loved, idolized, almost worshipped him. No
other man or men could supply his place to them. He was their
favorite and all-powerful Apostle of the Gospel of Health; and
when they could not secure his visits they would fain, like them
of old to Peter, have brought forth their sick into the streets, that
at least his shadow, in passing, might fall upon and bless them.
And this great Physician is dead!

Hering was the unrivalled champion and advocate of the Eternal
Law of *Similia Similibus Curantur.* Sincere, intelligent, high-
cultured, profound, original, bold and eloquent, he lifted his banner from the dust of popular contempt, and challenged, for its
insignia, the admiration and gratitude of the nations. All his interests, all his prejudices, the bent of his education, the pride of
championship, the heat of conflict, the hopes of his friends and
admirers—all forbade him to embrace the new and despised Heresy.
Yet embrace it he would and did, with all the fervor of his hero-
heart, simply, because upon investigation, not impartial, but
prejudiced, he found it true. The wave of conviction which rolled
into his mind, from the vast Ocean of Truth, washed every stain of
prejudice from its shores, and left them shining with the calm light
of certainty.

And his was so emotional conversion, born of a moment's frenzy
and destined to perish with the passing furor. It was not because
the New School saved that right arm which the Old had doomed
to excision, that he devoted its energies, with such consistent and
efficient fidelity, to the redemption of a pledge wrung from him
in an hour of insupportable anguish. It was because, with all the
exhaustive thoroughness of his grand and luminous intelligence, he

had previously investigated, tested and proved, until his whole nature was rife with conviction, that the healing touch of homoeopathy had power to kindle the long prepared train, and dedicate him, in an explosion of feeling, to the perpetual championship of its incomparable merits. Thenceforth, all his previous attainments became but the stepping-stones by which he ascended to the serene heights of Culture, and stood on their loftiest professional pinnacle, alone.

Hahnemann became his friend, intimate, and teacher; and from this Sage the hungry Neophyte drew all the accumulated treasures of his lore. Thence, girt with the commission of Royalty, under the stellar light of the Magellan Clouds, he sought the secret of nature in her most affluent home, and, fast as they accumulated, turned these treasures to the light of public advocacy of the cause he had so earnestly espoused. Farseeing, patient and profound, as broadly and highly cultured, he rested not on any yielding soil, but digged, and digged, until he reached the rock of ultimate truth; so that he may be said to have stood, with his head among the stars, catching the earliest and latest gleam of heaven's light, and with his feet planted upon the immovable foundations which support the world. With this gigantic reach and grasp of truth, he could not but be original. With the constituents of sincerity, earnestness, and self-sacrifice, he could not but be bold. With the freshness and enthusiasm of the youth, joined to the knowledge and culture of the philosopher, and the sage, he could not but be eloquent. All these he was. And this invincible Champion is dead!

Hering was par eminence the inspired Teacher. "Poeta nascitur non fit" had never truer application than to him. He was born for the vocation, and his high and incomparable gift of original genius he supplemented by the most careful training. Always he taught *con amore*. At home, on the street, in the sickroom, in his study, in the clinique, from the chair of the lecturer or the rostrum of the orator—wherever auditors could be found—he was their wise, patient, and delighted instructor. This was the purpose of all his learning. He gained but to impart. His whole capital of mental wealth was free to all comers. Of his illimitable gains he hoarded nothing. The fountain of his instruction was perennial, and had its source in the everlasting springs of Genius, Labor and Love. And, though he sought not this end, the paradox of Scripture was fulfilled to him; all of his gifts were gains. By the operation of a changeless law, what he gave to others was doubled to his own bosom. This was the secret of his unfailing readiness and fulness. Knowledge, he deemed a universal heritage, to which every willing and capable mind had an indefeasible right; and whereever he found such minds, it was more blessed for him to give than for them

to receive. Yet these gifts, widely and lavishly as he flung them
forth. were but the small change of his thought and his mind was
rich in massive ore, in ingots and gems. And with all this priceless wealth he dowered Humanity with his pen.

He was the father and maker of our Medical Literature; for
what he did not produce, he inspired. His own thought products,
completed, begun and designed, are so many and so intrinsically
great, that admiration loses its flippant eloquence, and sinks into
wonder and awe before the processes of so vast a mind. No such
writer on Popular Medicine has ever lived. His *Domestic Physician* still teaches the multitudes, in many languages and editions,
the secret of health at home; and his *Analytical Therapeutics*, and
Guiding Symptoms are of a quality which might satisfy the aspirations after fame of many first-class minds, and will require the
labor of many such to complete them, with the materials already
gathered and prepared by their great Author. All these precious
instructions to the world are couched in terms the most simple and
direct, and distinguished by an entire absence of style. He wrote
but to expound his thought; and his words are that thoughts
simplest and strongest vehicle. Of him it may be said, with truth
and emphasis, that, not only to our own school, but to the whole
world of Medical Thought and Culture, "He was a Teacher sent
from God." And this matchless Teacher is dead!

Hering was an unexampled Laborer. In boyhood, his sport was
toil. In maturity, his recreation was creation. In age, his repose
was application. He took no rest, and needed none. Work was his
pleasure and his passion. Each day of his life was too brief for the
busy ends he assigned it; each hour of every day, though beginning with the third after midnight and ending only with the tenth
after midday, too short for his toilful purpose. To the very last
day, and almost the last hour of his life, his unresting exertions
never ceased. And yet his energies never flagged. He did not toil
on doggedly and dully, the reluctant slave of a cruel purpose; but
with such warm, earnest and cheerful interest as made him dread
the hour of necessary suspension of his task. The sustained fire of
his energy was simply marvelous. There is nothing in the correla-
tion and conservation of material forces which can at all account
for it. It did not lie in the food he ate, or the sleep he took.
Rather, it would seem to have been the result of such an uncom-
mon affluence, in the original endowment of his vital forces, as the
world has seldom, if ever seen. Instead of losing, as is the case with
other men, this rare mind seemed rather to accumulate fire and
force by its own progress. And it was no unregulated and disorderly energy, which thus found its necessary expression in ceaseless
action. Every mental impulse had a method—every intellectual

ebullition poured its forces into a prescribed channel—every molten
thought settled into its previously prepared mould, and hardened
into the shape which it was predestined to take and wear forever.
It was labor with such method as economized and utilized every
particle of mental energy; as if the worker had been the poorest of
the poor, instead of the wealthiest of earth, in intellectual endowments. And the method was no clumsy, fanciful or grotesque con-
trivance of idle revery, perverted taste, or passionate prejudice, but
the highest and most finished product of original genius, guided by
intelligent and cultivated skill. It was such a method as may be
seen a sample of in the *Analytical Therapeutics;* a method to fill
the mind with wonder and joy, and to fall upon the world of
Medical Thought and Culture like the benediction of the Most High.

And all this measureless strength, indicated by such unrivaled
labors, was dedicated to the grandest objects, and justified by the
highest results. Its products, crystallized in print, admirable and
wonderful as they are, are but a small part of these results. The
walls of Hering's study, from floor to ceiling, are filled with manuscripts, in his own handwriting, all perfectly arranged and method-
ized, to carry on the complete and incomparable works which he
began and designed. Thus the matchless Worker, standing in his
study, built up around him that pearly palace of his thought, which
shall never know decay.

Alas! our Ulysses has departed on his travels, and there is none
left at Ithica strong enough to bend his bow! Atlas has gone to
the Hesperides, and there is none to bear up the skies. And this
incomparable Laborer is dead!

Above all, Constantine Hering was a man. All the constituents
of mental character was his. Strength, courage, force and constancy distinguished him above other men. In ability to grasp, and
firmness to hold, all that he recognized as truth, he had no peer.
In adventurous daring, supported and justified by the tremendous
momentum of his mind, he was simply sublime. His principles
were pure, unselfish and high, and his loyalty to conviction un-
wavering. A better or truer man never lived. And this strong
base of noblest manhood was overlaid with the fine gold of all
gentle and attractive qualities. He was susceptible, appreciative,
affectionate, constant, tender and forbearing. His heart was open
as his hand, and the clasp of the one was warm with the pulse of
the other. His tastes were cultivated and refined to that degree,
that his house was the house of Art and Culture, and the refuge
of struggling genius. His friends were statesmen, artists, scientists
of worldwide reputation and renown; and of these, once gained,
he never lost one. All who loved him, loved him to the end, either
of their own lives or his. He was gentle as a child, pure as a

snowflake, and warm as a sunbeam. In a word, the "grand old
name of Gentleman" was his, by right of eminence in the essential qualities which constitute that character. In the words of one
of our sweetest modern poets:

> "To him were all men heroes, every race noble,
> All women virgins, and each place a temple:
> He knew nothing that was base."

And this peerless Gentleman is dead!

Dead! Aye, even as the mollusk, the builder of the seashell
dies, leaving his soul crystallized in forms of imperishable beauty
which still ring with the sound of life's eternal sea.

Hering is not dead. He does not even sleep. His waking spirit
walks abroad, through all the realms of thought. For such as he
was there is no death. He lives, must ever live, in Memory, in
Blessing and in Hope. In the hearts of many, rich and poor, high
and low, his deeds have built a shrine whereon Gratitude will lay
her morning and her evening sacrifices, until the hearts which
cherished him as a Physician have ceased to beat; and even in
dying, they will bequeathe his memory as a rich legacy to their
children. The disciples and lovers of the cause he espoused and
defended will never cease to hear the all-eloquent Champion of
homoeopathy. The Student of Medicine, in the remotest future,
will bless and revere the name of Hering, as the great Bringer of
Order out of chaos of Materia Medica. The immediate and remote beneficiaries of his life-work will join hearts and hands in
gratitude for his benefactions and in emulation of his industry.
Ennobled by his name and fame, ever and forever, "his children
and his children's children, will rise up and call him BLESSED."

After the eulogy the following ode was sung:

> How sleep the brave who sink to rest,
>   By all their country's wishes blest!
> When Spring, with dewy fingers cold,
>   Returns to deck their hallowed mold,
> She there shall dress a sweeter sod
>   Than fancy's feet have ever trod.
>
> By fairy hands their knell is rung;
>   By forms unseen their dirge is sung,
> There honor comes, a pilgrim gray,
>   To bless the turf that wraps their clay,
> And freedon shall await repair,
>   To dwell a weeping hermit there!

A benediction was asked by the Rev. John Snyder and
the meeting adjourned.

MEETING IN KANSAS CITY, MISSOURI

A meeting was held in Kansas City, Missouri, from which a preamble and resolutions were presented and approved.

UNIVERSITY OF MICHIGAN MEETING

Prof. E. C. Franklin of Ann Arbor spoke as follows:

The early history of Dr. Hering finds him a bitter opponent of homoeopathy. Born with the beginning of the century, in Oschatz, Saxony, at an early period he began his student-life under the immediate charge of his father. Here we observe him as a diligent and faithful pupil; developing those sterling qualities of head and heart that made him so attractive to his teachers while pursueing his studies in the High School (Gymnasium) of Zittau, then under the rectorship of his father. His remarkable powers of observation and analysis, his centering application, marked him out as no ordinary individual. In his twentieth year he matriculated as a student of medicine at the University of Leipzig, and during his pupilage here was singled out by his preceptor, on account of his superior literary attainments, to prepare a monograph in opposition to that medical heresy that was at this time agitating and unhinging the medical mind of Germany and other parts of the Continent. Elated with the prospect of a scientific tilt with the sage of Coethen, he began a review of Hahnemann's writing, hoping to obtain an easy victory in his medical contest; but his reading only impressed him the stronger with the doctrines of Hahnemann, and scientific as he was, he became so thoroughly convicted with the depth of reason, and glow of genius, of the great medical reformer, that his criticisms were turned into laudation of the teachings of the author, and he became a convert to their strongly impressed truths.

About this time, and while pursuing his anatomical demonstrations, he inflicted upon his hand a poison-wound from the keen edge of the dissector's knife, which subsequently gave him no little solicitude and anxiety. He sought medical counsel of his old friends, and in spite of their best directed efforts he grew daily worse, and the gloomy alternative was given him of amputation of the hand. Chagrinned and discomfitted, he accepted the proffered aid of a friend, a disciple of Hahnemann, and had the proud satisfaction of seeing his hand daily grow better, and finally saved from the dreaded prognosis pronounced by his attending physicians. With this his conversion to homoeopathy was secured, and he left

Leipzig strong in the faith of *Similia* and entered the University of Wuerzburg. After attending lectures here, he graduated, in 1826, and returned to Saxony to practice his profession on his native soil.

He accepted the position of teacher of natural sciences and house-physician in a prominent school under the charge of Director Blochmann.

Wearied with continued application along the old groove of medical thought, disgusted with the endless jargon of medical theories and changing dogmas, and soured with the intolerant bigotry of that old school that is "broken down in council and in fight, in hospital and in camp, yet brokenly lives on," his active and restless spirit, imprisoned no longer by the bonds of state medicine, sought new and unpent fields for its scientific longings. He saw in the profession of medicine a system of castes of corporations, not of individual, but of collective castes. He saw that a man can be anything he can be, but no man can be anything out of the caste. He longed to be free, and like the imprisoned bird sought freedom in the boundless continent of beautiful fruits and flowers. An opportunity was soon presented, and he eagerly accepted the position that was the fulfilment of his daydream of usefulness, and which gave us the bright realization of his long-cherished hopes and made him a hero in the new world of progressive knowledge.

A distant relative had just returned from South America, whose vivid descriptions of the beauty and splendor of the natural curiosities of that far-off tropical region, where "nature wears her sweetest smile and sings her lovliest notes," inspired his young heart to woo fickle fortune in the distant lands of the occident.

By the aid of influential friends he procured an appointment from the King of Saxony to accompany the accomplished naturalist (botanist) Weigel, and in 1827, with rosy hopes and elated spirit, he set sail for his far-off western home and arrived in Dutch Guiana soon after. Hopeful and buoyant, with a soul full of ardor for his cherished work, he entered upon his new field of labor and made many friends and converts to the faith that animated all of his labors. Still keeping up his medical studies, *pari passu* with his zoological enquiries, he attracted considerable attention, both to himself, and to the system of medicine by which he was continually bequeathing rich legacies to suffering humanity. While upon the very tip-toe of encouragement and merited commendation from those who were the almost daily recipients of his kindly care and thoughtful consideration, and while pursueing with diligence and earnestness his chosen field of study, a message was handed him from the Fatherland reprimanding him for daring to extend and popularize the hated science of homoeopathy, afar off though it be, in lands beyond the sea. His noble spirit, no longer fettered by the chains of that medical despotism that had bound him to the care of a hated propagandism during the earlier period of his student life, was stung to the quick, and chagrined at the unlooked for result to his chosen mission, he resigned his office and devoted himself to the practice of medicine in the city of Paramaribo.

Soon after this (six years in all) he accepted an invitation to come to Philadelphia, where he arrived in January, 1833.

From here—

> "Out of his self-drawing web he gives us note,
> The force of his own merit makes his way;
> A gift that Heaven gives for him,"

we see him always intent upon his grand mission and entering upon his new work with renewed purpose. His enthusiasm for the theme of his chosen life-work overcame every opposition, and we see him ere the mantle of citizenship draped his manly form, lecturing in his native tongue to the few but earnest disciples of the new system gathered together to do homage to their distinguished countryman. From that time to the day of his death, animated by the noble purpose of improving, as far as he could, his cherished science, he labored constantly and enthusiastically for its advancement. He was the first physician who taught homoeopathy publicly, at Allentown, Pa., and in 1835, in conjunction with Dr. Wesselhoeft, and others he organized "The North American Academy of the Homoeopathic Healing Art," which flourished for a season and accomplished a great amount of good to those interested in its work. This institution temporarily succumbed to the pressure of pecuniary embarassment, but soon after was revived on a larger and more extended scale as "The Homoeopathic Medical College of Pennsylvania."

It was the master spirit of Dr. Hering, the liberal, energetic and enthusiastic admirer of a broad and liberal education in the arts and sciences, that gave birth to our own American Institute, the first national medical organization in the United States. His contributions to the homoeopathic literature, coeval with the *Archives*, even at that early day, secured for him an honorable position in the world of letters and established him as a worthy standard-bearer of our exclusive law of cure. I will not speak of his many and interesting contributions to our Materia Medica in which he was, of all others in this country, its most diligent and faithful contributor. I will leave that with one more competent to do the subject justice. He was truly the pioneer of our school of medicine in the United States, and by his labors on our Materia Medica he has added more wealth to our school of practice than any other man living since the days of the immortal founder of our school.

"The great joy of his late days," says a distinguished scholar and contemporary, "was the reading of the address delivered by the President of the American Institute of Homoeopathy, in which the methods of Hahnemann and the immutable principles governing our school were so earnestly laid before our National Institute, as were also the proceedings of its members."

A close student, an able teacher and an indefatigable worker for more than half a century, he furnished valuable and often brilliant articles to the periodical literature of America and Germany. In his social life he possessed a fund of anecdote and humor that made him a genial companion and an agreeable friend. He enjoyed in turn a good joke, and laughed heartily at its recital. Of late years his bodily vigor gradually failed, in consequence of his mature years and frequent asthmatic attacks which prostrated him severely. I remember him well at Centennial meeting, during my visit to Philadelphia at that time. I was invited to his house and became one of his few guests at a supper given on that memorable occasion.

He died as he lived, a firm friend, a devoted student and an uncompromising disciple of the truths taught by the immortal Hahnemann. He was borne to his last resting place at Laurel Hill by friends and colleagues who had shared his toil, and who gave him "Tears for his love, joy for his fortune and honor for his valor."

Prof. T. P. Wilson spoke as follows:

The glory of the Roman Empire and the name of Julius Caesar are inseparably connected. The grandeur of the American Republic and the name of George Washington are almost one and the same thing. And so I turn to the name of Constantine Hering, but I need not ask to what system of philosophy, to what department of knowledge, or to what great enterprise that name is indissolubly joined.

Constantine Hering and American Homoeopathy have grown together, the one from infancy to old age, crowned at last by the laurels of death, and the other, from infancy toward a matured youth; and so closely have they been joined that nothing but the searching hand of death could put them asunder.

Yet, in a certain sense, Hering is not dead. In the highest sense in which he lived, he still lives; and will continue to live; and his acts will be repeated—

"In states unborn and accents yet unknown."

When Hering was born, medical science and art were "without form and void, and darkness was upon the face of the deep." As night upon the seas enfolds the boundless waters in her jetty wings, so in those days, chaos covered and clouded all. Scarce one department of our present system of medicine had more than a local habitation and a name. Anatomy had achieved some progress, and the human body had itself undergone some rude and imperfect explorations—no more; but physiology was as a dream to the human mind, and its beauties had not reached the point of conception, much less had they been born. Pathology was an inextricable mass of facts and fancies, and upon these sat superstition enthroned, threatening divine vengenance to all who had the temerity to question their real character. Surgery, with its rude implements, was staining the earth with human gore; and while ignorantly striving to relieve, it added ,indefinitely to the sum of human misery. As for the general practice of medicine, it was "confusion worse confounded." Empiricism reigned supreme, and being without law or order, it was without success. It was then that the great Frenchman Bichat said of medical practice, "It is an incoherent assemblage of incoherent ideas, and is perhaps of all the sciences that which best shows the caprice of the human mind. It is a shapeless assemblage of inaccurate ideas, of observations often puerile, of deceptive remedies, and of formulae as fantastically conceived as they are tediously arranged."

It was into this age that Constantine Hering was born. And when he had come to mature life, it must have been a strange infatuation that led him to select medicine as his life's work. Perhaps it was in the vain hope that he might amend its broken ways. Perhaps it was under the delusive teachings of his preceptors, that taught him that:

1st.   Medicine was a great and perfect art.

2nd.   It had some few minor imperfections which might be improved; and

3rd.   That he that would attempt to improve it would in all human probability be eternally damned.

Passing out of the deleterious influences of the schools into a wider arena of thought, young Hering heard of the writings of one of his fellow-countrymen, a distinguished German physician, by the name of Samuel Hahnemann. He went to the store and bought his books. He took them home to read and to try to understand them.

Like another, in later years, he might have used those books for wadding to load a rusty ancient gun, and leaving to others to fire the train, he might have escaped across the seas to await the result of the explosion—and he might have returned to find no damage done worth speaking about. Hering did sincerely expect to overthrow Hahnemann's argument; but was himself overthrown. He had read Hahnemann's writings, caught such glimpses of the truth that thenceforth, like the children of Israel wandering in the desert, he had ever before his eager gaze the divine Shekinah which led him out of darkness and out of bondage into the land that flowed with milk and honey.

For more than fifty years he was a faithful follower of Hahnemann's teachings. If he had a creed it was a short one and to the purpose: "I believe in the one great law of cure."

With him that was not a blind faith. He brought that declaration to the test of experience, applying it with infinite patience to multitudes of suffering men, women and children—for let me say here that Constantine Hering was no idle dreamer. He never attempted to evolve truth out of his own consciousness; but he gave to this new doctrine the only test by which it may be proven, namely, demonstration.

I do not think his mental constitution led him far into the rationale of the law. He was no speculator. He looked at this truth as being thoroughly a practical one; and it was his life's labor to increase the facility of its application. And in that life there was wrought the labors of two score of the ordinary men of the profession. I think I may safely say that Constantine Hering was chiefly great because he was an incessant toiler. I do not think he ever grew weary of his task.

If you will go back to the time when he landed on the shores of this new country, with this new truth burning like a sacred fire on the altar of his heart, you will see him, an alien and a stranger, looking in vain amid a people whose language he did not understand, for kindred spirits, with whom he might commune, and for temples of science to whose altars he might bring his spotless offerings. There were medical schools and journals and societies, and there were thousands of medical men, but they had no sympathy with his thought. But, ah! his was a heroic soul! He knew the truth; he loved and worshipped it, and he resolved to give it to the world.

In a little town, in Pennsylvania, he laid the foundation of his work. I have never been at Allentown, but I would walk its streets today, if I could, with reverence. The rostrum and the press were the agencies he chose for his instruments. And how well they did their work, let the record of the past half century testify.

But another great secret of Hering's success lay in the masterly power of his inspiration. Himself endowed with inexhaustible inspiration, he seldom failed to inspire all with whom he came in contact.

It was no more idle to think of touching fire without being burned, than of meeting Hering and not catching some of the enthusiasm that warmed his breast. Nay, believe me, it was inspiration which made his face radiant with light, and caused his halting tongue to adorn the English language, which he never quite mastered, with new beauty.

It was not my privilege to know him intimately, but I have known many of his scholars; I have met many men who sat at his feet, and God bless his memory. I do not know that he ever sent out a halting or a doubting principle. However some of them who may have become broken pitchers in subsequent years, came from Hering's hands without flaw or blemish.

Constantine Hering was a true homoeopath. With his whole heart and mind he believed the truth as expressed in *Similia*. The power to demonstrate its universal application to all forms of disease, was greatly limited in his earlier days. The needed agencies were few. There were no schools to teach Hahnemann's doctrines. There were no books to promulgate this new-born truth. There were no journals in which to show the results of experience, and there was as good a chance of finding paintings by the old masters on this new continent as of finding drugs, of any sort, for homoeopathic prescribing. In some obscure corner of Philadelphia, in some hidden recess in New York, there might, perchance, be found a few remedies prepared after the formula laid down by Hahnemann; and these, when found, were mostly in the 30th centesimal attenuation.

But in those days they knew no better than to give such things to people who were sick. They had not heard of the Milwaukee Academy or of the revelations of the Boston microscope. And so the 30ths were given, and as the sick recovered, the name and fame of Homoeopathy was spread abroad.

From Allentown, Hering went to Philadelphia, and on a broader stage, surrounded and aided by ardent and able disciples, he found his cause growing with great rapidity.

It is not too much to say that the sceptre of command which he first took, on coming to America, did not fall from his hand until he was stricken by death. He fell at his post of duty, and upon the day of his death he was no less ardent and devoted to the truth of Homoeopathy than when he first espoused the cause.

We have seen some attempted changes within our school within the past few years. Our fabric has been rocked by the baleful influence of the spirit of reaction toward the chaos of eclecticism and the discarded errors of Allopathy; and while our future, in this respect may be clouded in doubt, we have the proud satisfaction of knowing that upon the fair escutcheon of Hering's name, this cloud can never rest, for never did he bow the knee to Baal.

The heroic old man is dead. Here ends one of the grandest epochs of medical history. Henceforth, on her fair pages shall stand fourscore years marking the life of Constantine Hering. What a magnificent spectacle is the production and completion of such a man! What a crown of glory it places upon the brow of humanity! What a priceless gift is such a life to the human race! What a harvest of intellectual wealth is now gathered in by the death of this great man! Like some choice ceramic he passed unharmed through the fires and became more and more beautiful as the flames of adversity burned deeply into his moral and mental nature the immortal colors of a deathless life.

Constantine Hering was a born leader of men because of his high intellectual endowments and his whole-souled devotion to truth. Tradition tells us, that, in the far East and in ages long since gone by, an elder Constantine, while at the head of his imperial army, saw in the clouds a vision of the cross and over it these words: *In hoc signo vinces.* And by that sign he went forth to conquer, and laid the foundations of a great and lasting empire.

So, in after times, this young Constantine, saw in his imagination, the fair temple of medical science rising till its golden spires were kissed by the clouds of heaven, and over its fair portals he saw deeply graven by the Divine hand these trenchant words: *Similia similibus curantur;* and he exclaimed—"By that sign we shall conquer," and like a true prophet he prophesied and then fulfilled his own prophesies. It is a supreme happiness to us who live today, that we have seen such a spotless life completed. He lived and worshipped at the shrine of nature; and when his days were numbered, he fell into the arms of the All-*Natura* which had cradled him in his infancy, and in that great bosom, the love and power of which no man knows, Constantine Hering sleeps the sleep of the just.

Professor H. C. Allen then said:

It is a remarkable fact that the efforts of the opponents to our system of practice, to prove the law of *Similia* a "humbug" by the writing of a work that should thoroughly expose it, completely uproot the heresy, and thus prevent its dissemination, should have resulted in giving to our school two of its strongest defenders and ablest champions—Dr. Quin, in Great Britain, and Dr. Hering in America. Commissioned to strike the budding truth a death-blow in its infancy, they were themselves convicted and became enthusiastic converts.

The former, as President and one of the founders of the British Homoeopathic Society, has done yeoman service in his native land—the land of Harvey, Jenner and Sydenham; while the latter, as one of the founders of the oldest medical society in America, and its first President—the American Institute—as one of the founders of the first Homoeopathic College in the world, and its first Professor of Materia Medica, has not only rendered heroic service to the Homoeopathic School, but has left a name, honored and revered wherever scientific medicine is known.

Hering's labors in the field of Materia Medica have been of a two-fold character, viz., his personal contributions—second only to those of Hahnemann in number—and the contributions which through his magnetic enthusiasm, that brilliant coterie of co-laborers by whom he was surrounded, were induced to make.

To Hering, more than to any other man, are we indebted for the Materia Medica contributions of Carroll Dunham—which are some of the clearest expositions and ablest differentiations of the mode of action of some of the remedies, to be found in our literature. Dunham has said: "In Constantine Hering I gained the most helpful, genial friend I have ever made;" and few men were more capable of judging than Carroll Dunham.

But it is not so much the number of remedies which he has added to our Materia Medica, great as they are, as the manner in which they are added, for which we should be most thankful. Like Hahnemann, Hering grasped the basic principle upon which, alone, an enduring Materia Medica can be constructed, viz., that the positive facts of the prover shall be recorded in plain, un-technical language, free from theoretical speculations. Provings thus made are of the nature of lasting observations, as fixed and unchangeable as the law of cure. This is the reason why the simple, pure record of observed facts, which Hahnemann and his disciples recorded in the Materia Medica Pura, fifty years ago, free from theories and speculations of a physiological and pathological character, are today as intelligible, as available, as well adapted to meet our wants in practice as when they left the Master's hand.

Hering, in our day, had the same material from which to con-struct a physiological theory of a drug that Hahnemann and his disciples had; in fact, the great advances made by the progressive sciences of physiology and pathology in the last fifty years, gave him a vast advantage over Hahnemann. But, like Hahnemann, he confined himself simply to the recording of the fact, thus leaving each observer free to place his own construction upon the action of the drug. This is a work which cannot be delegated to another; because, as Dunham says: "The significance of a fact is measured by the capacity of the observer."

Next to Hering's tireless, never-flagging industry, the "capacity to measure the significance of a fact" has been equalled by but a few men our school has as yet produced, and excelled by none, save Hahnemann himself. That rare quality of the student of Materia Medica, possessed by Hering in such a remarkable degree, viz., the ability to detect the individual characteristics of a drug—those finer points of difference not to be found in the provings of any other—

is what has rendered his labors of such lasting benefit to his fellows. It is this quality which has made his *Condensed Materia Medica* the best work of ready reference yet produced in the Homoeopathic School, for the busy practitioner. This also is the first work, of a standard character, in which the general anatomical divisions of our Materia Medica, adopted by Hahnemann as a basis for the classification of symptoms, has been departed from. The rubrics, it is true, are increased in number, but they are admirably arranged to meet a twofold object: the condensation of numerous provings, and the classification of symptomatology for ready reference, a want long felt in practice.

The introduction of the serpent poisons, in the magnificent proving of *Lachesis*, marked an era of advance in our Materia Medica. It was violently assailed by the pathologico—physiological branch of the school, both in this country and in Germany, and the author accused of "manufacturing the symptoms," etc. The old view, entertained by toxicologists "that the poison of serpents is digested by the gastric fluids, and cannot manifest any poisonous properties when introduced into the living organism through this channel," was first disproved by the proving of the attenuated poison of *Lachesis*, and abundantly verified since.

Hempel's *Materia Medica*, first edition, page 1143, says: "The provings of the *Lachesis* virus have been instituted with very small quantities of the poison, mostly with the hundreth up to the infinitesimal portion of a drop. It has, therefore, become questionable with a great many, and indeed, as far as Germany is concerned, with almost all thinking homoeopathic practitioners, whether the almost interminable array of symptoms which Dr. Hering alleges to have been produced by the *Lachesis* poison, is not the work of fancy rather than actual observation. In spite of every effort to the contrary, the conviction has gradually forced itself upon my mind that the pretended pathogenesis of *Lachesis*, which has emanated from Dr. Hering's otherwise meritorius and highly praiseworthy efforts, is a great delusion, and that, with the exception of effects with which this publication is abundantly mingled, the balance of the symptoms is unreliable."

The above was written in 1859, and it certainly was some gratification to Dr. Hering to have seen the verification of his proving in the succeeding twenty years, and his character of accuracy maintained.

The verifications of the Provings of *Lachesis* opened the door for all of the other serpent—as well as insect poisons; the principles involved being the same. Hence *Crotalus, Naja, Apium virus*, etc., have been accepted as proven.

As Hering was far in advance of his colleagues and cotemporaries in the demonstration of the power of the attenuated remedy

to produce genuine and reliable pathogeneses, so he was in practical
therapeutics, when he published his *Analytical Therapeutics* and
Guiding Symptoms. He lived long enough to see his *Lachesis*
proving verified in practice; and from Pisgah's height he viewed
the Canaan which the general profession may see in the next
generation, when there may be a demand for those two works.

Let us emulate his virtues, and practice his never-tiring industry,
so that we may be able to contribute our mite to the common stock
of knowledge.

MEETING IN CLEVELAND, OHIO.

On this occasion Dr. D. H. Beckwith made the following remarks::

We are called once more to bow with submission to the in-
scrutable will of Him, in whose hands are the issues of life and
death, to mourn the loss of one, who, during a long career, has
distinguished himself in our profession as a writer, a translator, a
teacher, a practitioner of medicine, and a prover of drugs.

That mysterious roll of human fate slowly unfolds her book,
page after page, guided by the unerring hand of time, and calls
us, one by one, to a sphere of higher existence. It would be a
strange neglect on the part of the medical profession if we would
give no formal expression of our grief and sorrow at the death of
one who has done so much for us all, and, while we mourn the loss
of this great man, we may also rejoice that such a man lived in our
day. No future can rob him of his history, and for many years
his name shall be cherished, and his works be emulated.

Like the falling leaves of this beautiful October day, many of
our physicians pass from the stage of existence, and no public
record is made of them, while, on the other hand, history takes up
our great men and holds them as precious jewels on her pages,
embalms them in their records, and perpetuates their memory to
generations yet unborn.

The profession will agree with me, without a dissenting voice,
that Constantine Hering was a man of application to that science
he loved so well. In his writing he had a keenness of vision, a
power of observation accorded to few. He was devoted to his
profession for over half a century, studying it always as a science,
and practising Homoeopathy as taught by Samuel Hahnemann.

When I call up the name of him whom we eulogize tonight, it
seems to me that he was an old good friend of mine, and that he
was one of my teachers of Homoeopathy thirty years ago. At that
time his name was familiar to all Homoeopathic physicians of the

West. In the year 1850 and 1851 there were but few homoeopathic publications and books in the English language.

Among those in my library were:

1st. "Hering's Domestic Physician."

2nd. "Samuel Hahnemann's Organon of Homoeopathic Medicine"

translated in the year 1849 from the last German edition. with suggestions and additional introductory remarks by Constantine Hering.

3rd. "How to Study Materia Medica," and the "Effects of the poison. of Serpents."

4th. "Chronic Diseases, their Specific Nature and Homoeopathic Treatment," with a preface written by Constantine Hering.

5th. "Jahr's Manual of Homoeopathic Medicine," in two volumes. with improvements and additions by C. Hering.

Also "Jahr's New Manual of Symptomen Codex" of over 2000 pages. in two volumes, with a preface from Hering, written in 1848. I regard this work of great value to the practitioner, as well as to the student of medicine.

In February, 1851, the first number was issued of the *North American Homoeopathic Journal*, a Quarterly magazine of 148 pages. devoted to practical and to scientific articles. Constantine Hering was the editor-in-chief, and each number contained several articles from his pen.

From book acquaintance I had formed an exalted idea of Hering, as a writer and teacher of Homoeopathy. He was regarded as a practitioner of medicine, second to none. In the year 1863 I formed his personal acquaintance, and since that time have often met him. He was a ripe scholar, refined by study, cultivated by extensive foreign travel. and familiar with most of the leading Homoeopathists of the Old World. He was, at all times, able and willing to instruct those who were thrown in contact with him.

I regarded him as a man of positive qualities, untiring in his labors for his profession and true to the principles of Homoeopathy.

I well recollect a call at his office several years ago; he was not in his usual social mood, but seemed very indignant that so many homoeopathic physicians, in Philadelphia. had deviated from the teachings of Hahnemann and were practising a mongrel system of medicine.

He exhibited to me a list of homoeopaths, on one page, and the other class on the opposite one. He was so positive in his remarks in regard to their practice. that I yet recollect the names as they appeared on the different pages. It was a source of deep regret to him that so much eclecticism was practised by those who were so intimately associated with him. in college, and in other work.

Mr. President, we all might have asked that a man so intellectual, so gifted in character, so true to his profession, might have been spared a little longer to have finished the work he was engaged in, and so near completed, but the, Great Physician called him to a nobler and higher sphere for his future labors.

Waiving, on this occasion, all utterances of private sorrow, we unite this evening with our brethern in other cities, at this hour assembled, in placing high on the roll of professional honor, the name of Constantine Hering.

MEETING IN DENVER, COLORADO.

Dr. Burnham spoke as follows:

Fourteen years ago, last August, I first met Dr. Hering, in his home in Philadelphia. I found him a genial, generous-hearted, painstaking man, whose ambition and highest aspirations pointed to the present and future growth of the principles and practice of Homoeopathy.

AS a man, of the noblest types of his nationality, by birth, and whose life career has adorned and made illustrious the nationality of his adoption.

AS a scientis,t the genius of his superior abilities numbered him among those of the largest attainments.

AS a theorist, he largely possessed the ability to prove, and practically apply, in science and in medicine.

AS a writer and author on medical subjects, he was one of the ablest and most industrious of his time.

AS a practitioner of the healing art, his eminent success gave him a world-wide reputation.

AS a pioneer of Homoeopathy in America, he has lived to see it rise from small beginnings, when its practitioners could be counted upon his fingers' ends, to be numbered by thousands, and whose patrons are found among the most cultured, refined and wealthy of the land, and whose literature, limited though it was in the primitive days of Homoeopathy, yet founded upon a principle as fixed and as potent as the fiat of its creation, has grown with its growth, and strengthened with its strength, until it occupies no inferior place in the annals of medical science; whose institutions of learning, started first by his enterprise, nurtured by his care, as a lone representative for the teaching of the principles of the new science and art in medicine, are now to be found in nearly all of the large cities of the continent.

Of all the names of the worthy few of the pioneers, none have contributed to render the literature and the practice of Homoeopathy more illustrious than Constantine Hering.

I consulted him on one occasion with reference to a patient in whom I had an especial interest (it being my other, and better half), and after making a careful and critical examination, he invited me to his private study to review the case further, and proceeded to make an exhaustive investigation. His manner of study, his thoroughness in analyzing a case (so in contrast with many whom I have met in the profession possessed with more of assumption than wisdom, who would deign to study a case only as a marked exception) impressed my mind forcibly as to the necessity of a thorough and accurate knowledge of pathological condition, symptoms, and remedy, before prescribing. In the course of that investigation he remarked to me: "Let us apply the tri-angular test, and if we can find three important, or characteristic symptoms, pointing to one remedy, let me assure you that we can prescribe it with almost unerring certainty. I have tested its application in hundreds of cases, and when clearly defined, it seldom fails to fulfil its mission. As an aid to my investigations, I have kept faithfully in view the illustration of the triangle, the trinity of symptoms, in the selection of a remedy, with the motto inscribed within the boundaries of its lines, and angles, so appropriately expressed—By this sign we conquer."

And now, fellow-members of the profession, let us one and all strive more fully to emulate the example of him in whose memory we have assembled here tonight, illustrious in not only a few, but in many things; working so faithfully in the cause so self-sacrificingly espoused, even to the very day and hour when his spirit was summoned to leave this earthly tabernacle, to come up higher; inscribing his name among the highest on the triangular pyramid of fame, wreathed with a galaxy of time-honored achievements, whose lustre shall brighten as the days wear on and the years roll by, to be crowned with immortal inheritance.

While thousands are assembled in their respective places of abode, on this day, and this hour, throughout the length and breadth of the land to do honor to his name—fitting tribute to one so noble and worthy—I will gladly express, in the language of another, the sentiment: "May his memory grow green with the years, and blossom through the flight of ages."

Dr. A. L. Cole made the following remarks:

The spirit of man takes its departure from the body, the lifeless tissues return to the elements from which they originated; the atomic rearrangement of these elements convert them again into living organisms, and man once dead again lives.

The transitory stage from life to death is not one of fear, pain or agony; not of anguish or regret, but calmly the vital forces ebb away, the combination of vital organs cease to perform their functions, the vitalizing fluid ceases to circulate, respiration is suspended, and all that was once a living animate being is transformed to a lifeless structure.

Man is but a mass of matter, the feeblest in nature; yet how mighty when compared with all else of the animal creation. This element we see in men like Hering, feeble in muscular development as compared with others, yet yielding an intellectual power which commands the respect, love and admiration of their strongest brothers. He will live in the minds of men; although literally dead, his memory is always fresh, his career bright, beautiful and pure, like the rich sparkling diamond.

He lived for the good of man, in order that this world might be beautiful for his having lived in it, and to this end a greater portion of his life was given up to the work for the benefit of others. He lived an honest, upright, modest life, temperate in his habits, pleasant and gentlemanly to those who sought his acquaintance, and aiding many without remuneration, to the great detriment of himself.

His home was in his study, the ornaments of which were volumes of manuscript; there he loved to devote his hours in gathering the products of thinking minds the world over, of ascertaining their accuracy, and arranging them into convenient form for us to digest.

And so he succeeded admirably; the products which from the result of his great mind are to be found in the libraries of his fellow-laborers of every land, cherished by their possessors as only the works of Hering can be cherished, and more valued than the wealth of gold and jewels.

For the noble work, performed by him, we, this day, assemble to commemorate his life, and may his memory be cherished by all. May we spare one moment in thought for him, and when in our libraries we ponder over master-work in search of knowledge that will enable us to save the life of some poor creature entrusted to our care, let us praise Hering for his great work.

Dr. Emma Eastman followed with these remarks:

Examining a placer mine and hearing a miner say that he wanted its gold, but that it would not pay to work it, reminds one of American scholars who bend all of their energies to the test question—will it pay?

If it pays they will burn the midnight oil and use their brain-power without stint or measure; but if not, the Yankee seizes upon the results of others and often robs the laborious student of his hardly won honors.

It is not so with the Germans. They are willing to delve for the grains of golden truth until their accumulations are the envy of all nations.

Preeminent among such miners was Dr. Constantine Hering. While a student he became so renowned for his profound scholarship, and for his bitter hostility to Homoeopathy, that he was appointed to expose the fallacy of the doctrine *Similia similibus curantur*. Like a true scholar he investigated, and experimented for himself, until he was won over to the new theory of medicine and wrote a thesis, *De Medicina Futura* in which he expounded and maintained the doctrine of Hahnemann in the great University of Wuerzburg, where he graduated.

Thus was the seed sown which will make the name of Hering go down the ages, growing brighter and brighter unto the perfect day.

———————

Dr. L. J. Ingersoll addressed the meeting in the following words:

A great and a good man has fallen. Dr. Hering was great as a student, as a scientist, and as a benefactor. He was great as a leader in a most beneficent profession; great as an organizer of a comparatively new school of medicine; great because he made few mistakes; great because, while he excelled others in breadth and exactness of knowledge, he was held as an enemy by none. He was great by nature, and great by culture.

Dr. Hering was good, because, while "cultivating earnestly the best gifts" for himself, he strove "through good and through evil report" to lead all men up into a higher and a better life; good because, while he acquired all the knowledge he could that would relieve the suffering, and keep the well from sickness, he used his skill, not for self, but for the good of all who would receive.

And now that Dr. Constantine Hering has gone from among us, we shall do well to gather up what of wisdom he has left us, remembering that he has written nothing that ought to be forgotten.

While we lament that one so great and good should have been called up higher from so needful a work, I am most thankful that he lived so long and did so much for his race—how much we can never know. As physicians we can never cease to cherish his memory, or forget the gracious heritage he has left us in his unsurpassable Materia Medica.

Hering is dead, but his words and works live to bless mankind. The stream that rose from the hills of Germany so many years ago, and which for half a century blessed our Western continent, has peacefully found its way back to its source. That life that sent sunshine and joy into so many sick-rooms, and brought health to so many, has at last gone out in the still brighter glory of the redeemed. He, who saved so many from the destroyer, could not save himself. Hering cheerfully passed away as one conscious of having dried many tears, and of having turned sighs into joy.

Who of all the thousands, that remain, will take the place of this fallen chief, this great and good "Master of Homoeopathy" in America?

I can say to every brother physician and to every patient, "I have lost a teacher today."

Dr. Ambrose S. Everett then said:

I have known Dr. Constantine Hering, whose genius and whose life-work they meet, tonight, all over the world to commemorate; personally, for nearly fifteen years, and since my first acquaintance with this Hercules of our school of medicine, I have never allowed myself to visit Philadelphia without calling upon him.

While I do now realize that he has gone from the scenes of his earthly labors, and that the place that once knew him shall know him no more, forever, yet I have no doubt, that when I come to visit Philadelphia again, I shall miss him, and his absence from the field of battle and the bivouac of professional life will come home to me in language far more eloquent and pathetic, than I can conceive, or express.

Of this I can assure you, that I never called upon him that I did not find him the same affable, courteous and hospitable gentleman. He always addressed me in terms of respect, and in language that showed that I was not only a welcome guest at his house, but that he bore for me an affection born of a true and lofty manhood. I have also seen him entertain others, and can say, for, and of him, that he always made his visitors feel at home, and all that he had in the way of entertainment was theirs. No matter how young, or humble his visitor in professional rank, that visitor was made to feel before he left, that in Dr. Hering's character, and make-up there was no such thing as caste or rank. In manner he was simple and unostentatious. He never paraded his knowledge, or displayed his learning for the mere sake of show, nor did he try to impress one with the greatness of his character or genius.

He spared no pains or expense in showing his admiration for and his attachment to his medical confreres.

While there is much in his life and character to respect, admire and venerate, yet there is one trait that strikes me with peculiar interest, and that is his life-long devotion to a single object and a single purpose. This trait stands out more boldly and more pronounced than all others.

What he accomplished in the field of Materia Medica, by this oneness of aim, proves that the first great law of success is concentration. He bent all his energies to one point, went directly to that point, and looked neither to the right nor left. He showed great wisdom in daring to leave many things unknown, and practical common sense in leaving other things untouched. If I study this trait of his character aright, he was impressed with the fact that life was too short and art too long, and too valuable for universal scholarship. The range of medical thought and knowledge is so vast and extensive that no one brain can encompass it, or grapple with it as an entirety. Therefore, if we would know one department of medicine well, we must have the courage to be ignorant of some others, however attractive or inviting they may appear. If we would succeed as did Hering, we must single out our specialty and pour the whole stream of our lives into it. No name has been longer or more intimately connected with homoeopathic interests and homoeopathic literature than that of our deceased brother, Dr. Constantine Hering. Certainly none is more widely known, more generally honoured, or more universally beloved.

For nearly the whole period of his life, he has devoted and consecrated all the energies of his mind, and body, to the unfolding of homoeopathic truth, and to the dissemination and elevation of its principles.

Even in old age he did not seek the rest and retirement which his years justified and his health demanded; but he, full of love for and devotion to his chosen school of medicine, worked on with such well directed zeal as to merit the highest respect and admiration of all succeeding generations. Although dead, he still lives in the books and works which he has left, and which are ours to inherit, and to enjoy. These are his voice, coming to us out of the grave of the past, floating on the tide of time, and breathing forth the fire of his youth, and the wisdom of his riper and more matured years.

Dr. Piepgras, of Loveland, made the following address:

Providence has called one of our dearest and greatest members to eternity, and we wish to express the deep grief which wells up from the depths of our hearts.

The name of Constantine Hering will be spoken with reverence by every true homoeopath down to remotest time, since he was a champion of truth in medicine, and one of the chief pillars of our school, in Europe as well as in America. I am sure that every advocate of the truths of Homoeopathy will love his memory until the time when he joins him above.

I have never enjoyed the honor of a personal acquaintance with him, but knew much about him through my master, Dr. Arthur Lutze, now deceased, and also through his writings.

I may be permitted to mention a little anecdote, which may be new to you, and which will give a pleasant remembrance of our dear departed.

"Whilst travelling in Germany,"—says Dr. Hering,—"I one day came to a village, the proprietor of which invited me to spend the night at his house, in place of putting up at the inn. He was a rich old gentleman, a great original; always an invalid, having *ennui* and good wine in plenty. On learning that I was a young medical man, about to commence my travels, he told me that he would sooner make of his son a hangman than a doctor.

"On my expressing surprise at the observation, he produced a large book, saying that it was now twenty years since he became ill in body, but not in mind; that doctors of celebrity, whom he then consulted, had quarreled about his diease and that, consequently he had not employed any of them, nor taken their medicines, but that he had registered the affair in his book. Then after finding that his sickness did not improve, he set out on his travels, resolved that if he could find three doctors who perfectly agreed upon his case, without hesitation, he would allow himself to be treated by them, but by none other. For this purpose, he had, first of all consulted physicians of reputation, but afterward others whose names were less known; but having, in spite of his sufferings never abandoned his first resolution, and while keeping an exact account of every consultation, in his book, he had never found any to agree upon his case.

"Accordingly, not having followed the advice of any, although an invalid, he was still alive. As may well be supposed the book had cost him a pretty sum of money.

"This book had the appearance of a ledger, in large folio, and was kept in tabular form. In the first column were the names of the physicians, amounting to 477 in number; in the second column the names of the disease with explanations concerning its nature, of which there were 313, differing radically; in the third column were the proposed names of the remedies, in all 1097, included in 832 prescriptions.

"The man now took up a pen and coolly requested me to prescribe something for him. Having no great inclination to do so, I asked if Hahnemann was on his list. With a smile he turned to number 301, name of disease 0; remedy prescribed 0; 'he was the wisest of the lot' he said, 'for he said that the name of the disease did not concern him, nor the name of the remedy; but that the cure was the essential point.' 'But why' I inquired, 'did you not allow him to treat you?' 'Because,' he replied, 'he was but one, and I must have three to agree.'

"I asked him if he were willing to sacrifice some hundred francs for an experiment, in which case I would be able to mention, not three, but thirty-three physicians, living in the neighborhood, and in countries and parts of the world widely separate, who would all be of one opinion. He expressed his doubts, but at the same time resolved to undertake the trial. We then made out a description of his symptoms, and when the copies were finished, sent them to thirty-three homoeopathic practitioners. He enclosed a *louis d'or* in each letter, begging each physician to name the remedies which were capable of curing, or at least of alleviating his disease.

"A short time since, I received a cask of Rhenish, of the vintage of 1822. 'I send you wine of the year 1822,' he wrote, 'because twenty-two physicians agreed upon a remedy respecting my case. I hereby perceive that there is certainty in some things in this world. I have gotten various works upon the subject, in order to get further information. From about two hundred medicines, twenty-two physicians have fixed upon the same remedy. One could not expect more. The physician nearest me has me under his care, and I am sending you the wine that I may not be tempted to drink too much of it from mere joy at seeing my health improving from day to day."

Dr. C. N. Hart spoke as follows:

There is a beautiful and ancient custom in the land of my ancestors, which causes each person on the highway to uncover his head as a funeral procession passes, whether the deceased be known or not.

This evening, we, with thousands of our brethren, assembled in all parts of the world, have met to pay a tribute to the memory of a great and good man who has passed away—Dr. Constantine Hering.

Let us rejoice that his life upon earth was one of social and intellectual enjoyment, and that upon passing onward he has left to us, and to future generations, such works as time cannot destroy.

After a long period of highest service to his Maker, and to mankind, both in Germany and in America, he has passed onward to a higher and brighter sphere, *ossa bene qui encant*. In the words of the great and lamented Dunham, the study of his life has been, "not fabrics, nor wares, nor stocks, the works or machinations

of men, but the noblest of God's creation—that which He made in
His own image—the body and mind of man."

He was, to both old and young, kind and affectionate, and alike
teacher and friend. Envy and malice had no part in his career,
but with his one hand as an index pointing onward, and his other
as a support to those acquiring knowledge, he lived and died. And
thus may all of us strive to emulate this noble man, who lived and
died in love and honor.

MEETING IN MINNEAPOLIS, MINN.

Address by Dr. S. P. Starritt:

It is customary upon the death of an individual, however humble,
to present some form of testimonial, recounting the relations of the
individual to society.

Naturally, the more noted the individual, the more public and
demonstrative the tribute.

The idea is primitive and general. We see it even among sav-
age and barbarous peoples, where skill, courage and prowess of
the fallen is cited to the surviving for emulation, and as special
traits of distinction.

Among the semi-barbarous and semi-civilized, we find these
relations embodied in fervid and glowing apostrophe, the lay of the
minstrel, the rude but heroic song.

Among civilized and cultivated nations, witness the sermons,
biographies, the finished and studied epic verse, the "towering
monument, sculptured bust, and storied urn."

Tonight, friends, without pomp, we come to an humbler, but
no less sincere way, to pay our tribute to the life and services of
one of earth's greatest sons, who has recently been called to another home, to a higher and ampler sphere.

Abraham was accounted worthy to be called the "Father of the
Faithful," because, at God's call, he left country, kindred and
home to go into a strange land, which was yet to be shown him,
having faith in Him who promised that he was to be the "father
of a great nation."

Him whom we honor tonight, God called in no less audible
voice, "Get thee out of thy country, and from thy kindred, and
from thy father's house, unto a land that I will show thee, and I
will make of thee a great nation, and I will bless thee, and make
thy name great."

The lives of both these great men have become historic, and
history has but proved the truth of prophecy.

Father Hering, as he was truthfully and affectionately called
by a great army of co-workers, in his early youth was taught how

to think, and no higher enconium, through his long and studious life, could be found, than he knows how to think.

Graduating with distinction from one of the Great German Universities, he first essayed to teach mathematics, but a fondness, or an instinct for medicine, led him to acquire what was taught in the schools.

Like all men of great force, profound conviction and energetic will, he espoused the established and so-called "regular practice", the school which was wont to prosecute what he afterward with great zeal embraced and advocated. From the versatility of his acquirements he was selected by his confreres to controvert and annihilate a new and progressive system of healing, which was forcing its way into recognition, and favor. Investigation led to wonder, wonder to admiration; while still doubting he became a sufferer, and after trying the appliances of the old system without relief, he sought the new and was healed. Thus, through suffering, he became a believer, was converted, and, after practically demonstrating the truth of the new art, he became the great apostle of Homoeopathy to the Gentiles.

Eminent for his attainments in science, his government appointed him naturalist of a scientific expedition bound for the southern continent of the New World.

Ostracised at home for his new faith, and possessed with the divine instinct of emigration, he eagerly embraced the offer tendered by the government, and with the characteristic ardor of young manhood, he discharged the duties to which he was assigned.

Meanwhile, not content with the knowledge already acquired by the New School of Medicine for healing the sick, he began to inquire how he could add to the list of remedial agents, and best disseminate their mode of application.

While rendering signal service to his country, he, perhaps, rendered his greatest service to mankind, by introducing into medicine, with its indications, the virus of the *Lachesis trigonocephalus*, which, from its healing properties in the hands of our great army of practitioners, has become one of the greatest of our mighty polychrests.

On his return home, while visiting some of the largest cities of the North, it is said that in Philadelphia he received the diviner impulse, which led him to conclude that there was indeed the "promised land".

The Old World may boast that it gave us a Hering, but the New World can reply, his potentiality only became reality under the inspiration and progressiveness of the New. Here, cut off from the peculiar bent of the European mind to follow custom and precedent, he strikes out boldly upon a new course, and with the intrepidity of an explorer he never deviates, but so amplifies, and gives so many fixed and reliable data, that it makes it comparatively easy for his successors to follow the same route.

There is ever an element of moral courage and greatness in those who discover or follow new truths, or paths of which the general mind is ignorant. The investigator is always a brave man, full of the spirit of sacrifice.

History is full of the sublime examples of men who have breasted the tides of opposition arising from ignorance, superstition, custom, envy and malice, in giving to the world new and progressive ideas and truths. History has always given to men their meed of praise, has placed the laurel upon their brows, and crowned them the world's heroes.

The mind sits enchained at the daring and hardihood of the navigator sailing a new and unknown expanse, from the rugged Norsemen of earlier times down to those of the present, who plow the icefloes of the Arctic seas. The blood is enkindled at the tales of Spartan and Roman heroism, and the sanguinary conflicts of Dane, and Pict and Scot. The sublime lessons of patience are taught over the achievements of Galileo, Kepler, Newton, Faraday, Miller, Fulton, Morse and hosts of others, who, through great toil, have added to the knowledge wrung from Nature and her slumbering forces. What monuments shall we rear to the world's martyrs and reformers, who, in the domain of mortal, civil and religious conflict have purchased for us that liberty which has made all other achievements of men possible?

He whom cardiac paralysis has just stricken down, in the full splendor of his hoary age, is not one whit behind the greatest of those to whom we have just referred, for he possessed their spirit, was actuated by the same motives, and spent his life in the same, or a kindred cause—the amelioration of his fellow-men.

Though not the Columbus of Homoeopathy, he followed faithfully the chart of the great discoverer. He extended and amplified in almost every particular the boundaries of Hahnemann. He confirmed every fact that Hahnemann had given to the world as such, while the theories of his great Master he tested and passed upon their validity. He analyzed and systematized where Hahnemann had only generalized; Hahnemann introduced Homoeopathy, but it was reserved for the genius of Hering to raise it to the sublime degree of a distinctive science. Both were great and original explorers.

It has been indeed always the pride and boast of Homoeopathy that it is invested with a gift of prevision, that is, given a picture of a certain malady, the remedy is at once forthcoming, already provided for. The only limit is one—human capacity— inability to prove all of the medicinal agencies of nature, and to retain their special therapeutic range. So true is this gift that it matters not whether the disease is obscure or known, or whether it be present or remote. Thus Hahnemann was enabled by our law of cure, to point out remedies curative for even the Eastern Plague, and robbed it of its terrors before he had ever seen a case, or even before it had spread to his own country.

In like manner could, and did Hering for our Southern Plague, the yellow fever. Both these great minds went further than this, they indicated the remedies preventive, so as to render even contagion powerless.

Come now, and admire with me the moral courage and greatness of the man, who, from adherence to known law and principle, not only called down upon himself the odium of the great minds that had given him his diversified instruction, and from merit elevated him to confraternity, but also in his emigration to the New World, the same odium precedes and attaches to him, emanating from kindred sources. The Cholera from the distance is advancing, and Hering, true to his convictions, points out a simple and efficacious prophylactic, but which only excited ridicule. In the streets of his own city and home, see the rabble and street-Arabs pursue him with jeer and scoff, prompted by those holding the same distinguished positions as those who had cast him off in the Fatherland. The quiet shrug, or the curious look of the more cultivated was no less cruel than the open scoff of the slums. But the fatal scourge is come, depopulating the city, and "Sulphur Hering" is remembered, and men now, through fear, begin to try the efficacy of wearing a spoonful of the milk of sulphur (Lac Sulphur) in their stockings, and receive immunity from contagion.

Friends, it requires the highest order of both physical and moral courage, to risk life calmly in trying to succor others. Witness the heroic act of a man alone in a room, whence all the attendants have fled, with a box he has just opened containing the most venomous serpent, the largest of its species, from whose glands after the most mature deliberation, he is about to abstract the deadly poison. See the nerve of the man, who, alert as is the snake, seizes it just below the head with firm grasp, when with folds uncoiled, with reared head and flaming eye, forked tongue and naked fang, it is poised to strike the intrepid soul, who, at the risk of his life, seeks from its venom the healing balm for earth's sufferers. Watch him adjust the pointed stick between the opened jaws of the serpent whose bite is certain death, and whose impotent rage secretes the deadly saliva, while he tantalizes it till it can distil no more poison, when into a jar of alcohol he thrusts the monster, nor relaxes his grip of steel till life is extinct. The poison, caught in a watch glass is transferred to a mortar and rubbed with sugar of milk, till his purple and bloated face, and swimming brain, suspend his eager operation. He swallows the preparation with measured regularity to produce upon himself the effects of the venom. Observe him toss in his fever, note the loquacious delirium as he flits from subject to subject, note the suffocation, the frantic struggle for breath, while he clutches and tears from throat and breast all clothing; mark his mental condition, the anguish and apprehension, and ask yourselves for whom, for what purpose he does this and then answer—is he not a hero?

Or friends, can you imagine the sensation of standing before a rabid dog, bent upon getting the frothy *hydrophobinum*, for the sole purpose of obtaining a remedy for healing the sick? How would you characterize the act—courageous, or not?

Does it not exhibit moral heroism to assert the truth of a scientific world? Scientists scoffed at the idea that the poisons he procured, and proved upon himself at the jeopardy of life had any remdial efficacy, because, forsooth, they had been preserved in alcohol! "Why", exclaimed they, "we drench an individual with whiskey when bitten by the *Crotalus*, and it antidotes and prevents systemic poisoning, and saves the life of the patient! Alcohol antidotes animal poison, therefore animal poisons preserved in alcohol are rendered harmless and inert"; and from the deductions of such logic the world hooted at his provings, and cures, produced by the use of alcoholic preparations of his animal poisons, most notably *Lachesis*, of which he had asserted much. But he was patient, knowing whereof he had affirmed, and the scientific world, after experimenting, demonstrated that the hypodermic injection of even the 3rd centesimal of *Lachesis*, and even the still higher dilutions were destructive of animal life, and, after many other and varied experiments, it was publically acknowledged that Hering was right, that animal poisons, preserved in alcohol, held still their poisonous qualities intact.

Again, think you it required no moral backbone to stand by the assertion that radiated heat was one of the most efficient agencies to antidote the poison in wounds, whatever their origin, when the world denied and disbelieved! Mark the courage of the test! A man (himself) with an inoculated arm (with venom from the fang of a rattlesnake) swollen, purple, throbbing, painful, threatening the loss of life, will not listen to the voice of friends and surgeons, but sits quietly down, in his kitchen, and thrusts his arm into the heated oven and holds it there until the poison is counteracted, or eliminated, and the member reserved for future usefulness, and now, the world, after experimenting, announces that radiated heat is antidotal to poisonous wounds. Hering was right again.

Still further, witness him walk with quiet dignity into the sickroom, where lies a girl in throes of severest agony, after the major operation of a lithotomy, and amidst the sneers of distinguished sur-

geons summoned in consultation, who had signally failed to miti-
gate her suffering, and had given her over to the king of terrors—
see him solicit symptoms from the sick, and from his inexhaustible
fund of knowledge, watch him pour a few pellets of *Staphisagria*
(in a high attenuation) into water and administer it to the sufferer.
To the gratification of the sick one and her friends, and to the
amazement of the scoffers, the pain is mitigated, finally assuaged,
and sleep comes gradually to restore strength, and a precious life
is saved.

NOTE: (In consequence of having called Dr. Hering, in
whose prescriptions he had reason to have confidence from previous experience, to the case, the
famous surgeon who had made the operation, was
in danger of losing his membership and standing
in the society of Old School physicians.)

These are but a few striking instances which serve to illustrate
the timber of the man, who, by courage and calm demeanor amid
trying scenes and sacrifices, won public and private esteem, when
Homoeopathy was not to the public what it is today, and forced
the popular recognition of his system of healing, obtaining for it
the sanction and protection of the civic law. It is now comparatively easy for the practitioner to dispense the blessings of an enlightened Homoeopathy, but what do we not owe to Father Hering,
who, by his skill, patience and learning, and above all his moral
courage, overcame the popular ignorance and prejudice, so that it
has passed into a proverb, that Homoeopathy cannot flourish among
the ignorant and unthinking, but numbers its adherents among the
cultured, thoughtful and educated.

As a scholar and student Hering stands unrivalled in his time.
He was authority in every branch of medicine, and so intimately
was he acquainted, not only with medical, but kindred sciences,
that his thoughts and ...terances became books. His habits and
methods were those of the student. Accustomed to rise very early
in the morning, at three o'clock, he was wont to take a slice of
zwieback and a cup of coffee or cocoa, when he would study and
write until breakfast, at nine. After breakfast he would pursue his
studies further, and attend to his professional duties till evening,
when he would either pass the time in continued study, or converse with those who desired instruction. I believe it was his custom to retire about nine in the evening unless so occupied. He
had preeminently the genius for hard and continuous study, and
this systematic and arduous course he pursued up to the time of
his demise.

The fruit of such labor is, of course, voluminous, and it is by
authorship that he will be best known to posterity. He is the author

of many books and monographs, and all of them are the acknowledged standards of our school. He devoted the greater portion of his studies to the proving of drugs, and he has enriched our Materia Medica more than any other author, Hahnemann not excepted. His "Guiding Symptoms" is characteristic, and no such full, complete and accurate work on Materia Medica was ever published. He esteemed it the crowning effort of his life. It is the fruit of advanced age, the product of a long life of rich and varied experience, united with the most profound research and learning.

One would naturally suppose that he would have fallen in with the prevailing system of German Philosophy, and that his works, like those of Grauvogl, would have been tinctured with theories founded upon philosophical speculation. But not so. He brought everything to the touchstone of scientific experiment, and he was wont to say "There is no such thing as belief in science. A property or thing is, or is not." His method was empirical; perhaps sciential would be the better word. It partook rather of the inductive system of philosophy than transcendentalism, which was to him a horrible word, which he gave with a prolonged, rough, guttural roll of the rrs.

Everything was subjected to trial, and if it did not stand the test of experiment, did not prove a literal fact, he never strove to bolster it up with a more plausible theory, but cast it off as one would a useless garment.

Just a year or two previous to death, while the writer, with a body of students sitting at his feet, as sat St. Paul at the feet of Gamaliel, he remarked: "Well, gentlemen, to-day I have lost one of my best beloved children! For more than twenty years I have been collecting facts and data to establish a pet theory of mine, and I was about to publish and give the results to the world, when today I have fully decided that it cannot stand the test of scientific experiment, and so I have buried it out of sight. Not without a pang, gentlemen; but, as my theory is not true, that is the end of it. His mind was both analytical and synthetical.

He was a tall man, sun-crowned in the light of knowledge; a man of capacious soul, gigantic brain, an intellect of colossal proportions. That which seemed veiled to other men was to him luminous with light. In his capacious mind truth alone was sought, discovered, seized upon, made incarnate and disseminated over sea, island and continent, till it became the common heritage. But it was as an instructor, or lecturer that he surpassed himself. Brimful, overflowing with knowledge he was just as eager to impart as to acquire. Give him respectful attention, and he would forsake every other duty and proceed to talk, or lecture without note of time, and I assure you he was as tireless as time itself. He has been known to forget fatigue and rest and sit up all night to instruct some practitioner who wished either to be led into, or receive more light in the sublime degrees of Homoeopathy. Even in the last years of his life his eye would kindle in the presence of a body of students, his mind unfold, and truth would come forth robed in beauty, and not till the long hours were passed, and not even then, unless soliciated to cease and rest, would he think of retiring. The totality of the symptoms, and the single remedy corresponding to that totality, were his two watchwords.

He was a kind and affectionate father and husband. a good citizen, but a citizen of no particular country. He owed allegiance to the world.

More given to imparting knowledge and ameliorating the sufferings of the race than to the acquirement of wealth, he laid up for himself the true riches. He achieved more than fame—he was great. His kind and beneficent deeds, the truths he discovered and established, the sacrifices he made, and the arduous toil, guide us in the divine art of healing.

He died full of years, honored and respected by even his adversaries. A long life of usefulness has been spent. We are left with greater and undimmed lustre in a fairer and boundless horizon.

Truly of him it can be said in the language of old: "And thou shalt be a blessing, and in thee shall the families of the earth be blessed."

Friends, the unfolding of the prophetic scroll shall fully establish history, for already has he become the "father of a great nation."

MEMORIAL ADDRESS TO KANSAS PHYSICIANS.

Dr. Henry W. Roby spoke as follows:

Friends: There is a pause in our labors; a break in our ranks; a shade on the Stygian river. Constantine Hering, the pupil and intimate friend of Hahnemann, the venerable Nestor of Homoeopathy in America; the unrivalled scholar, philosopher and author in the new school of medicine; the most successful practitioner, and the ablest medical counsellor of his age, has gone to his final rest at the age of eighty-one years. And yet, as was said of the great statesman, Thiers: "He died too young by a score of years."

Like Goethe's, his grandest works were the last. His massive brain and untiring hands had nearly finished the crowning glory of his life-work—the most masterly piece of medical authorship ever given to the world.

Like the immortal Lincoln, he died before God, or circumstances had created a successor large enough to fill his place in the world. But nature is rich in compensatory laws. The cause which creates a great leader, like a Luther, a Buonaporte, a Thiers, a Bismarck, a Washington, a Lincoln or a Hahnemann in one age or generation, will be carried forward through the succeeding ages or generations by their disciples and followers.

A great leader in the cause of the twin-sisters, Humanity and Homoeopathy, has but recently died in Philadelphia, and today physicians, by thousands, and their patrons by millions, scattered all over the world, sincerely mourn his death. But there is left to us this consolation, that the cause which he led is strong enough, at his death, and well enough officered, to march steadily forward to final and glorious triumph, without the further inspiration of a great individual leadership. So, a detachment buries the fallen leader and decorates his grave, while the great army marches on without halting, for the cause is greater than the leader.

As inductive philosophy no longer needs a Lord Bacon for leader, or astronomy a Galileo or a Copernicus, so Homoeopathy no longer needs the personal inspiration of Hahnemann, its original grand master in Europe, or Hering, his co-laborer in America. It now marches steadily on to the drum-beat of principle under the influence of a demonstrated and ever demonstrable truth. Whenever truth involves enough of human interest to start it on its march around the world, if it does not find in waiting a man sufficiently large for a captain-general, it takes one from the common walks of life, and enlarges him sufficiently for the great work of leadership.

And Nature seems to have no regular rule for the choice of men for leaders. She takes a tinker, a printer, a cobbler, a rail-splitter, a tanner or a student, and so sharpens his vision, that he can see the new truth which is marching along through his day and generation, so enlarges his intellect that he can grasp and hold the truth, and so shape and energize tongue and pen that he can show to the world the strength and beauty of the principle he has apprehended, and its correlations to other great truth in the world. In one case she takes a mechanic, puts him into a bathtub which overflows, and he straightway leaps out and cries "Eureka! Eureka!" In another she leads a dreamer into an orchard and drops an apple at his feet, and in the light of that falling apple he thinks the law of gravity.

She takes a schoolmaster of Padua, sets him stargazing and his trembling tongue informs an astonished world that all the heavenly bodies, our earth included, are wheeling through immense orbits, in immeasurable space, and also revolving on their own axes. And thus the science of astronomy is born even under the shame and humiliation of a compulsory recantation. Again, nature takes a poor humble student, leads him along the old paths of knowledge, through the labyrinthine mysteries and utter chaos of old medicine, and then leads him on into that clearer light which gives to the world a scientific, perfect guide to the choice of drugs for the cure of disease. And then she crowns him with leadership in a grand reformation of a human cause.

And thus, through the long reach of ages, one human interest after another, one great fact, or truth, or principle after another is developed and established in the minds and lives of men, of communities and races.

But Nature seems to be never in haste. It took twenty-two hundred years of the slow coaching of old medicine to develop a Harvey and to establish in the minds of men the fact of the circulation of blood in the human organism. And it took almost two centuries longer to establish nature's law of drug-action on the human system, and to give to the world the law of cure. The very discovery of that law had to wait for the discovery and develop-ment of inductive philosophy, for only by its processes could the law of cure be discovered and fully demonstrated. That law is now incontestably established on an absolutely scientific basis, and today it challenges all of the scientific tests known to men, to dis-prove its correctness. And Hahnemann its real discoverer, and Hering its wise elaborator, can be, and are, both, called from labor to rest. For years the profession has watched, with eager eyes, the progress of Dr. Hering's life-work, almost in fear and trembling, lest he should not live to complete it. But life held on its course, and the indefatigable worker, through days and nights, and years of incessant study and toil brought the work nearer and nearer to completion. And when at last his work was done, his manuscripts completed and the press began to turn out his volumes, the fiat of "well done" was issued from on high, and he was suddenly called away from his proof-sheets to everlasting rest.

Others could read the proof and he was spared that labor. His work was done. But he lived to write the master medical work of the world, which will soon issue from the press, fitly named *Guiding Symptoms.*

Unlike the *Mystery of Edwin Drood*, the hand of its creator guided the pen to the end of its last chapter, though proof readers, pressmen and binders have their work still to perform.

Homoeopathy, under the leadership of Hahnemann and Hering, reinforced by an already grand army of coadjutors, has wrought a grand and beneficent reform in medicine, and conferred inestim-able blessings upon the world. It no longer needs any champion defenders. It is a great and well established fact in the world. It has already become aggressive, has changed the field of conflict and the front of battle, has carried the contest into the enemy's country and put gouty old medicine on the defensive, and compelled it to adopt "so many changes and improvements, and abandon so many barbarities and cruel and dangerous devices in its methods, that could Galen, Paracelsus, Hippocrates, Paris, Cullen or Sydenham be called from their graves today, they would have a thousandfold more trouble to recognize their disciples than did Rip Van Winkle to recognize his daughter, or his dog, after his twenty years of sleep. Hahnemann and his followers have achieved a deeper and broader and sounder knowledge of Materia Medica in the past eighty years than old physic has done in eighteen centuries.

Still the world moves, and even now the sleepy disciples of Galen are walking up and announcing with a great flourish of trumpets to the world, as new discoveries in medicine, facts which Hahnemann announced over eighty years ago.

Fortunately the world is already astir in all the great camping-grounds of philosophy, science, art, theology, law and medicine; it is waking up the Rip Van Winkles all along the line, and demanding from them more intelligent and scientific methods, more light and better results. And when the masses demand better lawyers, better preachers, better doctors and more intelligent methods, the demand is sure to be responded to. If the people demand better quality in books, of food, of raiment, of merchandise, there will not be long wanting live merchants and tradesmen who will find, or create a way to supply the demand.

A hundred years ago there went up from an already long-suffering humanity a cry for release from old medical superstitions and barbarities, and for the introduction of a more humane and scientific medicine, one that could give a reason, not only for its existence, but its methods, and already the whole medical world—the most superstitious of all worlds—is revolutionized, and half a million of active brains and busy hands are toiling eagerly to fulfil the demand. Many of them are among the old sleepers, and we see, almost daily, some of them rubbing the scales from their eyes, dropping their shackles of prejudice, coming to the front and joining the ranks of Homoeopathy. Order is being evolved out of chaos, system out of confusion, light out of darkness, and the cry of the world for a safe and wise medical system is receiving its answer.

Let the good work go on, and when a veteran and hero finishes his work and is given his eternal leave of absence from our ranks, there will be a hundred willing hands, and heroic hearts, to take up and carry on the great work. Let us, one and all, make and hold ourselves competent and ready to take up and carry on successfully any part of the great work that circumstances, or Providence may assign to us.

MEETING IN WILMINGTON, DELAWARE.

The following address was read by Dr. A. Negendank:

While we are today assembled, representing the Homoeopathic physicians of the State of Delaware, to share in the general respect, and to show our high esteem to the departed master spirit of Constantine Hering, I feel that in honoring him we are conferring honor upon ourselves as being followers of the same principle in medicine—*Similia similibus curantur*—which our deceased veteran ever defended, and to the elucidation of which he devoted a large portion of a long life of eighty years.

Dr. Hering was a man *sui generis*, far above the grovelling propensities of ordinary human nature; he forgot, in his devotion to science the entity of worldly existence for which so many toil. Our profession has always claimed, not for the individual, but for the body collective, a high standard of honor and unselfishness, a position above those who know less of the frailties of humanity. Let everyone judge for himself if he deserves such a claim or not, but I say it without hesitation, that our departed friend deserved that claim, and that I believe him to have been the high priest of his profession.

There are men who seem to be sent into this world for purposes and action only. All their facilities are bent to toil and work; their spirits and their frames alike teem with energy. They pause and slumber like other men, but only to recruit from actual fatigue; they occasionally need quiet, though only as invigoration for renewed exertion; they investigate and reflect; their mission, their enjoyment, the object and condition of their existence is work; they would not be content to exist here without it, nor conceive of another life without it. Their vitality is beyond that of ordinary men; they are never seen idle; in repose they dream of work, and their pleasure is work.

A few years before his death, on a warm summer day, hot enough to lull the energy of the youngest, while sitting in his arm-chair smoking a cigar and sipping his coffee, the venerable old gentleman was overcome by fatigue, and rousing himself from slumber exclaimed: "If it was not for the work begun, the completion of which rests upon me, the frail and weary body might wish to be at rest." Such a man was our highly esteemed and distinguished Hering.

I had the privilege of living with the doctor for several years, as his assistant, and there is not a day of that time that I cannot recall with pleasant remembrance; at his frugal table he was cheerful, conversational and instructive, never dictatorial, always pleased to receive. If it was upon any subject with which he was not as familiar as the speaker, he would listen with grave attention, and a pleasant sparkle of the eye would indicate his gratification to learn. Humble people were cheerfuly entertained at his hospitable table, and the kindest attention and respect were shown them by the doctor, as well as by Mrs. Hering. If friends happened in in the evening before the doctor retired to his study, he was always ready for a social chat, full of good humor and wit. A cigar, rye bread, a piece of Swiss cheese, a glass of wine and plenty of time in prospect would furnish material for an enjoyable evening. But if our venerable sage came home overworked and fatigued, he preferred to be undisturbed and he retired to his study where quiet reigned, there to be in company with his books or pen.

To the young man he was full of encouragement; enthusiastic in showing him the way that would be sure to lead him of success; never oppressing him with his store of knowledge to learning, but ready to give to the fullest extent, all that he judged his hearer to be capable of receiving. A faint smile would be probably all the censure bestowed on a weak effort in literature; but for an able antagonist he had voluminous ammunition for battle, including a fair quantity of grape-shot. A good jest, even though at his own expense, or even against Homoeopathy he relished, but a cold or wilful expression against the sacred truth of Therapeutics he considered unpardonable. After the death of Dr. Watzke, in 1867, I expressed my regret at losing such an able colleague from our ranks; he knit his brow and answered: "I am not at all sorry; a man who, after finding a truth, can say 'that he is sorry for it', ought to die."

The patience of Dr. Hering in listening to the endless narration of a patient afflicted with a chronic disorder, was remarkable, and one might have thought that the master's day had no end, or that he had only the one patient to attend. The restlessness of all who were waiting in his office, did not in the least disturb him; they might wait, or go home to come back another time. He did not believe in hurry, and often said, "No one is in a hurry but the devil."

Dr. Hering was a power. But what was that power? Was it his learning? No doubt it was a part of it. Was it his industry? No doubt it was a part of it. But the great lever of his power lay in his character. He was modest, kind and open-hearted. Integrity and honor were his beacon-lights; a man in whom there was no guile.

I may be asked by some of our friends, did our sage never get out of humor, or could he scold? I am frank to say that he could get out of humor and scold too. Tell him that he promised, so and so, and you were sure to put him in bad humor; it was especially distasteful to his feelings, as would be a doubt against his honest character. "No; I never promise, never, never; no one makes promises but the Old Nick, and he never keeps them!" He had his own fashion of scolding, and it was done in full earnest, but never to hurt anyone, as he was always careful not to let its force descend directly upon the subject who had offended.

One stormy winter night, the coachman awaited the doctor before the house of a friend where he was calling and had become so interested in conversation, that driver, horses and storm were alike forgotten. About ten o'clock, John, not feeling very comfortable on his box, and perhaps thinking the doctor might have given him the slip by a side door, drove away to the stable. The old gentleman returned shortly after on foot, naturally out of humor, and John was soon hacked to pieces, hundreds, thousands, tens of thousands of pieces, roasted, fried and baked, the frying pan emptied out of the second-story window, into the dark, cold night. All of this time John slept soundly in his warm bed, and never heard any of these maledictions.

Dr. Hering's standing as a scientist, skilfulness as a physician, his special love and labor as a therapeutist I shall pass by in silence, knowing full well that ample justice will be done him, this day by our fraternity. Ages to come will appreciate his labor, which was done to free medicine and the medical profession from that vortex of endless speculation in therapeutics, which has been a labyrinth, as old as the history of medicine. The work of building up a true temple of science kept the tools of our mason bright. He was industrious to the last breath of his life when kind nature's signal called him for retreat.

In love, to the memory of the departed, I have given these few outlines of his character.

MEETING IN WASHINGTON, D. C.

A preamble and resolutions were adopted by the meeting commemorative of the departed.

MEETING IN SCHLESWIG—HOLSTEIN.

At a meeting of physicians and laymen the exercises included the following programme, in German:

1. Trauerweise, von Trautenfels.
2. Prolog, gesprochen von Frl. Boege.
3. Freunde schmueckt des Meisters Haupt; von Dr. Mossa.
4. Prof. Dr. C. Hering's Wirken in Amerika und Deutschland. Vortrag von Dr. Werner.

5. Es wird dereinst die Nachwelt blaettern; von L. Frankl.
6. Blau—Weiss—Gold. Vortrag.
7. Der Scmerzensschrei aus allen Ecken. Ein Volkslied mit homoeopathischen Randzeichnungen. Von Prof. Dr. Hering, und Dr. Werner.
8. Schlusswort.

MEETING IN PARIS, FRANCE.

An account of the proceedings of the Memorial meeting held in Paris, is copied from the Bibliotheque Homoeopathique:

La fatale nouvelle, venait a peine se repandre dans Philadelphia que le fils de notre confrere, M. Heermann, en informait son pere par le telegraphe. Le secretaire-general de la Societe Hahnemannienne Federative comprit aussitot que les homoeopathes francais devaient rendre un hommage public et collectif a ce veteran de l'homoeopathie, a celui qui, depuis Hahnemann, avait de plus enrichi la Matiere medicale. Aussi il invita sans plus tarder tous nos confreres presents a Paris a se reunir chez lui le 31 juillet 1880, pour aviser au meilleur moyen d'honorer la memoire de ce grand bienfaiteur de l'humanite. La plupart des membres de la Societe furent exacts au rendez-vous et la seance fut ouverte a 9 heures du soir, sous la presidence de M. Leboucher. M. Love, vice president de la Societe, et M. Cramoisy, etaient au nombre des assistants.

M. Heermann, apres un court eloge d'Hering, expose l'objet de la reunion. Ensuite chacun emet son avis et l'on adopte a l'unanimite les deux resolutions suivantes:

1. Une lettre de condoleance scra adressee a Mme. veuve Hering et signee non-seulement par tous les membres presents, mais aussi par le plus grand nombre possible de medicins homoeopathes a Paris.

2. M. Heermann, en qualite d'ami d'Hering, est charge d'ecrire son eloge avec tous les developpements que comporte l' importance de ses travaux.

The following eulogy, in French, read by Dr. C. Heermann, translated by Mrs. M. F. Green and Miss Emily Jones is here reproduced:

On the 23rd of July, at about ten o'clock in the evening, Dr. Hering departed this life, having passed his 80th year.

He had, for some time before his death, suffered from asthma, without, however, ceasing to attend to his daily duties. He retired to his study, on the evening of the 23rd, a little after 8 o'clock. About ten o'clock he called his wife, who found him suffering from much difficulty in breathing, but in full possession of his faculties. Doctors Raue and Koch were summoned at once, but before they came his soul had passed away.

To one of those around him, Mrs. Mertens, a friend of the family, he said, "Now I am dying." Upon other occasions, when he had been very ill, and given up by his friends, he had always refused to believe that he was dying, feeling sure that his hour had not yet come.

Constantine Hering was born in Oschatz (Saxony), Germany, January 1st, 1800. From his earliest childhood he evinced a great desire for knowledge, and finished with honor the studies preparatory to entering the college at Zittau, where he devoted himself to classical learning, from 1811 to 1817. He excelled in everything, especially in mathematics, and in all branches he went far beyond the average of his time. He had a decided taste for the study of medicine, which he followed first at the Surgical Academy at Dresden, then at the University of Leipzig where he was a pupil of the celebrated surgeon Robbi. His preceptor having been at the time requested to write an article against Homoeopathy, entrusted his pupil with the writing of it. The latter threw himself into it with ardor, studied the writings which he was to attack, and there found this expression, "Represent me, but represent me correctly." (Machts nach, aber machts recht nach). He decided to make a personal investigation of the matter in order to insure a more complete victory.

Hering, with this end in view, applied to a druggist, in Leipzig, for the bark of Cinchona; the druggist, who was a friend, said to him, after having heard his purpose, "Let that alone dear Hering, you are treading on dangerous ground;" but Hering replied that he did not fear the truth.

The pamphlet against Homoeopathy was not written.

About this time a dissecting wound produced upon him such serious effects, that not only did amputation seem necessary, but grave fears for his life were felt.

One of his friends, at this time, persuaded him to try against this malady the power of homoeopathic drugs. An entire cure was the result. His conversion to Homoeopathy was from that time complete, and his thesis written to obtain his degree contained a masterly defence of the homoeopathic law.

After he obtained his degree, March 23rd, 1826, at the University of Wuerzburg, he was appointed, by the King of Saxony to go to Guiana, for the purpose of scientific research, and to make a

zoological collection. There he pursued the study and practice of
the new doctrine, and cured the daughter of the governor of the
province of a disease which had been pronounced incurable by the
resident physicians. Having, besides, during his stay in South
America, contributed to the *Homoeopathic Archives*, thanks to the
influence of the court physician, he received "royal orders" to quit
the study of medicine and attend only to the duties of his position.

His independent nature rebelled at so much intolerance and
he immediately sent in his resignation, and continued the practice
of medicine in Paramaribo. One of his friends and a student, Dr.
Bute, who had formerly been a missionary there, and who had since
then established himself at Philadelphia, represented this city to
him as a useful field for his labors. Hering arrived there in January, 1833, but only remained a short time, having been asked by
Dr. Wesselhoeft, of Allentown, Pa., to assist him in founding there
a homoeopathic school of medicine, the first which had ever existed. The government of Pennsylvania accorded to the faculty the
right to confer the degree of doctor of medicine.

We next find Dr. Hering established in Philadelphia, with a
large practice.

So great was the variety of the doctor's acquaintance, and the
charm of intercourse with him, that his society was sought eagerly
by statesmen, and the most illustrious representatives of political
economy, science and the fine arts.

But the doctor reserved for the students, and younger practitioners, his Saturday evenings, during which he taught them from
his own experience, and shared with them the boundless treasures
of his knowledge. This kind custom was kept up during his entire
life, and even the most clever considered it a great honor to be
admitted to these intellectual feasts.

What witty nights, where science and manly enjoyment were
united to a hearty simplicity and native freshness! What delicious
love-feasts under his truly hospitable roof!

As to his works, let us at least give a list of them which will
serve to show the boundless activity of this fertile brain. Before
leaving the Saxony legation he had proven *Mezereum, Sabadilla,
Sabina, Colchicum, Plumb. ac., Paris quad., Cantharis, Sodium,
Antim. tart., Arg. met., Aristol, Clematis, Bellad., Caltha palust.,
Opium, Ruta, Tenacetum, Viola tric.*, etc., etc.

During his stay in South America his proving extended to
*Lachesis, Theridion, Askalabodes, Caladium, Jambos, Jatropha,
Solanum, Spigelia, Vanilla, Alumina, Acid phos.*, and *Psorinum.*

After his arrival in Philadelphia, he either himself, proved or
superintended the experiments and editing of the provings of the
following medicines: *Mephitis, Ictodes foetid., Crotalus, Hydrophobinum (Lyssin), Brucea, Calc. phos.* (acid and basic,) *Hippo-*

manes, Castor eqorum, Kalmia, Viburnum, Phytolacca, Gelsemium, Gymnocladus, Chlor., Brom., Fluoric ac., Thallium, Tellurium, Palladium, Platinum, Osmium, Lithium, Glonoine, Apis, Cepa, Aloes, Millef., Baryta carb., Nux mos., and *Formica.*

Besides his contributions to the *Homoeopathic News,* 1854, and to the *American Journal of Materia Medica,* 1867-1871, (the *Homoeopathic Quarterly* and other Journals) and the help which he gave to the translation of *Jahr's Manual,* we have many of his writings, large and small:

Rise and Progress of Homoeopathy, a pamphlet translated into Dutch and Swedish.

Proposition to Suppress Homoeopathy, 1846, a satire.

Logic of Homoeopathy, 1846, a satire.

Effects from the Poisons of Serpents, 1837.

Suggestions for Making Medical Provings.

The Domestic Physician, 1835, of which there have been edited seven editions in America, two in England, and fourteen in Germany; it has been translated into French, Spanish, Italian, Danish, Hungarian, Russian and Swedish.

American Drug Provings, 1853-1857.

Translation of Gross' Comparative Materia Medica, 1866.

Condensed Materia Medica, two editions, 1877-79.

Analytical Therapeutics, 1875.

The Guiding Symptoms of Our Materia Medica, in 10 volumes, the 3rd of which was in press at the time of his death (since completed from his manuscript by his literary executors).

The quantity of material gathered together by Dr. Hering, from which are drawn his Analytical Therapeutics and the Guiding Symptoms, is a marvel of activity, and the most careful and complete collection which exists upon Materia Medica.

Dr. Hering was an active member of the American Academy of Natural Sciences, in Philadelphia, to which he gave his large zoological collection (including the original *Lachesis trigonocephalus* from South America, from which were made the first provings).

He was one of the founders of the American Institute of Homoeopathy, of which he was the first President, and to which he lent his cooperation during his entire life.

He founded the American Publishing Society, whose shareholders obtained his medical works and other publications at greatly reduced rates.

He was the author of a number of satires written in defence of Homoeopathy and printed in the German language; (also a political pamphlet entitled *The Natural Boundary,* in German, which treats of the dividing line between France and Germany).

He was a co-founder of the American Prover's Union, co-founder of the Medical Academy at Allentown, Pa., co-founder of the Hahnemann College and Hospital where he taught for a long time the doctrine of Homoeopathy according to the *Organon*, which, as a true disciple, he himself honored in interpreting.

The Hahnemann College of Philadelphia was, when in danger of closing, saved and reorganized by Dr. Hering. It numbers at this time ten professors, seven lecturers and demonstrators; contains a large library, a collection of models and pathological specimens, a complete chemical laboratory and rooms for the study of anatomy and practical surgery. Medicine is taught here in all its branches, including toxicology, materia medica, general and special therapeutics, etc.

At his death Dr. Hering was Emeritus Professor of Institutes and Materia Medica in this institution.

Of medium height and athletic build, nature had fashioned Dr. Hering physically as a wrestler in a struggle, which he sustained during his entire life with ardor and dignity. Upon his broad shoulders was carried a grand head with the resolute look of one, who, without any pride, knows how to appreciate his own value, and without affectation, unless one might call such his beautiful hair, which he always wore long, like the Germans of the olden time. He had the well developed forehead of the observer, heavy eyebrows, shading the dark eyes of his race, and an expression in which played the anxiety of unwearied thought joined to a boundless kindness of heart. His step, noiseless and elastic in spite of his weight, pre-possessed all in his favor; his presence shed abroad an atmosphere of benevolence, and inspired the young with confidence in a superiority which might have crushed them, the sick with courage and all with sympathy, while to those who were fortunate enough to approach sufficiently near to appreciate him, his presence served to fill them with an admiration of the tenderest nature.

Of a happily tenacious memory, he was at home on all subjects, listening with attention to the young whom he was teaching, and of such affability, that giving, he seemed to receive and learn from them.

His faculties of a superior order, formed upon musical harmonies from birth (his father was an organist) and coordinated by the study of mathematics to a form of reasoning, and by classical learning to the very depths of philosophy, had been enriched by the study of natural science, of which he was a perfect master. His clear, precise enunciation; his sweet voice; his just, candid appreciation, where the severe logic of science was mingled with great goodness of heart, all united in showing a feeling of honest and irresistible conviction at the centre of which resounded, like an ever-vibrating echo, these words of Hahnemann: "Follow me correctly".

Scientifically speaking, his well-molded hand (soft as velvet) showed a depth of receptive sensibility capable of analysis, and, by its eastern form, the synthetic power well characterized. Humanly speaking it was like his heart, which, deeply affected, sympathized with all in the arduous contest of life, giving both of his support and charity. For it must be said, that slightly negligent of external forms, he seemed to be only the guardian of benefits received, which he scattered round him without any regard for riches; so to him was given the title of Father Hering.

To understand him thoroughly one must remember that he was brought up at a time of great effervescence. which accounts for his communicative enthusiasm. Perfectly balanced, his judgment did not allow his imagination to expend itself in any direction, save in the ardor which he lavished upon his studies; and his moral sense, or feeling of duty, sustained him in his great work, in which he never failed, in spite of the many meannesses of those who were jealous of the great stranger in a country which was not his by an accident of birth, but by adoption, and in spite of the bitterness with which those, who, not being able to reach the man, tried to disparage him and the truths to which he had consecrated his life. To these truths he was faithful to a degree which never lessened, neither when pursued by vexations. nor when struggling against the restraints of the age, for, a few days before his death, he returned thanks for all the good that he had received from Homoeopathy. He planned, even at that time, a new Materia Medica, in which the theory and practice should explain each other, to the great joy of the disciples of the school.

The results of his unheard-of work, and of his perseverence, are not only spread through the writings of many periodicals, but are recorded in volumes of extraordinary merit. One is astonished in becoming acquainted with this study, made so deep by comparisons, parallel quotations, by circumstances of time, of position, of direction, and of sides. And the question arises, why so much care, which no one before him had thought of any use, unless the compilation of Boenninghausen should be considered as something more than patient statistics. Dr. Hering brought to this work not only the minute exactitude of the naturalist, and the faithfulness of the homoeopathic believer, but the ardent perserverance of one who studies the laws of a living pathology. He thought that there should be a reason for the preference of certain remedies for this or that part of the body: is it the result of medical affinities, of idiosyncrasies, or the result of medical action and physical reaction? What law does the circulation of the nervous fluid follow? What reason, what course must be assigned for the vital wave? Through the statistic method, to which he was devoted, there came to him the suspicion of a law to be discovered. And do not let us criticize too severely this ambition. The measure of intuition and appreciation, which a mind thus exercised, makes use of, is not ours. The law of doses, and the law for which Hering sought, will both one day be added, like great luminaries, to the discoveries for the good of mankind. Hering, himself, knew that the hour of this revelation, a kind of promised land, had not yet come, and he contented himself to erecting a monument of facts and works, so that others might make use of it later on. Then seeing that the Materia Medica, worked in this way, would be almost too collossal a work, he began another, as fine, but much shorter, which the student might, if he wished it, rework. It is in fact more within our reach. Then, to define still more clearly the lines to be followed, in the practical way, he makes a resume of the whole, under the name of Analytical Therapeutics, the result of long years of observation, either by himself or of others; a work still incomplete, but of inestimable value.

At the time when Dr. Hering appeared upon the scene, our school, but just started, was like a fragile shell upon the waters, ready to be engulfed at the least movement of the waves. Hering came, incomparably eminent, fortified with vast knowledge, an unceasing activity, a boundless kindness, a feeling of duty to be done equal to every struggle. He started every movement for the good of our school, never allowed himself to be discouraged, was present everywhere upon the scene of action, encouraged and directed the students, stimulated the people to work, adding to his daily practice the work of a large correspondence, of medical provings and of a college professorship. To accomplish this he was often on duty twenty-one hours of the twenty-four.

Our school has gained in size, in strength, in consideration; it is no longer a shell, a plaything at the mercy of the waves, but a majestic ship, with its flag floating proudly on all shores, the joy of every land. And if we, the contemporaries of Hering have seen him and known his worth, posterity, on account of the imperishable monument which he has left us as the fruit of his labors, will place him, a worthy competitor, by the side of the Master himself, and bestow upon him the title of "great" which he has so richly deserved.

When Hahnemann attacked the old school at its foundations, by the denial, both of its fundamental principle and the efficacy of its therapeutic power, he did not content himself with a simple denial. For the denial, which may become the starting-point of an argument or a system, is not one in itself. Alone, and without reconstruction, if something has not been rebuilt upon the ruins of that which has been demolished, it is either the return to an unwholesome barbarism, foreign to our day, or the paltry confession of weakness of mind. Hahnemann, while making clean work of the old school, determined the rules which should govern the choice of a medicine in a case of sickness, reunited by his system the disavowed ties which exist between the maxims of physiology and therapeutics; for the untenable law of opposites, substituted the indisputable law of similars, and by means of provings on the healthy man, initiated us into the complicated study of the psychical and physical man, a close bond, by which, in every disease these double beings are united.

1. Physiological maxim. The parts of a whole are in the same conditions as the whole, the whole in the same conditions as the parts. All local treatment rests upon a disavowal of this maxim.

2. Examples of the law of similars. A frozen limb is cured by the application of snow, or the air of a cold room. Inflammation is reduced by the application of warm water. Purgatives are employed in cases of diarrhoea and dysentery. Vomiting is stopped by drinking of warm water or by an emetic of mustard, and lastly vaccine, which is not in any respect like smallpox is used, indeed legally enforced by the old school.

3. This law is deduced from the observation of facts; it is a general one, in so far as no cure is effected without its application.

4. The study of all our pathogeneses begins by that of the mental, moral, or psychical state in certain physical conditions. One of these conditions being given, the other is necessarily deduced from it. This study, applied to infancy, gives us the means of modifying its psychical tendencies, or of improving the race.

Strong in obedience to the law, and this science, we entered the arena, physicians of the body, physicians of the soul, apostles of the right, true benefactors and regenerators of the human race. It was from henceforth a question if the science of medicine should be material or spiritual. By its very constitution Homoeopathy is the realization in science of that which the Christian idea has already attained in art and literature, a vital influence which preserves from death.

To deny Homoeopathy we must either return to the singularly changeable—some say useless—medicine of the Academy, medicine of experiment, of quackery, and which, by the uncertainty of its course, tends to destroy all faith, or else we must invent new principles, the formula of which we do not suspect today. And it must be said, during the length of time that we have existed, nearly a century, in spite of the almost febrile mental activity of the times, no one has found this new way. After Hahnemann no denial is possible. In his system the connection of the different parts is so close, and binding, that it is not to be wondered at that a mind which sincerely tries to become acquainted with it should become seriously impressed. Hering, the medical student, his knife in his hand wished lightly to make this acquaintance; but he soon discovered that it was instead a study which one must follow carefully. At a single glance he was struck with the importance of this event in the medical world. He saw not only what we have said, but many other things besides, all the advantages of the position, a victory already acquired, which it was only necessary to organize. This life-work was spread out before him from that very hour.

Armed with the motto, "I can do nothing unless God helps me," he risked his career, and before the faculty which was to decide his fate he dared to throw down the gauntlet in the name of the medicine of the future. This faith never contradicted itself; it inspired him.

After a few preliminaries in the way of observations and controversy, he made his first appearance through the study of *Lachesis,* a production sufficient in itself to insure him the reputation of a master.

For many years he made personal confirmations of the provings made by Hahnemann, verifying them and adding to them new symtoms. His part in the great struggle was determined by the certainty which he thus obtained for the superiority of our Materia Medica, and of the great benefit which our school derives from it. He gave his life to add to the precious discoveries which are comprised in our Materia Medica. If a cure, or a new symptom was reported to him he made careful note of it, but subjected it to careful examination. When verified, it became new material. He adopted nothing which had not been subjected to positive proof. His horizon, always enlarging, widened by sure degrees. But so great success never caused a single fibre of his heart to contract. Whoever knocked at his door was welcomed kindly upon the threshold, for Dr. Hering joyfully opened to all the doors of the sanctuary of science. And everyone, receiving more than he had hoped to find, went away with his wishes gratified, and his heart ennobled by his great example. It is not because the American people were credulous, or lacked a practical spirit, but rather because they were so eminently practical, that they listened to this man, who was born a physician of full growth, and that he accomplished, under this influence, the results which we know. Either as advisor, or associated invisibly with all our struggles, which are crowned with success, Hering, in his turn, did full justice to his fellow-workers, attributing to himself but a small part of the results. And names of Dunham, Gosewich, Gray, Guernsey, Haynel, Hull, Jeanes, Kitchen, Lippe, Neidhard, Pulte, Raue, Wells, Wesselhoeft, Williamson, and many others were always mentioned by him with respect and enthusiasm.

Dr. Hering's conversation, accustomed as he was to write with precision and brevity, was not constrained in private life. It was enlivened by piquant and witty remarks, and he sometimes employed sarcasm, although he rarely made use of this weapon. He enjoyed a joke, and his easy and natural narration of different events, joined to a slightly bantering air, lent a great charm to a sweet and sonorous voice.

Thus, for a half century, Dr. Hering worked, gathering together treasures of science, which he has bequeathed to us, as if the duty of doing good was the only thing which kept him on this earth. A man of a profound and sincere religious faith; as a Homoeopath, having faith in the cause, and feeling himself endowed with a special mission, he has fulfilled his task, worthily, nobly, grandly, for the good of man and to the glory of God, in whose peace he is still living.

MEETING OF CANADIAN HOMOEOPATHIC INSTITUTE.

At the meeting resolutions commemorative of Dr. Hering, were read as also the touching memorial by Dr. Edward Bayard, printed in this volume under the transactions of the New York County Homoeopathic Medical Society.

MARYLAND STATE SOCIETY.

At a meeting of this Society, held on November 11, 1880, Dr. McManus spoke as follows:

Forty-three years ago, this very month of November, I had the pleasure of making the acquaintance of Constantine Hering, M. D., by calling upon him. I was then visiting Philadelphia preliminary to my investigation of Homoeopathy. I explained to him the object of my visit, and was listened to with kind patience and advantage to myself. I profited by the instructions I received from him. My visit having occurred during his consultation office hour, I noticed that he frequently made reference to his books for aid in selection of his remedies. I mentioned this to him, and he replied; "You will find out that no man can carry Homoeopathy in his head, every case being different, and a subject for study." I oftentimes, afterwards, derived aid from his suggestions and advice when consulting him about serious and obstinate cases.

By the splendor of his mind, and by his indefatigable labors in the cause of medical science, he has created his own monuments, to perpetuate his fame, and his worth to future ages, and a stimulus to ambition in all who are engaged in his high, honorable and responsible calling.

It has often been remarked—in religion, in medicine, in law, in politics, in the arts and sciences—of some distinguished individual, that "his place can never be filled as he filled it." If ever such a remark proved to be true, it may be proclaimed in regard to our late distinguished colleague, Dr. Constantine Hering.

WEST JERSEY SOCIETY MEETING.

This meeting was held on February 16th, 1881.
A preamble, and resolutions were adopted.

AMERICAN INSTITUTE MEMORIAL SERVICE.

At the thirty-fourth session of the Institute, held at Brighton Beach, N. Y., a special hour was set apart on the fourth day of the session, June 17, 1881, for a memorial service in honor of Dr. Constantine Hering.

The necrologist, Dr. Henry D. Paine, of New York, had presented the following memoir:

No memorial that can be embraced in the circumscribed limits of these brief chronicles of our departed colleagues, can adequately set forth the character and services of this eminent and venerable apostle of Homoeopathy, whose death, since the last annual session of the Institute has affected our whole fraternity with a profound emotion. Wherever Homoeopathy has any standing in the community, the name of Dr. Hering has been known, for a generation at least, as that of one of its most distinguished expositors and propogandists, while thousands who have shared the privilege of his personal acquaintance, or having received instruction from his lips, not only venerate him as a master, but loved him as a friend and father.

To give a full account of his honorable career, or even a summary of his great services to the cause to which the greater part of his life was devoted, would far exceed the object and the limits allowed to these reports, as well as the time and ability of the writer. An extended eulogium in this relation is unnecessary, in view of the memorial service which is to be held in his honor before the close of this meeting. All that will be attempted in these brief remarks is a brief sketch of the principal circumstances in the life of Dr. Hering, every turn of which must henceforth be of interest to every member of the Institute, with whose foundation and early history he was so closely identified. It was expected that in the preparation of this narrative, the compiler would have had the assistance of some one whose knowledge of these events, derived from a long and intimate familiarity of them, would have more thoroughly secured its accurate performance. Although disappointed in this expectation, it is hoped that the following compendium, though imperfect, is substantially correct.

Constantine Hering was a native of Saxony, and first saw the light in the town of Oschatz, on New Year's Day, 1800. His father was a man of liberal views on education, and an advocate of the system of instruction that has since become a characteristic of German educational policy. As may be supposed, young Constantine was given every advantage, and he worked his way through the successive grades of schools in a manner calculated to gain the highest praise of his preceptors. His inclination for the study of natural history was manifested at an early age. He even delighted in collecting, analyzing, and arranging specimens and examples from the different kingdoms of nature, some of which were thought worthy of acceptance by the public museums.

In due time he entered the University of Leipzig, intending to study especially with the view of becoming a physician. Having so strong a passion for the natural sciences, he soon became a favorite with some of the professors, who gave him every encouragement.

It was while resident at this seat of learning that his attention was first directed to the subject of Homoeopathy, by a request from a large publishing house to write a refutation of the doctrines of Hahnemann, which were already stirring up no little commotion among the medical profession. Under the belief that this would be an easy task, and encouraged by the assurances of his teachers, he set about the work with ready confidence. The better to qualify himself for his undertaking, he wisely began by an examination of the tenets and methods that he was expected to demolish, as promulgated in Hahnemann's own writings. The result of this preliminary investigation was such as to cause the abandonment of the engagement, after a struggle of several months, greatly to the chagrin of his family and the disgust of his former medical friends. Further examination satisfied him of the truth of the new ideas, and completed his conversion.

These proceedings sadly darkened his prospects at Leipzig, as they lost him the patronage he had enjoyed by the favor of his preceptors, and he became seriously embarrassed in the prosecution of his studies. Having, however, received from one of his family the means for the purpose, he removed to Wuerzburg, where, on the 22nd of March, 1826, he succeeded in obtaining his degree, notwithstanding that in his inaugral thesis, *De Medicina Futura*, he unhesitatingly espoused the cause of Homoeopathy.

For some time after graduation he was occupied in teaching; but after some months he was offered an appointment as a member of a scientific expedition to South America, of which the King was patron. His love for natural history induced him to accept the position. While absent upon this expedition he fulfilled his scientific duties with entire satisfaction to the promoters of the scheme. At the same time, however, he did not neglect his study of Homoeopathy—practising his art as opportunity offered—but especially in making and conducting provings of new drugs, in which work he had already done valuable service before leaving home. The accounts of his provings, etc., were sent to, and published in the Homoeopathic Archives. When this became known to the government an official intimation was dispatched that he should, in future, devote himself exclusively to the objects of the expedition. On receipt of this order he speedily resolved to sever his connection with the enterprise and devote himself to the practice and cultivation of Homoeopathy. He remained six years in South America, during which time he diligently prosecuted the work he had taken in hand. Especially in the number and thoroughness of the provings that he then conducted, his characteristic industry and perseverence were remarkable. His reports of *Lachesis, Theridion, Caladium, Spigelia*, etc., are among the classics of our Materia Medica.

When practising in Paramaribo, he had for a patient a Moravian missionary, Geo. Bute, who had been sent to Surinam. Bute was dangerously ill with spotted fever—exceedingly dangerous in that climate—but recovered under Dr. Hering's treatment. He was so amazed at his own unexpected cure, and so grateful withal, that he began to crave a knowledge of the wonderful medical system, and from being a patient he became a student of his preserver. After his return to this country, in 1831, Dr. Bute practised in Nazareth, Pa. On the outbreak of cholera in Philadelphia, in the following year, he went to that city to assist in the care of the sick.

Finding the demand of his services so great, he wrote to Dr. Hering, urging him to come and join him. The appeal was effectual, but Dr. Hering did not arrive until the spring of 1833. He associated himself with Dr. Bute in Vine St., Philadelphia, an arrangement which continued with mutual satisfaction until, from enfeebled health, Dr. Bute was obliged to retire to a country practise some years later.

Dr. Hering did not introduce Homoeopathy into Pennsylvania. This had already been done, before his arrival, by Drs. Detwiler. Ihm, Bute, Freytag, and others, and he found himself surrounded by a small, but intelligent and earnest band of adherents to the system. His reputation had preceded his advent, and he was welcomed with great cordiality and enthusiasm. In December of the same year he joined with a number of others in organizing the first school of instruction in homoeopathic therapeutics in the world, under the name of the "North American Academy of the Homoeopathic Healing Art", to be located at Allentown, Pa. Dr. Hering was to be president and principal professor. A charter was obtained, funds were raised, buildings erected, a faculty appointed, students taught and graduated, and a vast deal of other work in behalf of the great medical reform, which cannot even be alluded to here. In all of this the leading spirit and the valiant hand was Dr. Hering's. The history of Homoeopathy in this country cannot be fully understood without reading the narration of the "Allentown Academy," as it was generally called, of which an instructive sketch may be found in the second volume of the World's Convention, of 1876. The faculty continued its labors until 1842, when, after a useful, but brief career, the enterprise was discontinued. Dr. Hering returned to Philadelphia, but the same untiring zeal and industry never deserted him. He has ever striven with an earnest purpose and an intelligent judgment to develop and extend the resources of the Hahnemann therapeutics. In 1844 he presided at the organization of the American Institute of Homoeopathy, composed, at first, of a few but zealous converts, but which, he lived to see embracing many hundreds of members.

Apart from his scientific, literary and professional labors, his life, during the last thirty years presents but few incidents of prominence. With strong domestic habits, and a deep conviction of his duty and mission, he was content to carry on the work of his vocation without ostentation, enjoying the respectful deference of his disciples, as they sought information or advice, more than the applause of the noisy multitude.

Our venerable colleague lived to a ripened age, and had seen rich fruits from his unselfish and sometimes unappreciated labors, and he finally sank to his rest on July 23rd, 1880, with the calmness and composure of one who has performed his task with diligence and honesty of purpose.

The President, Dr. John W. Bowling, of New York, spoke as follows:

I cannot close without reference to the great loss the entire homoeopathic profession, throughout the world, has met with, in the death, since we last met, of Dr. Constantine Hering, president of the convention which originated the organization of the

American Institute of Homoeopathy. In the midst of labors from which, for over fifty years he had never rested, he quietly fell asleep. I could hardly feel that this was an occasion for mourning, for he had been with us for more than half a score of years beyond the allotted time of man; and this long, this spotless life had been one of usefulness and unremitting labor in the cause which he loved to the end. The results of the labors of his later years are living, and will live to aid us, and those who come after us in the work to which our lives are being devoted. We should rejoice that during his long and active life not a truthful word had ever been uttered that could reflect on his character as a man, as a Christian, and that at the last his death was peaceful, calm, and free from protracted suffering. We should rejoice that his troubles, for he had sorrows—sorrows hard to bear, too, are at an end, and that there is before him an eternity of happiness, for I believe that of such as he, is the Kingdom of Heaven. Others of us, noble men and true, dear to their families, friends and clientage, have died since we last met together, but this pioneer was dear to us all, honored by us all, and will be remembered by us all, and our children will be taught to honor his memory.

Dr. J. C. Morgan, of Philadelphia, then said:

Having already exhausted such reflections as seem worthy of our deceased colleague, Dr. Hering, in connection with our two Philadelphia meetings, I had thought to remain silent here. It may explain the backwardness of other Philadelphia members, perhaps, to say that this is the case with many of them: they feel, too, that they have passed the subject of his death into the more sacred precincts of the memory. The revival of it, here, by us, you will therefore understand, is attended with something like the pain that one has in the uncovering of an old and partly healed wound, or one, at least, which has become quiet; my colleagues from Philadelphia have, however, requested me to introduce this subject of national interest. Permit me, then, to make reference to my personal acquaintance with Dr. Hering. I will commence with one point, very important to me personally, by saying that in boyhood, when Dr. Hering was yet in the vigor of his youth, I was take. ·ɔ him for the purpose of medical treatment by a friend of his, one of his early supporters, and also a friend of my own, Mrs. Rev. Dr. Bedell; and my recollection of the prescriptions made by Dr. Hering is that they were eminently successful. We had no further personal relations for very many years. In the meantime I had become a physician of the old school, later of the homoeopathic school. Even then my acquaintance with Dr. Hering

was not renewed; this was partly owing to the fact that those from
whom I had just derived my impressions of Homoeopathy were
his opponents. They had disagreements in Philadelphia, the city
of brotherly love. It so happened that I learned my Homoeopathy
along with antagonism to Dr. Hering. I was taught to believe that
he was a visionary; to use the words of my informant 'an eccentric'.
I, therefore, in all the pride of my youth, and with my but half
regenerate allopathic mind, refrained from making his acquaintance, and I will add that I am heartily ashamed to have to say it.
I was, however, introduced to Dr. Hering without my own knowledge. and in a way most characteristic of himself.

My home was in Illinois, a thousand miles from his. I made a
two weeks' proving of *Gelsemium*, which was published in Dr.
Shipman's *Journal of Materia Medica*. Dr. Hering's peculiarity
was that he would seize upon provings wherever he found them,
and with the skill of the anatomist would dissect them, and de-
termine their essential points. It was my good fortune, therefore,
to meet Dr. Hering's skill in the discussion of my proving of that
drug. That is to say, he found therein, the now historical symptom,
viz., that depressing emotions produce a tendency to diarrhoeic
disturbance of the intestinal canal.

It was observed by me in April, 1861, on reading the telegrams
of the firing on Fort Sumpter; these so disturbed me that I gave
up the proving, and stated it a fact that the telegrams produced
the effect. But Dr. Hering, with the sagacity which was so
peculiar to him, with that keen eye and that analytical skill in
Materia Medica, in which he was *facile princeps*, seized upon the
very thing which I thought was vitiating the proving; said he,
"There is the grand characteristic of the drug." Years later, when
I had returned to Philadelphia and become acquainted with him,
and others associated with him, I found that it had been erected
into what is now called a key-note. He gave me back my finding;
and there are a thousand other such gems that we owe to Dr.
Hering. In this way, then, he had become acquainted with me,
and when I met him in the college, he was prepared, and I was
prepared to form, as we did form, a warm and sympathetic friendship. I soon found out that I had been utterly misled in regard to
the character—the intellectual character, I mean, of Dr. Hering; no
one dared breathe anything other than profound respect for his
moral character. I have to say here, ladies and gentlemen, that I
believe Dr. Hering has been unfortunately misunderstood in this
respect. He had his own peculiarities; to some he may have seemed
perhaps, sometimes disagreeable; those who have suffered from
that, have, no doubt, buried the recollection of it in his grave; but
the idea of Dr. Hering being backward in attending to the progress
of research and science, the idea that Dr. Hering was at all a

visionary, in the bad sense, is a great mistake, a great unconscious slander upon the memory of his intellectual greatness. As a matter of fact, Dr. Hering was always foremost, in our school, in recognizing every forward movement. There is not a single one of the recent advances in science of which he had not, before any of his co-laborers, learned something, and it has commonly happened, during the past fifteen years, that when something new came up, and I have come to his office, I found that he had already become cognizant of the details of the subject. Some of my first information in regard to the recent revelations of the spectroscope came, to my surprise, from his lips. Whatsoever had a bearing upon Homoeopathy had for him a religious savor, and appeared to him in all the sanctity of a Divine revelation; so that if he were ever intolerant, it was with the inspiration of the Crusader fighting for the Holy Sepulchre against the infidel, or of the Covenanter, defending his Bible in the mountain passes of his native land.

My acquaintance with Dr. Hering, in a social way, and more in relation to the college faculty, was exceedingly pleasant as a rule. We did not always agree; that could not be expected; but throughout we maintained that mutual respect and affection which I am glad to recall today. The faculty meetings, held usually in his office, in deference to his years, were really club-meetings in their social aspect. They were all that we desire in a social club, and he was the illuminator of the club, always ready with some matter of interest and novelty, always ready to give of his rich store of medical information, always ready with some new point in general science with which to interest our minds, and valuable, either in society or in our professional duties; many a key-note, as we call it in the Materia Medica, I received from him in this way. Indeed, it was my practice, in these frequent convocations with Hering, Guernsey, Lippe, Raue, etc., to have a little memorandum book and my leadpencil ready, and often as these golden nuggets of homoeopathic experience fell from the lips of these experts, I recorded them; I think no one furnished them more frequently than Dr. Hering. This note-book became part and parcel of my capital in professional work.

The matter I am speaking of I would not part with for any consideration. Such then, was our relation in the faculty. We all looked upon him, as a master of course, as our pater-familias, and so he regarded himself; would sometimes, indeed, claim a little supremacy, and thought that he might be privileged to talk to the rest of us as to the "youngest of the family."

Once it was said to him, "Dr. Hering, these youngsters are all about forty years of age and upwards." "Boys of forty!" he exclaimed, in jocular contempt, and so gained his point; we were always willing enough to be considered, by him as "boys of forty."

and in this way we got along happily, yielding to his supremacy and always profiting by it. In his last days, fellow-members of the Institute, Dr. Hering's heart-life seemed to undergo a special development; the Philadelphia members here present understand what I mean.

He was born with the century; the first day of January, 1800, witnessed his advent into the world; and as the year 1880 dawned he reached his eightieth anniversary. Dr. Hering realized now that the end of his time was nearing. He made all arrangements in regard to his literary work—and that work, let me assure the profession, is in able hands, and will be issued as he would have it. This done, he seemed to cling, as never before, to those who had surrounded him during the past years. He desired that we should often come to see him; to some, as to me, he said, "Here is my study (many of you know it, on the second floor of his house), you have the entree at all times—come right upstairs and knock." This was, of course, a great privilege, of which we were not slow to avail ourselves, and to myself they were occasions of great satisfaction. The clinging of the dear old man to these friends, and to me among the rest, at this time, was touching, and, I for one, tried to be faithful to his last days, my only regret being that I had not seen him for three weeks at the time of his decease. I think that everyone of our members from Philadelphia will bear me out in saying that the kindliest recollections of Dr. Hering are those of the last six months of his life.

Dr. J. P. Dake, of Nashville, next spoke as follows:

Mr. President: I desire to say a few words in regard to the character and labors of our deceased brother, the father of Homoeopathy in America, Dr. Constantine Hering. And in speaking with regard to him it is understood, perhaps, by all who are present, that I was among those who differed with Dr. Hering, pointedly, and decidedly, upon several matters, and I feel that it is therefore the more fitting that I should, upon this occasion, say something.

In Dr. Hering I recognized, as I doubt not that everyone here present recognized, a genius in medicine, and not only a genius in medicine, but a master-workman in medicine. Rich in new thoughts, he was industrious in the application and the working out of these thoughts. Dr. Hering has added to our Materia Medica many things of great value. These things will remain, and the passing years will increase their importance. They will be comprehended more and more. But Dr. Hering was mortal; Dr. Hering was fallible; not all of his opinions can we accept, nor can we appreciate the value of all that he has added to the Materia

Medica; but we, in the homoeopathic school, have been taught to think independently, to think for ourselves, to weigh all things and form our opinions in regard to them. We learned early, as did Hahnemann, who taught us to disregard authority when authority was not in accord with facts, and with science. Therefore, in taking the works and products left by Dr. Hering, it becomes us not to accept them as revelations from above, as perfect in all respects, but to accept them as contributions to truth, and opinions put before us for our consideration, and our use, in the light that is given us from all quarters. We are not expected, therefore, to accept all of Dr. Hering's works, and all of his teachings as authoritative, not to be differed from at all. What was defective and erroneous in the opinions and works of Dr. Hering will pass away. No amount of veneration of him, no amount of appreciation for his genius, nor his industry, will require us to hold on to those things which experience and increasing light and knowledge do not endorse and sustain.

Dr. H. M. Smith, of New York City, said:

Dr. Dake seems to have been cut short in the expression of his feelings in regard to Dr. Hering. When he moved that the time be limited to five minutes to each speaker, he must have known that he could not have expressed his feelings in so short a time. I could not imagine any occasion on which I could not have something to say about Dr. Constantine Hering, but in five minutes I do not know where to begin, any more than I know where I shall end. I can only give expression to my feelings and my veneration for that man.

As a young man in the profession, I cannot but think kindly of the many happy and instructive interviews I have had with him. When the *American Homoeopathic Review* was in existence, we received a great many contributions and a great deal of assistance from Dr. Hering, and it was our custom to spend one or two days with him every summer. Dr. Carroll Dunham and Dr. P. P. Wells, and myself, went on there to meet the homoeopathic physicians from various sections of the country, and in his study, that Dr. Morgan speaks of, the recollections come back to me of many pleasant and instructive hours, and it is pleasant to recall the merry laugh and cheery face of Dr. Hering, when giving us some information, or relating an anecdote. I went in one day to see him especially in regard to *Digitalis*. He had written an article in the *Review* on *Digitalis*, the second part of which was never published. He was never ready to publish it because some proofs were wanting he was to get from a convent, or monastery in Italy. After some casual remarks I said, "Dr. Hering I came to see you especially in regard

to that article on *Digitalis;* when can you give me half an hour?"
"Quarter of four tomorrow morning," said he. Accordingly, the
following morning I was in Dr. Hering's library. The old gentleman slept there. He had arisen from his couch, and was reading.
He directed me to sit down, and to write what he dictated to me.
That was the way that Dr. Hering worked, careful to obtain sufficient proof before making statements as facts, and always ready to
assist everybody who sought information.

Dr. F. R. McManus, of Baltimore, said:

I wish to state a little incident that occurred in the early part
of my homoeopathic investigation and career. I went from Baltimore to Philadelphia in search of an allopathic physician who had
practised both systems, and I found one; I went to another
physician afterwards, who was Dr. Hering. I introduced myself to
Dr. Hering as Dr. McManus, of Baltimore. I told him the object
of my visit, and he said: "I am very glad to see you, but you have
happened to call at a time when I am attending to my consulta-
tions; take a seat there for a few moments, when I will talk to you."
Well, I waited until he got through, and I said to him: "Doctor,
I noticed you referring to your books and volumes of your library in
every case in which you prescribe. "Yes," said he, "and no man
will be the right kind of a homoeopathic physician who does not do
it, for there never was a brain, in my opinion, that could ever
contain the one-hundredth part of what it ought to hold to enable
one to practise without studying every case; for every case is a
new one." I told him it seemed to be a great deal of labor. "Well,"
said he, "when you come to study Homoeopathy, you will find out
the difference in the two schools, in regard to the means and the
facility to practise, because an allopathic physician can prescribe
for forty cases where a homoeopathic would be hardly able to
prescribe for two or three, or perhaps one."

I merely mention this because it may stimulate the younger
members of the profession to individualize and study their cases
closely, as it has always stimulated me in my forty-three years of
homoeopathic investigation and practise. It has been to my advantage to do so, and, of course, much to the advantage of
Homoeopathy. I hold his memory in the sweetest recollection, and
I am glad that I cannot say anything that will throw the slightest
cloud upon his efficiency as a physician, or to his adherence to
Hahnemann as a homoeopathist.

Dr. T. C. Duncan, of Chicago, spoke as follows:

I cannot let this opportunity pass without presenting my deep regret for the death of our distinguished father of Homoeopathy in the United States, and the impression made upon me by his loss will deepen as the years glide on. I think the one thing that will impress the profession, more than anything else, is the inexhaustive power of Dr. Hering in gathering together the fund of information that was scattered here and there in our medical writings. He was the one individual in the whole world of Homoeopathy that gathered together all facts, and it is perfectly wonderful what he has accumulated, and it seems to me very proper that some one should take this up and continue it.

Various facts are coming out bearing upon Materia Medica and on Therapeutics that will be lost except some one gather them together as did Hering. Dr. Hering has made a noble beginning. He has, I believe, in his library, or did have them at the time of the Centennial, every fact bearing upon Homoeopathic Materia Medica extant. His memory will be bright forever; I hold him in high regard, and his influence upon the cause, in the United States, I think we cannot too highly appreciate.

Dr. Fisher, of Montreal, said:

I will not take up the time very long, but still, while we are on the subject, I may mention that before I commenced practise on this side of the Atlantic, on my way back from Europe I called at Philadelphia and saw Dr. Hering, and one of the things which he then mentioned, and which I thought characteristic, I was very much struck with, and have often thought of since—he said, "When I come to the bed-side of a patient I often feel like a fool." Now, such has been the result of my own experience on many occasions. I have often looked back and thought of that fact, which has encouraged me to go on, notwithstanding that I felt for the moment like a fool. There was another thing struck me at the time. We were speaking about somebody else, another medical man. "Well," said he, "He is a queer fellow, but we are all queer." Well, that also struck me, and I have often thought, since, that most men are dreadfully frightened by what the world calls eccentricity. Now, it has often occurred to me that no man can be really original without being more or less eccentric. He may be eccentric without being original, but the effect of that eccentricity, no doubt, keeps a good many of us from doing things which we would otherwise like to do.

Dr. I. T. Talbot, of Boston, said:

I cannot let an occasion like this go by without dropping one tribute of memory to a great man, for I believe Dr. Hering was really great. The memory of his kindness to students and young men, the memory of Dr. Hering's kindness to myself, who had no special claims upon him, in any way, is pleasant to contemplate. Soon after I had graduated, and about to visit Europe, I was recommended, by Dr. Carroll Dunham to get some letters from Dr. Hering to physicians living abroad, and assuring me that he would be willing to give them, I called upon Dr. Hering in Philadelphia. He was busy at the time, and said: "Come to me tonight and I will be happy to see you." At what time shall I come? "Well, I shall get through with my work about 10 o'clock; come then." I went there. He had two friends with him who were also acquainted in Europe, and whom he had brought there for the special purpose of seeing me. From 10 p. m. until 3 a. m. was spent in talking of European affairs—of what could be of benefit to me in my trip abroad—a sacrifice, on his part, of sleep, of rest, for an entire stranger, which we could hardly suppose any one would make on such an occasion. Having made a list of letters which he proposed to give, he the next day sent me six, to prominent persons in Europe, old Dr. Stapf, being one of them. The letters were of great service to me, and the kindness extended through each of them I place as a tribute to the memory of Dr. Hering, and I venerate that great heart, that noble spirit that could give so much to a young man without any claims upon him.

Dr. P. G. Valentine, of St. Louis, then said:

It seems that what has been spoken of Dr. Hering this morning has been mostly of the nature of personal reminiscences of him. I think that but once it was my pleasure to meet him, and that was when attending the Centennial meeting in Philadelphia. As he entered the door, and passed down the aisle he was cheered by all the members present. He came upon the stand and took his seat by the others there; the English gentlemen, etc.

But my acquaintance with Dr. Hering was entirely through the Materia Medica. I wish to say that through that work I have learned to admire and to venerate him. The question with us, in St. Louis, when any point in Materia Medica is raised, is, what does Dr. Hering say?

I have no other personal recollections of him. The only way I learned to love him was through the Materia Medica.

Dr. M. M. Eaton, of Cincinnati, said:

It has not been my privilege to have had a personal acquaintance with Dr. Hering, and I can only say that I feel that one of our greatest men has passed away. I feel that he has left a record behind him worthy of emulation, and it struck me that we should profit by the example which has been set, that we should each endeavor to do something to add to the store-house of knowledge for those who may come after. It strikes me that upon occasions of this kind we should make such resolves as to our future course as may benefit mankind.

Dr. Wm. von Gottschalk, of Providence, said:

I wish to speak a few words of Dr. Hering as a German. As there are no Germans present to speak about him, or in his memory, I think it finally to be my duty, after so many different Americans have spoken in praise of that most peculiar man, to give my tribute to his character, in a different way.

I first saw Dr. Hering in 1852, when I was an old school practitioner in the city of New York. I was then induced to try Homoeopathy. I still looked upon Homoeopathy as a peculiar quackery, and I wanted to see the greatest quack of them all. Dr. Hering being a countryman of mine struck me peculiarly as I visited him. He encouraged me in Homoeopathy more than any other man I had ever met, and probably he was the sole cause of my becoming a complete homoeopath to whom I owe my position in Homoeopathy today.

What I wish to allude to now, in particular, are his distinguishing German characteristics. As a scholar he was a thorough German. This I knew at the moment in which I entered his house, in 1876, when he called me by name. He called me the Yankee-Dutchman, and asked me to sit down and take a glass of wine with him. Then, in response to his request, I went with him to his garden back of the house where, in a small arbor, was spread a table for his family, and here we sat down for a friendly chat. On the table were familiar German dishes, and the hospitality of a German was extended. It was a delight to be there and to receive the hospitality of this man. He was a true German, in all his habits, to the very last moments of his life. I wish that an abler man, better qualified in the use of the English language, were here to pay a more proper tribute to him in this regard. Other Germans mostly become Americanized. Hering always adhered to the ways of the Fatherland, a thing which I have not done. But I respect him for this peculiar characteristic, that in all of his life he remained, as he was born—a German.

A TRIBUTE FROM ITALY.

Dr. Pompili, of Rome, on behalf of the Italian practitioners of Homoeopathy, has requested the publication of the following tribute, to which is appended a translation furnished by Dr. Horace Howard Furness:

Constantine Hering
Artis Medicae Doctori Eximio
Post Hehnemannium Magistrum
Suae Scholae Principi ac Decori Praecipuo
Qui
Doctrina Editisque De Homoeopathia Voluminibus
Ubique Terrarum
Veri Cupidos Docuit, Docet Et Docebit
Joachimus Pompilius In Urbe M. D.
Suo Itallesque Homoeopathicorum Nomine
Or Tantum Virum Amissum Moerentissimus
Honoris Memorlesque Ergo
Inscribit Et Dicat.

Translation:

To
Constantine Hering
The Excellent Doctor Of Medicine
Next After The Master Hahnemann,
The Chief And Preeminent Ornament Of His School
Who
In Word And In Print By His Discoveries In Homoeopathy
Teaches, Has Taught And Will Teach
All Who Are Desirous Of Truth Throughout The World
This Tribute
To The Honor And T The Memory Of A Man Thus Lost
And
Most Deeply Mourned
Is By
Joachim Pompili, M. D.
In His Own Name And In The Name Of
The Practitioners of Homoeopathy In Italy
Inscribed And Dedicated.

Of the numerous Obituary Notices which appeared in the daily papers and in the various medical journals throughout the world, only a few of the foreign ones are published as indicating the esteem and veneration in which the subject of this Memoir was held in other than the two great English-speaking nations, and especially in his own dear fatherland.

Of these may be mentioned:

La Reforma Medica, Mexico,
The Allgemeine Homoeopathische Zeitung, Leipzig,
The Homoeopathische Monatsblaetter, Stuttgart,
The Populaere Zeitschrift fuer Homoeopathie, Leipzig.

PEACE TO HIS ASHES, and Honor To His Memory.

PART - V

INDEX

PART V

INDEX

21.-